ACSM's
Exercise for Older Adults

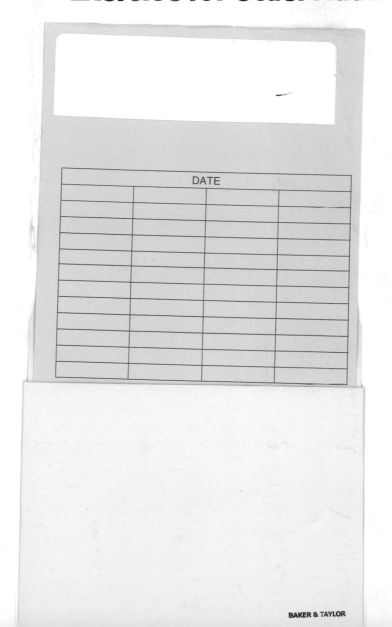

DATE			

ACSM's
Exercise for
Older Adults

Edited by

Wojtek J. Chodzko-Zajko, PhD

Professor and Head
Department of Kinesiology and Community Health
University of Illinois at Urbana-Champaign
Urbana, Illinois

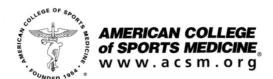

AMERICAN COLLEGE
of SPORTS MEDICINE
w w w . a c s m . o r g

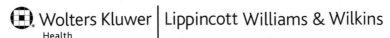

Wolters Kluwer | Lippincott Williams & Wilkins
Health

Philadelphia · Baltimore · New York · London
Buenos Aires · Hong Kong · Sydney · Tokyo

Publisher: Chris Johnson
Acquisitions Editor: Emily Lupash
Product Director: Eric Branger
Senior Product Manager: Heather A. Rybacki
Product Manager: Michael Marino
Production Project Manager: Marian Bellus
Marketing Manager: Sarah Schuessler
Manufacturing Coordinator: Margie Orzech-Zeranko
Design Coordinator: Stephen Druding
ACSM's Publications Committee Chair: Walter R. Thompson
ACSM's Group Publisher: Kerry O'Rourke
Compositor: S4Carlisle Publishing Services

First Edition
Copyright © 2014 Lippincott Williams & Wilkins, a Wolters Kluwer business

351 West Camden Street   Two Commerce Square
Baltimore, MD 21201   Philadelphia, PA 19106

Printed in China

9 8 7 6 5 4 3 2

Library of Congress Cataloging-in-Publication Data
INSERT CIP DATA HERE

DISCLAIMER

Care has been taken to confirm the accuracy of the information present and to describe generally accepted practices. However, the authors, editors, and publisher are not responsible for errors or omissions or for any consequences from application of the information in this book and make no warranty, expressed or implied, with respect to the currency, completeness, or accuracy of the contents of the publication. Application of this information in a particular situation remains the professional responsibility of the practitioner; the clinical treatments described and recommended may not be considered absolute and universal recommendations.

The authors, editors, and publisher have exerted every effort to ensure that drug selection and dosage set forth in this text are in accordance with the current recommendations and practice at the time of publication. However, in view of ongoing research, changes in government regulations, and the constant flow of information relating to drug therapy and drug reactions, the reader is urged to check the package insert for each drug for any change in indications and dosage and for added warnings and precautions. This is particularly important when the recommended agent is a new or infrequently employed drug.

Some drugs and medical devices presented in this publication have Food and Drug Administration (FDA) clearance for limited use in restricted research settings. It is the responsibility of the health care provider to ascertain the FDA status of each drug or device planned for use in their clinical practice.

To purchase additional copies of this book, call our customer service department at **(800) 638-3030** or fax orders to **(301) 223-2320**. International customers should call **(301) 223-2300**.

***Visit Lippincott Williams & Wilkins on the Internet*: http://www.lww.com.** Lippincott Williams & Wilkins

RRS1307

To my mother, Ewa Maria Zofia Chodzko-Zajko

In the chapters of this book, you will learn about the many reasons why older adults should engage in regular physical activity. The world renowned group of researchers and practitioners selected as chapter authors have presented a compelling case for physical activity, summarizing the physiological, psychological, social, and other benefits that accrue to people of all ages who are able to maintain a physically active lifestyle. You will be exposed to a substantial body of scientific evidence that indicates that regular physical activity can bring dramatic health benefits to people of all ages and abilities and that these benefits extends over the entire life-course. Simply put, physical activity offers one of the greatest opportunities to extend years of active independent life, reduce disability, and improve the quality of life for midlife and older persons.

Unfortunately, despite a wealth of evidence about the benefits of physical activity for mid-life and older persons, there has been little success in convincing Americans older than 50 years to adopt physically active lifestyles. For example, the Centers for Disease Control and Prevention estimates that between one-third and one-half of Americans older than 50 years get no leisure-time physical activity at all. *ACSM's Exercise for Older Adults* will assist you to identify and understand some of the barriers faced by older adults when they attempt to increase their physical activity and to outline specific strategies for helping them to overcome these barriers.

For those of us who make our living advocating for healthy and physically active lifestyles, it may come as a surprise to realize how little many older adults know about physical activity. However, most older adults were educated at a time and in a culture in which little was known about the health benefits of physical activity, and professionals and members of the public were skeptical about the need to remain physically active after retirement. In the pages of this book, you will find a succinct and easy to read summary of the current evidence base in the area of exercise and physical activity for older adults. As an exercise professional, one of the most important things you can do for your clients is to help them to understand that there are different ways to be active. By following some of the strategies and suggestions presented in this book, you can help your older clients realize a lot of benefits associated with a physically active lifestyle.

FEATURES

Chapter Introductions and **Chapter Outlines** at the beginning of each chapter provide an overview of important concepts. **Key Point** boxes illustrate terms, definitions, and ideas. **Real Life Stories**, or vignettes, describe older adults who have successfully implemented physical activity programs. **Questions for Reflection** help students review what they have learned and encourage students to engage in critical thinking.

SUPPLEMENTAL MATERIALS

Supplemental materials for students and instructors are available at http://thepoint.lww.com/activate. Instructors can access:

- Power Point Lecture Outlines
- Image Bank, including all figures and tables from the text.
- Full Text Online

Students can also access the Full Text Online.

Acknowledgments

Foremost, I would like to acknowledge the contributions of my colleagues who have willingly agreed to share their expertise and experience by writing chapters for this book. Your hard work, enthusiasm, and dedication to this project are greatly appreciated. You have been a joy to work with! Next, I would like to thank the American College of Sports Medicine and all of its staff and officers for your commitment to our profession and your dedication to the dissemination of the scientific evidence about the benefits of physical activity. Finally, I would like to express my personal thanks to my colleague and partner, Dr. Andiara Schwingel.

Contributors

Wojtek J. Chodzko-Zajko, PhD
Professor and Head
Department of Kinesiology and Community Health
University of Illinois at Urbana-Champaign
Urbana, Illinois

Jennifer L. Etnier, PhD
Professor and Director of Graduate Studies
Department of Kinesiology
University of North Carolina at Greensboro
Greensboro, North Carolina

Ellen M. Evans, PhD
Associate Professor
Department of Kinesiology
University of Georgia
Athens, Georgia

Bo Fernhall, PhD
Dean and Professor
College of Applied Health Sciences
University of Illinois at Chicago
Chicago, Illinois

Dolores D. Guest, PhD, RD
Clinical Research Assistant
Department of Clinical Research
The Parkinson's Institute & Clinical Center
Sunnyvale, California

William B. Karper, EdD
Associate Professor
Department of Kinesiology
University of North Carolina at Greensboro
Greensboro, North Carolina

Abbi Lane, MS
Department of Kinesiology and Nutrition
University of Illinois at Chicago
Chicago, Illinois

Elizabeth K. Lenz, PhD
Assistant Professor
Department of Kinesiology, Sport Studies, and
    Physical Education
The College at Brockport — SUNY
Brockport, New York

Pamela "Pommy" Macfarlane, PhD
Professor Emeritus
Kinesiology and Physical Education Department
Northern Illinois University
DeKalb, Illinois

James R. Morrow, Jr, PhD, FACSM, FNAK
Regents Professor
Department of Kinesiology, Health Promotion and
    Recreation
University of North Texas
Denton, Texas

Anne E. O'Brien, PhD
Temporary Assistant Professor
Department of Kinesiology
University of Georgia
Athens, Georgia

Michael E. Rogers, PhD, FACSM
Professor and Chair
Department of Human Performance Studies
Director
Center for Physical Activity and Aging
Wichita State University
Wichita, Kansas

Nicole L. Rogers, PhD
Assistant Professor
Department of Public Health Sciences
Wichita State University
Wichita, Kansas

Agnes F. Schrider, PT
Nelson Physical Therapy and Wellness Center
Roseland, Virginia

Andiara Schwinge, PhD
Assistant Professor
Department of Kinesiology and Community Health
University of Illinois at Urbana-Champaign
Champaign, Illinois

Scott J. Strath, PhD
Associate Professor
Department of Kinesiology
University of Wisconsin-Milwaukee
Milwaukee, Wisconsin

Rudy Valentine, PhD
Post-Doctoral Researcher
Diabetes and Metabolism Research Unit
Boston University School of Medicine
Boston, Massachusetts

Jakob L. Vingren, PhD, CSCS, FACSM
Assistant Professor
Department of Kinesiology, Health Promotion and
  Recreation
University of North Texas
Denton, Texas

Mary Frances Visser, PhD
Professor
Department of Human Performance
Minnesota State University, Mankato
Mankato, Minnesota

Diane Whaley, PhD
Professor, Applied Developmental Science & Director,
  Lifetime Physical Activity Program
Curry School of Education
University of Virginia
Charlottesville, Virginia

Anne-Lorraine T. Woolsey, BA
Department of Kinesiology, Health Promotion and
  Recreation
University of North Texas
Denton, Texas

Huimin Yan, MS
Department of Kinesiology and Community Health
University of Illinois at Urbana-Champaign
Urbana, Illinois

Reviewers

Helaine Alessio, PhD, FACSM
Miami University
Oxford, Ohio

Stephen D. Ball, PhD
University of Missouri
Columbia, Missouri

Marybeth Brown, PhD, FACSM
University of Missouri
Columbia, Missouri

Meredith Butulis
Globe University/Minnesota School of Business
Richfield, Minnesota

Carol Cole
Associate Professor
Sinclair Community College
Dayton, Ohio

Angela Fern, MS
Beaumont Health System
Royal Oak, Michigan

Eric J. Fuchs, ATC, EMT
Director, Athletic Training Education Program
Associate Professor
Eastern Kentucky University
Richmond, Kentucky

Matthew J. Garver, PhD
Assistant Professor
Abilene Christian University
Abilene, Texas

Greg K. Kandt, EdD
Fort Hayes State University
Hays, Kansas

Raymond Leung
Graduate Deputy
Brooklyn College of the City University of New York
Brooklyn, New York

Sarah MacColl
Personal Trainer
Cape Elizabeth, Maine

Marilyn K. Miller, PhD
Associate Professor
Bloomsburg University of Pennsylvania
Bloomsburg, Pennsylvania

MaryAnn Molloy
Personal Trainer
Healthy Body Fit Mind
South Portland, Maine

Jeffrey L. Roitman, EdD, FACSM
Rockhurst University
Kansas City, Missouri

Karin Singleton
Personal Trainer
Fitness Personified
Raleigh, North Carolina

Pam Soto
Department Chair, Professor
Health & Kinesiology
Austin Community College
Austin, Texas

Lucille Sternburgh, MS
Beaumont Health & Wellness Center
Rochester Hills, Michigan

Contents

CHAPTER 1

Understanding Human Aging

Andiara Schwingel

CHAPTER OUTLINE

INTRODUCTION

Aging is an experience that every human being shares but no one fully understands. Human aging is associated with a wide range of physical, psychological, and social changes that impact our everyday functioning, leave us more vulnerable to a number of diseases and conditions, and make us more susceptible to death (1). This chapter examines some of the underlying processes thought to be responsible for structural and functional decline with advancing age. The chapter begins with a brief discussion of different definitions of age and the aging process. Although aging is usually defined with reference to the passage of time, even the most rapid examination of the gerontology literature reveals that chronological age alone is an inadequate measure of senescence and that more complex definitions of both age and aging are needed if we are to increase our understanding of the complex biological and psychological processes accompanying human aging.

Furthermore, this chapter examines the underlying biological mechanisms responsible for the aging process. Despite more than 50 years of research and the concerted efforts of many researchers, little progress has been made toward the identification of a single, cohesive theory of biological aging. Indeed, current research suggests that it may be more appropriate to consider aging as an umbrella term covering a wide variety of changes that occur at molecular, cellular, and systemic levels, all of which together have the effect of decreasing the body's ability to respond to internal and external stressors. Although structural decay and associated functional decline appear to be an inescapable consequence of advancing age, there are often considerable individual differences with respect to both the rate and the extent of this decline. It is now well established that it is possible for individuals to deviate from expected patterns of aging and, at least for some time, postpone the consequences of aging. The chapter will conclude with a discussion around successful aging regarding some of the lifestyle modifications that have been proposed to influence the time course of human aging.

DEFINITIONS OF AGE AND THE AGING PROCESS

For the average person, it may seem unnecessary to have to define aging. Most of us are used to thinking of age as simply the number of years, months, or days that we have lived. The most commonly accepted measure of aging is the passage of calendar time. It is very clear, however, that we do not all age at the same rate and that definitions of aging that focus exclusively on calendar time are incomplete. More complex and sophisticated definitions of both "age" and "aging" are needed if we are to understand the intricacies of human aging. To understand the aging process, it is important to consider a broader perspective that combines biological, psychological, and social aspects of growing older.

Chronological age

Chronological age refers to the length of time a person has lived. It is usually expressed by the number of years or months since birth, and its measurement is independent

Real Life Story 1-1   Jeanne Calment — Profile of a Chronologically Remarkable Older Adult

In 1965, Jeanne Calment, aged 90, signed a deal, common in France, to sell her condominium apartment to François Raffray (then aged 47) on a contingency contract. François agreed to pay her a monthly sum of approximately US$550 until she died, an agreement sometimes called a "reverse mortgage." At the time of the deal, the value of the apartment was equal to 10 years of payments. This would have been a good business arrangement for François; however, he was dealing with the world's longest lived person. In fact, Jeanne survived for more than 30 years after the deal, and François died before her of cancer at the age of 77, leaving his widow to continue the payments for 2 years. Jeanne Calment lived until 122 years and 164 days, and she stands as a remarkable illustration of long chronological aging.

of physiological, psychological, and sociocultural factors. However, because it cannot differentiate between individuals who share the same age but differ markedly along physiological and/or psychosocial parameters, chronological age alone does not tell us much about how a person is doing as he or she grow older. Most gerontologists accept that in order to increase our understanding of individual differences in the aging process, it is necessary to supplement chronological age with other measures of aging that are designed to differentiate between individuals of the same chronological age. These alternative measures of senescence are sometimes described as indices of functional age. The most common measure of functional age is biological age, although gerontologists have also identified other functional ages, including psychological age and social age.

Biological age

Rather than focusing on elements of calendar time as the principal measure of aging, biological age focuses on age-related changes in biological or physiological processes. A wide variety of approaches have been adopted for the measurement of biological age (2–4). A common goal of all biological age inventories is the determination of relative age of an individual, or the extent to which an individual is aging faster or slower than an average person of the same chronological age. For example, an individual who is aging successfully may have a biological age that is substantially less than his or her chronological age, whereas a person who is suffering from multiple medical complications in old age may be found to have a biological age that is greater than his or her chronological age.

There have been literally dozens of approaches proposed for the calculation of biological age. Biological age assessment usually involves a number of tests that measure biological variables known to deteriorate with advancing age. An overall score on a test battery is generated for each person taking the test, and this score is then compared with scores for other persons of the same chronological age. Unfortunately, little consensus has developed with respect to exactly how biological age should be

Real Life Story 1-2   David — Profile of a Biologically "Younger" Older Adult

David has been physically active for virtually his entire adult life. He started his lifelong activity program shortly after leaving the navy, having seen action in the Pacific Islands during World War II. He retired as paymaster of a large pharmaceutical company in the mid-1990s, but retirement did little to slow him down. At 83, he is far more active than most persons half his age. Every Monday through Friday, 52 weeks a year, David runs 5 miles through the streets of his small northern Illinois town. On weekends, he takes time out from his running schedule to join his wife Elaine and their walking group on long, not so leisurely, hikes throughout the Illinois countryside. I have had the distinct pleasure of sharing several enjoyable runs with David. I never cease to be amazed at what an exquisitely trained older athlete he is. Waneen Spirduso of the University of Texas has described elite older athletes like David as a measure of what it is possible to achieve in old age. They serve as an inspiration to individuals many years their junior, and they remind us that aging need not necessarily result in physical decline and decay (6).

measured (5), and recent years have shown a reduction in the number of papers published using biological age as the primary measure of senescence.

Psychological age

Psychological age refers to person's capabilities along with a number of dimensions of mental or cognitive functioning, including self-esteem and self-efficacy, as well as learning, memory, and perception. In much the same way that people of the same chronological age often differ biologically, it is now recognized that it may be possible for people to have different psychological ages. Birren (7) suggests that some older persons demonstrate psychological adjustments that are typical for their chronological age, whereas others behave as though they were psychological younger (or older)

Real Life Story 1-3   Charles — Profile of a Psychologically Vibrant Older Adult

Charles is professor emeritus of physics at a large Midwestern University. Officially, he retired from the university in 1989; however, I doubt that anybody noticed. For the first 8 years of his retirement, he continued to teach half-time for the physics department, while increasing his involvement in numerous local organizations and philanthropic groups. Charlie also served on the local School Board and Environmental Council. Despite this busy schedule, he is a committed exerciser, enjoying hiking and gardening in the summer and cross-country skiing in the winter. There are few weekends in the year when he cannot be found outdoors, enjoying the fresh air. Recently, at the age of 83, Charlie signed a contract with a publishing company to start work on the seventh edition of his highly successful high school physics textbook. When asked where he finds the energy to be so intellectually active, he simply shrugs his shoulders and explains he cannot imagine doing anything else.

than their contemporaries. As with biological age, there is no consensus with respect to how to measure psychological age (8); nonetheless, it is apparent that psychological health and adjustment is an integral component of successful aging and that the assessment of psychological integrity is at least as important as the assessment of physical status in experimental gerontology (9).

Social age

Social age refers to the notion that society often develops fairly rigid expectations with regard to what is considered to be appropriate behavior for a person of a particular age. As a result of these societal norms, we are sometimes uncomfortable when we encounter individuals who are behaving in a manner that is viewed as unorthodox or inappropriate for their chronological age. In these instances, we sometimes wish that people would "act their age." Although socialization and the development of "age-appropriate behavior" patterns is a complex topic, it is apparent that social roles and expectations can play an important role in the lifestyle choices of older persons. For example, a number of recent studies have shown that later life physical activity choices are dependent on an individual's perception of what is, or is not, age-appropriate behavior (10, 11). As physical activity professionals, many of us will have encountered older persons who grew up believing that it is undignified for older women, in particular, to be seen exercising in public. We will need to break these stereotypic misconceptions if we are to be successful helping some of our older clients to be more physically active.

In 2008, the U.S. Department of Health and Human Services issued Physical Activity Guidelines for Americans (12) that strongly encouraged Americans of all ages to adopt physically active lifestyles. The guidelines actively encourage clinicians, health professionals, and older persons themselves to break away from stereotypic

Real Life Story 1-4   Alice — Profile of a Socially Engaged Older Adult

Alice retired as dean of a college of arts and sciences at Midwestern Liberal Arts University in 2005. She is a trained gerontologist. In her capacity as dean, she was instrumental in the establishment of an undergraduate gerontology program at her university. The program has trained hundreds of professionals who are currently serving older adults throughout the Midwest and beyond. When she left her paid employment at the university, she forgot that retirement was supposed to be a time for disengagement and taking it easy. Instead, she has continued to serve in an advisory capacity to many local groups and organizations. While serving on one of these committees, she met a widower almost 20 years her junior, whom she married for the first time last year at the age of 78. Alice and her new husband Ed are committed exercisers. Alice and Ed have decided to divide their time between their Indiana home and their winter retreat in Florida. Alice has confided in me that Ed is a big hit with the ladies when he leads them in impromptu calisthenics sessions on the beach near their Pensacola home.

perspectives about aging. Instead of encouraging seniors to follow expected patterns of behavior and "take it easy," the guidelines urge us to promote a more vigorous and healthful model of aging in which older persons are invited to play a more active role in their own aging.

Despite many years of research, there is no consensus with respect to how best to quantify any of these alternative measures of aging. Thus, although it is apparent that chronological age is an incomplete measure of senescence and that alternative definitions of aging are both useful and necessary, no single unified definition of biological, psychological, or social aging exists. Nonetheless, it is clear that an appreciation of chronological, biological, psychological, and social perspectives on aging is essential if we are to grasp the true essence of aging.

BIOLOGICAL THEORIES OF AGING

The highly complex nature of human aging is reflected by the large number of theories that have been proposed to account for the underlying biological mechanisms of aging. However, despite the efforts of many dozens of investigators (13–15), little progress has been made toward the identification of a single, unified theory of biological aging. Indeed, it seems increasingly likely that aging is not caused by a single mechanism that can be easily identified and understood and that aging occurs in response to a wide variety of mechanisms.

It is well beyond the scope of this chapter to provide a detailed summary of the many theories of aging. However, it is useful to present an overview of the major types of theories that have been proposed. One of the most useful classification schemes was proposed by Leonard Hayflick (16) who argued that aging theories can be subdivided into three major classes: cellular theories, genetic theories, and control theories. However, Hayflick cautions that these theories are seldom mutually exclusive and that many of the proposed mechanisms are likely to be operating simultaneously.

Cellular theories of aging

Cellular theories of aging focus on degenerative changes that occur at the microscopic level of analysis. One of the most commonly proposed mechanisms of cellular aging is *free-radical oxidation* (13). A free radical is a molecule of oxygen with an uneven number of electrons in its outer shell. Because the odd number of electrons in its outer shell makes the free radical molecule highly unstable, the free radical attempts to link up with other molecules to regain the electron it needs to achieve stability. However, this process results in the creation of another free radical and can initiate a series of destructive oxidative chain reactions that can be many thousands of events long. In healthy individuals, free radicals coexist in a state of equilibrium with a series of *mixed function oxidases* that neutralize their destructive effects.

In aging and disease, the state of balance between free radicals and mixed function oxidases is often disrupted. The disruption of this equilibrium can occur as a result of a wide variety of internal biological changes as well as environmental factors such as exposure to radiation and chemical carcinogens. There is some evidence to suggest that aging results in a decreased expression of mixed function oxidases, which disrupts the biological equilibrium and results in an increased likelihood of free-radical attack. Among the damage attributed to free radicals are alterations to the structure of collagen and elastin, the destruction of DNA, and a progressive breakdown of the immune system.

Bjorksten (17) has proposed that aging at the cellular level is caused by age-related breakdowns in the structure of cells because of the formation of *cross-links* between adjacent molecules. The bonding together of adjacent molecules alters their configuration and often has significant functional consequences. Cross-linking disrupts the structure of cells by promoting DNA damage, cell mutation, and eventually cell death. Bjorksten suggests that the formation of cross-links is the precursor to most age-related changes at the cellular level. He further notes that since free radicals are effective cross-linking agents, free-radical oxidation can be considered a special instance of the cross-link theory.

Genetic theories of aging

There is considerable evidence from twin studies to support the notion that a significant portion of age-related changes can be attributed to genetic mechanisms (18, 19). A Russian scientist named Medvedev has proposed that aging occurs as a result of the progressive destruction of DNA sequences by randomly occurring mutations (20). This loss of DNA sequences disrupts the ability of the cell to reproduce and continues progressively throughout the life cycle.

Leonard Hayflick (16) has proposed that the genetic control of senescence is not simply regulated by randomly occurring mutations, but rather, cell death appears to be due to a programmed, purposeful sequence of events written into the genetic code. Hayflick has shown that cultured human and animal cells exhibit a finite limit with regard to their ability to reproduce. The "Hayflick limit" has been replicated in numerous tissues from a wide variety of species (21). The "Hayflick limit" presents strong evidence to suggest that cells age in an orderly and programmed manner. However, this research has not been able to identify a single mechanism that is responsible for cell disruption and death.

In recent years, considerable attention has focused on the role that telomeres play in the regulation of biological aging (22–24). A telomere is a region of repetitive DNA at the end of a chromosome, which is thought to protect the chromosome from deterioration. Olovnikov has shown that aging is associated with a systematic shortening of telomeres, which results in a decline in the cell's ability to reproduce (25). In 2009,

Elizabeth Blackburn, Carol Greider, and Jack Szostak were awarded the Nobel Prize in physiology or medicine for their work that has helped to explain the process by which telomeres influence the viability of human cells and provide insights into some of the mechanisms underlying human aging (26, 27).

Control theories of aging

A third class of theories attempts to explain aging in terms of the function of specific physiologic systems known to be vital for controlling our bodies' ability to respond to stressors. An example of such a system is the immune system. There is strong evidence to suggest that both the quality and the quantity of immune system responses to stress systematically decrease with advancing age. Older adults not only exhibit a significant decline in *T-cell activity*, but also are more susceptible to autoimmune disease.

The principal genetic control of the immune system occurs in a complex series of genes known as the *major histocompatibility complex* (MHC). The MHC is thought to govern the expression of antigens, or chemical markers, that tag each of our cells and to cause the body to spot and reject foreign tissues and invading germs. The integrity of the MHC has been shown to deteriorate with advancing age. Interestingly, the MHC not only controls immunologic functioning, but is also responsible for the genetic expression of the mixed function oxidases, which, as previously mentioned, protect cells against damaging free-radical oxidation. The MHC role in immune functioning is thus an example of how an important regulatory system can provide a viable link between the cellular, genetic, and control theories of aging.

The immune system is not the only regulatory system implicated in the control of the aging process. In recent years, attention has also been paid to the importance of the endocrine and the neurocognitive systems in control of human aging. It seems likely that future research will confirm the importance of numerous different control systems in the regulation of aging at the molecular, cellular, and system levels.

To summarize, our current understanding of the biological mechanisms responsible for aging strongly suggests that aging is a complex process in which multiple biological mechanisms acting at the molecular, cellular, and system levels result in a progressive and inevitable decrease in the body's ability to respond appropriately to internal and external stressors. Because biological aging is apparently regulated by many redundant mechanisms, there is little reason to believe that experimental science is likely to afford us a miracle cure for the aging process in the foreseeable future.

SUCCESSFUL AGING

Although structural decay and functional decline are an inescapable consequence of aging, there are often considerable differences between individuals with respect to both the rate and the extent of this decline. It is now clear that it is possible for individuals to deviate from expected patterns of aging and, at least for some time, postpone or minimize the consequences of aging. A recent review of the physical activity and aging literature (28) concludes that regular physical activity appears to be one of the few lifestyle behaviors identified to date that can favorably influence such a broad range of physiological systems and chronic disease risk factors, and may also be associated with better mental health and social integration.

Over the past 20 to 30 years, a substantial body of evidence has accumulated regarding the benefits that accrue to older adults who participate in regular physical activity (12, 28). This book provides an overview of the substantial evidence that links physical activity participation to successful aging. The WHO has proposed an organizational schema that can be used to categorize the benefits of physical activity for older adults into two broad categories (29): (a) benefits of physical activity for the individual persons and (b) societal benefits of promoting physically active lifestyles among older persons. Under the WHO schema, the individual benefits can be summarized into three general areas: physiological benefits (Table 1-1), psychological benefits (Table 1-2), and social benefits (Table 1-3), as well as the benefits for society (Table 1-4). The WHO physical activity guidelines recommend that virtually all older persons should participate in physical activity on a regular basis and that society has a responsibility to advocate broad-based participation in physical activity whenever possible. The WHO guidelines conclude that regular physical activity

Table 1-1 Physiological Benefits of Physical Activity for Older Persons

IMMEDIATE BENEFITS

Glucose levels: Physical activity helps regulate blood glucose levels.

Catecholamine activity: Both adrenalin and noradrenalin levels are stimulated by physical activity.

Improved sleep: Physical activity has been shown to enhance sleep quality and quantity in individuals of all ages.

LONG-TERM EFFECTS

Aerobic/cardiovascular endurance: Substantial improvements in almost all aspects of cardiovascular functioning have been observed after appropriate physical training.

Resistance training/muscle strengthening: Individuals of all ages can benefit from muscle strengthening exercises. Resistance training can have a significant effect on the maintenance of independence in old age.

Flexibility: Exercise that stimulates movement throughout the range of motion assists in the preservation and restoration of flexibility.

Balance/coordination: Regular activity helps prevent and/or postpone the age-associated declines in balance and coordination that are a major risk factor for falls.

Velocity of movement: Behavioral slowing is a characteristic of advancing age. Individuals who are regularly active can often postpone these age-related declines.

The WHO guidelines have been placed in the public domain and can be freely copied and distributed (29).

Table 1-2 Psychological Benefits of Physical Activity for Older Persons

IMMEDIATE BENEFITS

Relaxation: Appropriate physical activity enhances relaxation.

Reduced stress and anxiety: There is evidence that regular physical activity can reduce stress and anxiety.

Enhanced mood state: Numerous people report elevations in mood state after appropriate physical activity.

LONG-TERM EFFECTS

General well-being: Improvements in almost all aspects of psychological functioning have been observed after periods of extended physical activity.

Improved mental health: Regular exercise can make an important contribution in the treatment of several mental illnesses, including depression and anxiety neuroses.

Cognitive improvements: Regular physical activity may help postpone age-related declines in CNS processing speed and improve reaction time.

Motor control and performance: Regular activity helps prevent and/or postpone the age-associated declines in both fine and gross motor performance.

Skill acquisition: New skills can be learned and existing skills refined by all individuals regardless of age.

The WHO guidelines have been placed in the public domain and can be freely copied and distributed (29).

Table 1-3 Social Benefits of Physical Activity for Older Persons

IMMEDIATE BENEFITS

Empowering older individuals: A large proportion of the older adult population voluntarily adopts a sedentary lifestyle that eventually threatens to reduce independence and self-sufficiency. Participation in appropriate physical activity can help empower older individuals and assist them in playing a more active role in society.

Enhanced social and cultural integration: Physical activity programs, particularly when carried out in small groups and/or in social environments, enhance social and intercultural interactions for many older adults.

LONG-TERM EFFECTS

Enhanced integration: Regularly active individuals are less likely to withdraw from society and more likely to actively contribute to the social milieu.

Formation of new friendships: Participation in physical activity, particularly in small groups and other social environments, stimulates new friendships and acquaintances.

Widened social and cultural networks: Physical activity frequently provides individuals with an opportunity to widen available social networks.

Role maintenance and new role acquisition: A physically active lifestyle helps foster the stimulating environments necessary for maintaining an active role in society, as well as for acquiring positive new roles.

Enhanced intergenerational activity: In many societies, physical activity is a shared activity that provides opportunities for intergenerational contact, thereby diminishing stereotypic perceptions about aging and the elderly

The WHO guidelines have been placed in the public domain and can be freely copied and distributed (29).

Table 1-4 Societal Benefits of Promoting Physical Activity for Older Persons

Reduced health and social care costs: Physical inactivity and sedentary living contributes to a decrease in independence and the onset of many chronic diseases. Physically active lifestyles can help postpone the onset of physical frailty and disease, thereby significantly reducing health and social care costs.

Enhancing the productivity of older adults: Older individuals have much to contribute to society. Physically active lifestyles help older adults maintain functional independence and optimize the extent to which they are able to actively participate in society.

Promoting a positive and active image of older persons: A society that promotes a physically active lifestyle for older adults is more likely to reap the benefits of the wealth of experience and wisdom possessed by the older individuals in the community. A large proportion of the older adult population voluntarily adopt a sedentary lifestyle that eventually threatens to reduce independence and self-sufficiency.

The WHO guidelines have been placed in the public domain and can be freely copied and distributed (29).

provides substantial health-related benefits; it is cheap, safe, and readily available; and physical activity interventions have a major role to play in the prevention, treatment, and management of noncommunicative diseases and conditions associated with advancing age.

In the United States, societal interest in promoting physical activity has been recently underscored by the decision of the Department of Health and Human Services (DHHS) to develop, for the first time, official U.S. Government Physical Activity Guidelines (12). The recently published DHHS Physical Activity Guidelines Advisory Committee Report concludes that there is strong evidence that, compared with less-active persons, more-active men and women have lower rates of all-cause mortality, coronary heart disease, high blood pressure, stroke, Type 2 diabetes, metabolic syndrome, colon cancer, breast cancer, and depression. In addition, strong evidence also supports the conclusion that, compared with less-active people, physically active adults and older adults exhibit a higher level of cardiorespiratory and muscular fitness, have a healthier body mass and composition, and have a biomarker profile that is more favorable for preventing cardiovascular disease and Type 2 diabetes and for enhancing bone health. The report concludes that there is also evidence indicating that physically active adults and older adults have better quality sleep and health-related quality of life (QOL). Although no amount of physical activity can stop the aging process, there is now compelling evidence that a moderate amount of regular physical activity can minimize the physiological effects of aging and increase active life expectancy by limiting the development and progression of chronic disease and disabling conditions.

S U M M A R Y

A brief reflection on the present status and future direction of research and clinical practice in the area of physical activity and successful aging concludes this chapter. The past quarter century has seen a tremendous expansion of interest into the physical activity needs of older persons. This interest is reflected in an increase in scientific journals, scholarly publications, and academic meetings focusing on physical activity and aging. During this time, we have learned a great deal about the role that regular physical activity plays in successful aging. It is now well established that significant physiological, psychological, social, and societal benefits accrue from participation in physical activity and that the benefits of a physically active lifestyle extend throughout the lifespan. The WHO, the U.S. Surgeon General's Office, and U.S. Department of Health and Human Services are among the many organizations that have officially endorsed physical activity as an integral component of healthy aging.

These positive developments notwithstanding, there is clearly much that remains to be done. Despite the apparent benefits of remaining physically active, the proportion of older individuals who participate regularly in physical activity is disappointingly low. For example, in the United States, only about 25% of older adults exercise at or above recommended levels of physical activity and as many as one-third of American seniors engage in no physical activity at all (28). In this book, you will learn about some of the complex factors that help motivate individuals of all ages to begin and to continue to participate in regular physical activity.

Although it is widely recognized that physical activity is a necessary component of active aging, there is little agreement with respect to the optimal structure and content of physical activity programs for seniors. Indeed, because the older adult population is characterized by tremendous diversity, it is probably unrealistic to expect that we will ever be able to identify a single optimal physical activity program for older persons. Rather, it is likely that physical activity programs for older adults will need to be highly individualized if they are to meet the diverse needs of the older adult population. Most researchers and practitioners do agree that effective physical activity programs will need to be multidimensional, including a combination of cardiovascular endurance, muscle strength, flexibility, balance, and coordination activities.

In recent years, a consensus has emerged among physical activity and aging researchers that a key objective of physical activity participation in older adults is the preservation and/or restoration of acceptable QOL. Although QOL is difficult to define precisely, most researchers agree that QOL is dependent on a complex combination of factors including physical health, psychological well-being, social satisfaction, and spiritual contentment. It is increasingly clear that physical activity alone is insufficient for the promotion of high QOL in old age. In order to age successfully, older persons will need to be not only physically active, but also socially, intellectually, culturally, and (for many seniors) spiritually active (30, 31). One of the challenges for our profession in the future will be to learn how to integrate physical activity into the wider social, cultural, and economic context of active ageing as a whole. In this chapter, I have provided brief descriptions of four individuals who have followed remarkable paths with respect to the direction taken by their aging process. Our challenge as exercise professionals working with older adults is to find ways to assist others to follow similar paths — growing old as healthy, independent, productive, respected, and valued members of our society.

 QUESTIONS FOR REFLECTION

1. How do you define aging?

2. What do you understand by chronological, biological, psychological, and social aging?

3. Why do we age? Please explain the biological theory of aging that makes most sense to you.

4. Why is it so difficult to establish a precise age in which old age begins?

5. The rate and extent of biological, psychological, and social changes experienced in old age vary considerably from person to person. Why?

6. Can the aging process be slowed? Please explain.

7. What does it mean to age successfully?

8. Discuss ways to promote successful aging.

9. What are some benefits of physical activity on health status in older adults?

10. What are some societal benefits of physical activity?

REFERENCES

1. Ashford JW, Atwood CS, Blass JP, et al. What is aging? What is its role in Alzheimer's disease? What can we do about it? *J Alzheimers Dis.* 2005;7(3):247–53; discussion 255–62.
2. Demongeot J. Biological boundaries and biological age. *Acta Biotheor.* 2009;57(4):397–418.
3. Bhanot SM, Naik P, Gopalakrishnan R, Salkar DM, Nagashabandi K. Biological age vs. chronological age. *Eur Urol.* 2005;48(1):168; author reply 168–70.
4. Jackson SH, Weale MR, Weale RA. *Biological age — What is it and can it be measured?* Arch Gerontol Geriatr. 2003;36(2):103–15.

5. Fallin MD, Matteini A. Genetic epidemiology in aging research. *J Gerontol A Biol Sci Med Sci.* 2009;64(1):47–60.

6. Spirduso WW, Francis KL, MacRae PG. *Physical Dimensions of Aging.* 2nd ed. Champaign (IL): Human Kinetics; 2005. ix, 374 p.

7. Birren JE. Research on the psychologic aspects of aging. *Geriatrics.* 1963;18:393–403.

8. Springer KW, Pudrovska T, Hauser RM. Does psychological well-being change with age? Longitudinal tests of age variations and further exploration of the multidimensionality of Ryff's model of psychological well-being. *Soc Sci Res.* 2011;40(1):392–8.

9. Lacruz ME, Emeny RT, Bickel H, et al. Mental health in the aged: Prevalence, covariates and related neuroendocrine, cardiovascular and inflammatory factors of successful aging. *BMC Med Res Methodol.* 2010;10:36.

10. 1Brawley LR, Rejeski WJ, King AC. Promoting physical activity for older adults: The challenges for changing behavior. *Am J Prev Med.* 2003;25(3 Suppl 2):172–83.

11. Seefeldt V, Malina RM, Clark MA. Factors affecting levels of physical activity in adults. *Sports Med.* 2002;32(3):143–68.

12. U.S. Department of Health and Human Services, editor. *2008 Physical Activity Guidelines for Americans.* Washington (DC): U.S. Department of Health and Human Services; 2008.

13. Rattan SI. Theories of biological aging: Genes, proteins, and free radicals. *Free Radic Res.* 2006;40(12):1230–8.

14. Troen BR. The biology of aging. *Mt Sinai J Med.* 2003;70(1):3–22.

15. Masoro EJ, Austad SN. *Handbook of the Biology of Aging.* 7th ed. (The handbooks of aging). Amsterdam, Netherlands: Elsevier Academic Press; 2011. xx, 660 p.

16. Hayflick L. Theories of biological aging. *Exp Gerontol.* 1985;20(3–4):145–59.

17. Bjorksten J. The crosslinkage theory of aging: Clinical implications. *Compr Ther.* 1976;2(2):65–74.

18. Lee T, Henry JD, Trollor JN, Sachdev PS. Genetic influences on cognitive functions in the elderly: A selective review of twin studies. *Brain Res Rev.* 2010;64(1):1–13.

19. Christensen K, Frederiksen H, Vaupel JW, McGue M. Age trajectories of genetic variance in physical functioning: A longitudinal study of Danish twins aged 70 years and older. *Behav Genet.* 2003;33(2):125–36.

20. Medvedev ZA. Age changes of chromatin. A review. *Mech Ageing Dev.* 1984;28(2–3):139–54.

21. Shay JW, Wright WE. Hayflick, his limit, and cellular ageing. *Nat Rev Mol Cell Biol.* 2000;1(1):72–6.

22. Friedrich U, Griese E, Schwab M, Fritz P, Thon K. Telomere length in different tissues of elderly patients. *Mech Ageing Dev.* 2000;119(3):89–99.

23. Collerton J, Martin-Ruiz C, Kenny A, et al. Telomere length is associated with left ventricular function in the oldest old: The Newcastle 85+ study. *Eur Heart J.* 2007;28(2):172–6.

24. von Zglinicki T, Petrie J, Kirkwood TB. Telomere-driven replicative senescence is a stress response. *Nat Biotechnol.* 2003;21(3):229–30.

25. Olovnikov AM. [Aging is a result of a shortening of the "differotene" in the telomere due to end under-replication and under-repair of DNA]. *Izv Akad Nauk SSSR Biol.* 1992;(4):641–3.

26. Szostak JW, Blackburn EH. Cloning yeast telomeres on linear plasmid vectors. *Cell.* 1982;29(1):245–55.

27. Greider CW, Blackburn EH. Identification of a specific telomere terminal transferase activity in Tetrahymena extracts. *Cell.* 1985;43(2 Pt 1):405–13.

28. American College of Sports Medicine, Chodzko-Zajko WJ, Proctor DN, et al. American College of Sports Medicine position stand. Exercise and physical activity for older adults. *Med Sci Sports Exerc.* 2009;41(7):1510–30.

29. World Health Organization, editor. *Heidelberg Guidelines for Promoting Physical Activity Among Older Persons.* Geneva, Switzerland: World Health Organization; 1996.

30. Depp CA, Jeste DV. Definitions and predictors of successful aging: A comprehensive review of larger quantitative studies. *Am J Geriatric Psychiat.* 2006;14(1):6–20.

31. Rozanova J. Discourse of successful aging in The Globe & Mail: Insights from critical gerontology. *J Aging Studies.* 2010;24(4):213–22.

CHAPTER 2

Physical and Psychological Benefits of Physical Activity and Exercise for Healthy Older Adults

Jennifer L. Etnier and William B. Karper

■■■ **CHAPTER OUTLINE**

- **Introduction**
- **Physical benefits**
  - Effects of physical activity on aerobic capacity
  - Effects of physical activity on cardiovascular function
  - Effects of physical activity on body composition
    - Effects of physical activity on bone health
    - Effects of physical activity on muscle strength, power, and endurance
    - Effects of physical activity on balance
    - Effects of physical activity on flexibility
    - Effects of physical activity on physical functioning and activities of daily living
- **Psychological benefits**
  - Effects of physical activity on psychological well-being
  - Effects of physical activity on quality of life
  - Effects of physical activity on depression and mood
  - Effects of physical activity on cognitive performance
- **Summary**

INTRODUCTION

The information in this chapter broadly covers the physical and psychological benefits that healthy older adults can gain from engaging in physical activity and exercise on a regular basis. For the purpose of this discussion, an older adult is defined as anyone 50 years old or older, and the term *physical activity* is characterized as "any bodily movement produced by the contraction of skeletal muscle and that result[s] in a substantial increase over resting energy expenditure" (4). Also, two major types of physical activity, aerobic exercise and resistance exercise (strength training), will be considered in regard to all of the outcomes that are reviewed. Range-of-motion exercise (flexibility training) will be discussed relative to the outcome of flexibility, and certain types of exercise that may be particularly important for balance will be addressed.

In 2009, the American College of Sports Medicine® (ACSM) released an extensive position statement entitled, "Exercise and Physical Activity for Older Adults," which provided an up-to-date, comprehensive review of the latest research available on this topic (18). Much of the information discussed in this chapter is bolstered by the work presented in various parts of that report and is framed in a similar way. This was done so that readers who are interested in obtaining more in-depth information or additional references can go to the ACSM position statement and easily locate them under headings similar to those used in this chapter. In addition, evidence from meta-analytic reviews is presented. Meta-analytic reviews provide a statistical synthesis of data from studies conducted to test the same research question, and are particularly useful for summarizing well-developed bodies of literature when the results of the studies are not consistent. According to Tricoci et al. (85), results from meta-analyses provide the highest level of evidence to support clinical practice. Thus, these findings are considered in conjunction with the ACSM position to support the conclusions.

It is generally acknowledged that increasing age in humans is associated with a steady functional decline in numerous systems of the body. However, people can make conscious decisions to alter certain lifestyle factors, which can slow down some of this decline. Most exercise- and health-related professionals agree that participating in regular physical activity is an important lifestyle factor that both directly and indirectly connects to successful aging because of the many positive effects physical activity has on numerous physiological systems in the human body. In general, research demonstrates that regular exercise accompanied by adequate amounts of leisure-time physical activity can avert the physiological effects of inactivity and can keep a person active longer in life by affording significant protection against numerous chronic diseases and conditions that cause disability (18). Therefore, it is safe to say that almost everything about ongoing engagement in almost any type of physical activity for older adults is positive.

PHYSICAL BENEFITS

Effects of physical activity on aerobic capacity

Aerobic capacity (how well a person transports and uses oxygen) is best expressed in terms of maximal oxygen uptake (VO_{2max}), which is the greatest amount of oxygen a person can use while exercising as hard as possible (see Key Point 2-1). VO_{2max} can be increased in many older men and women with appropriate exercise training. For example, recent research shows that combined aerobic endurance and strength training increases aerobic capacity in older men (44), as does cycle training alone.

> ### KEY POINT 2-1
>
> VO_{2max} (the amount of oxygen the body uses during maximal physical effort) is the measure used by most exercise professionals to denote cardiorespiratory fitness level. During exercise, there is a close relationship between VO_2 and heart rate — both increase nearly linearly with increasing intensity of exercise. The rating of perceived exertion (a self-perception of how hard one is working — RPE) is also generally correlated with exercise heart rate and the amount of work being performed during exercise and can be used during exercise testing as a way to know when the person will fatigue and become exhausted. RPE values can also be used to predict VO_{2max}. It is generally accepted that physical training decreases RPE and heart rate at any given intensity of exercise and increases VO_{2max} (57).

The extent to which VO_{2max} is increased is influenced by three factors, which together determine exercise volume: intensity (how hard the person exercises), frequency (how often the person exercises), and duration (how long the person exercises). Greater exercise volume is directly related to larger increases in VO_{2max} (34). This principle is true even in the oldest elderly (those people older than 75 years); however, the improvements may not be as great in very old people as they are in younger adults (59). Importantly, there is evidence to suggest that changes in aerobic capacity in response to exercise differ between men and women. In particular, women seem to be somewhat more sensitive to increases in the volume of exercise than do men. In addition, the physiological mechanisms in the cardiac, pulmonary, vascular, central nervous, and muscular systems that cause increases in VO_{2max} in older people may be different for men and women. More research will be necessary to fully understand these differences.

Concerning potential health effects related to changes in aerobic capacity, it is significant that aerobic exercise (see Key Point 2-2), which markedly increases aerobic capacity, appears to decrease oxidative stress in previously sedentary older women. Oxidative stress occurs when physiological stressors (*e.g.*, exercise, dietary patterns, and smoking) are introduced and cannot be adequately repelled by the body's immune system. Free-radical oxidation can damage human cells, and this damage is

> **Real Life Story 2-1   Carol**
>
> Carol was 80 years old and had not been a regular exerciser. Lately, when she was working in her garden, she noticed that she felt tired much sooner than she thought was normal. So she decided to push herself harder, but very soon she was not able to continue because of fatigue and running out of breath. She decided to join an older adult exercise class at a local recreation center to get into better shape. The class turned out to be a dance/exercise class with music. After participating in the class for 12 weeks, Carol noticed that she could push herself a lot longer and harder while gardening without becoming breathless or tired. Apparently, the exercise class had increased her aerobic capacity. Following her latest treadmill exercise test at her doctor's office, in which the test lasted until she could not continue, she was told that her ability to deliver and utilize oxygen had increased since her last test and that her participation in the dance/exercise class was probably the reason for the increase. Most importantly, Carol found that she was able to work longer and harder in her garden, and her yard looked lovely.

considered by many researchers to be a causative factor in numerous underlying chronic diseases, such as heart disease or diabetes. Interestingly, the positive changes in aerobic capacity and oxidative stress outcomes occur with very little change in body fat or muscle (15).

KEY POINT 2-2
Aerobic exercise is physical activity performed at an intensity that is supported by oxygen utilization. It improves cardiovascular health.

Effects of physical activity on cardiovascular function

Aerobic exercise performed regularly over a period of 3 months or more lowers heart rate at rest and during physical activity performed at less than 100% effort (31). People who participate in regular aerobic exercise also experience a smaller rise in blood pressure during submaximal physical activity (76), have various biochemical and hemodynamic improvements in trained muscles (43, 61, 93), and demonstrate cardioprotection (*e.g.*, healthier cholesterol levels) (81) as compared with those who are sedentary.

Effects of physical activity on body composition

Regularly participating in moderate-intensity aerobic physical activity has been shown to reduce the amount of fat on the bodies of older adults (46, 83). It is possible that this fat loss may be related to the number of activity sessions in which a person participates. Logically, participating in more sessions should be associated with greater fat loss. Importantly, it seems that it is the fat carried around the midsection of the body that can be reduced (37). This is a positive effect because it is fat weight around the middle of the body that has been related to risk of ill health (41). Although aerobic physical activity does not usually cause an increase in the size or strength of

> ## Real Life Story 2-2   Paige
>
> Paige thought she was too heavy. Specifically, she felt that she carried too much fat weight as compared with the weight she carried from bones and muscle. She never liked physical activity very much because she was not very coordinated. Her friend Dave suggested that they go for a walk every evening. He said that walking would be a good activity for two older people like them. Because she liked Dave and thought she would enjoy talking with him while they walked, she agreed. Over time, they reached the point where they were walking for about an hour, five evenings each week. Paige noticed that her clothes were beginning to feel increasingly loose, and she mentioned this to Dave. He told her that she was probably losing fat weight as a result of their evening walks.

muscle (83), resistance exercise training (strength training) performed at a reasonably high intensity can increase muscle strength in older men and women (9, 35, 36). In addition, resistance exercise training at moderate-intensity levels or higher appears to reduce fat at various places on the body in older men and women (9, 35, 36, 38, 42, 84). Exactly where the body fat will be lost with this type of activity is unclear. Lastly, new research supports that resistance training actually prevents weight gain and limits the negative changes in body composition that occur in postmenopausal women (11).

More generally, it is important to know that modest amounts of numerous types of physical activity (*i.e.*, physical activity broadly defined) have been reported to slow down undesirable age-related weight loss by as much as 25% in older people. Higher-intensity physical activity does not appear to offer any additional benefits in this regard (79).

Effects of physical activity on bone health

Results from numerous meta-analytic studies show that both resistance exercise and aerobic exercise may have positive effects on the density of bone in women and men at various ages (47, 48, 92). Most of the investigators doing physical activity research on bone health have used women as subjects because of concerns about bone deterioration as women age. In this regard, it is important to recognize that engaging in low-intensity, weight-bearing physical activities (*e.g.*, casual walking and certain types of social dancing) for 3 or more days a week may have very little or a modest effect on bone mineral density in older women (49). Of course, these types of activities may be useful in preventing other age-related problems (8, 49). But other physical activities engaged in at higher intensities (*e.g.*, walking fast, walking with weights, jogging/running, and walking up and down stairs) may produce a larger bone mineral density effect in older women (49). Research also indicates that resistance training, and particularly high-intensity resistance exercise, can have a positive effect on bone mineral density when compared with no training (47–49, 92). Future studies are necessary to provide information about the relative benefits of different modes of physical activity, the effects of physical activity on the bone health of older men, and specific dose-response guidance concerning exactly how much exercise is needed to strengthen bone in the hip, spine, and wrist areas for older men and women.

Effects of physical activity on muscle strength, power, and endurance

Results from numerous studies support that older adults (men and women) can increase muscular strength (defined as maximum force that can be exerted in just one or a few muscle contractions) when they engage in resistance training (16, 26, 27, 30, 32, 54). It is possible that some older adults may actually increase their muscular strength (measured as a percentage of change) as much as younger people. Of course, how hard and how often a person trains and the length of each training period will be the strongest predictors of the amount of change. However, a person's gender may also influence the magnitude of these increases (39).

KEY POINT 2-3

One repetition maximal effort is defined as the maximum amount that a person can lift in a single repetition for a particular exercise (*e.g.*, bench press and biceps curl).

Regarding muscle strength and power, research supports that older adults who engage in strength and power training show significant improvements in knee extension and the one repetition maximal effort (see Key Point 2-3) leg press (60). In addition, research has shown that older people are able to increase muscle power (defined as the amount of muscle force or torque applied multiplied by the speed of the movement) to a significant degree when they engage in appropriate resistance exercise (40, 64, 86). Even though few investigators have studied muscle endurance (defined as producing muscle force or power repeatedly over a period) in older adults, it appears that muscle endurance gains can be accomplished by older adults with the use of adequate exercise intensity (2, 30, 89). This conclusion is further supported by evidence that cycle training increases leg strength and power and upper leg muscle size in older men (57).

Effects of physical activity on balance

Engaging in physical activity, especially that which directly conditions a person for better balance, muscle strength, flexibility, and walking skill, appears to prevent falling (13, 14, 65). Also, aquatic exercise (along with fall prevention education) improves fall risk factors in older people with osteoarthritis (7). Research results also support that tai chi (an activity growing in popularity with older adults) reduces falls (55). In fact, balance can be improved after 6 months of specific tai chi training (82). Therefore, numerous dry land and aquatic activities have been shown to produce positive outcomes in those older people who are at high risk for falling.

Effects of physical activity on flexibility

Healthy older adults have been shown to improve their range-of-motion (flexibility) using various types of range-of-motion exercises (77). Logic dictates that this is probably true for most of the joints in the body. However, there is a lack of published, data-based studies concerning this research question. For instance, there is not a large body of research that addresses the specific number of stretching exercises or how long a certain static exercise or position should be held to most positively affect range-of-motion in older adults. The same is true regarding how often an older person should engage in these exercises to achieve a satisfactory outcome relative to becoming more flexible in different joints. In addition, it is very difficult to find studies on the safety of such exercises for older adults. Given the potential importance of flexibility for functional fitness (50) and the prevention of falls (22), future research exploring ways to effectively improve flexibility is warranted.

Effects of physical activity on physical functioning and activities of daily living

This is another area where more research is needed. Numerous clinicians and their clients report, anecdotally, that resistance exercise training appears to positively impact certain types of physical function related to activities of daily living (ADLs). Most physical activity professionals intuitively believe this is true. However, more research is needed to completely understand all of the relationships between engagement in various types of physical activity, various types of physical functioning, and ADLs. Recent research connects leisure-time physical activity (broadly defined) with relative gains in survival and years of healthy life, and reports that these gains are largest for those older than 75 years (33). One factor that may affect the magnitude of these gains is the potential increase in ADL-related functional capacity, which results from habitual physical activity, and its subsequent contribution to older people remaining independent. In addition, new research supports that regular engagement in aerobic physical activity (especially walking) reduces chronic disease factors in older people (73). Any reduction in chronic disease factors and the many symptoms that accompany chronic diseases would be expected to positively affect ADLs.

PSYCHOLOGICAL BENEFITS

In addition to physical benefits that result from physical activity, there is also evidence that physical activity has psychological benefits for older adults. Psychological outcomes that have been studied most include psychological well-being (broadly defined), quality of life, depression and mood, and cognitive performance. A number of psychological and physiological mechanisms have been proposed to underlie the psychological benefits of physical activity. The psychological mechanisms include self-efficacy (a person's confidence that he or she can successfully complete a given task) and social support. The physiological mechanisms include effects on chemicals in the brain that transmit messages (*e.g.*, dopamine and serotonin), chemicals in the brain that contribute to its overall health (*e.g.*, brain-derived neurotrophic factor and nerve growth factor), brain blood flow, and brain structure (*e.g.*, gray and white matter density).

Effects of physical activity on psychological well-being

Psychological well-being is a multifaceted construct that includes four components: emotional well-being (*e.g.*, depression, anxiety, and mood), self-perceptions (*e.g.*, self-efficacy and body image), bodily well-being (*e.g.*, perception of physical symptoms and experience of pain), and global perceptions (*e.g.*, life satisfaction) (63). By applying meta-analytic techniques to summarize the findings from numerous studies testing the effects of physical activity on these components in older adults, Netz et al. have shown that the overall effect of physical activity on psychological well-being is small. However, effects are larger for perceptions of physical symptoms and for overall well-being, self-efficacy, and positive affect (or mood). By looking more closely at the studies that produced the largest effects, Netz and colleagues determined that aerobic exercise has the largest effect, with resistance exercise a close second, and that moderate-intensity exercise results in the greatest benefits. In this review, larger effects were also apparent for participants who were initially sedentary than for participants who were already physically active. Thus, the existing literature suggests that the psychological well-being of older adults can be positively affected by participation in moderately intense physical activity and that the greatest benefit can be obtained by participants who are currently sedentary.

Effects of physical activity on quality of life

Quality of life has been defined as a global indicator of one's conscious satisfaction with life. However, with regard to physical activity, researchers have typically been more interested in health-related quality of life (HRQL), which refers to a person's

Real Life Story 2-3   Lewis

At 65 years of age, Lewis has just begun an exercise program after years of being inactive. He has joined the local YMCA and is attending strength training sessions on Tuesdays and Thursdays and a swim aerobics class on Mondays. He is really enjoying the new friendships that are developing at the YMCA, and he has been pleased to notice that he is able to climb the stairs in his home without losing his breath. Most importantly to him, however, he has noticed that he feels better in general — he wakes up feeling energized and positive and experiences fewer nagging pains in the mornings. In addition, Bill is pleased to recognize that his overall sense of well-being has improved steadily since beginning his exercise program, and he feels like a new man.

perception of the effects of health on physical, cognitive (or mental), emotional, and social functioning, and on perceptions of pain and vitality (17, 69). Individual studies testing the effects of physical activity interventions on quality-of-life outcomes have been inconsistent, but generally show that physical activity has a positive effect on HRQL (68). When reviewed meta-analytically (21), results of studies testing the effects of physical activity on HRQL in participants with chronic illness indicate a small positive gain resulting from the intervention. Evidence from a series of randomized controlled trials conducted with frail older adults to test the effects of physical activity on HRQL indicates that there is a positive effect for older frail adults for emotional functioning and social functioning and that physical activity did not exacerbate perceptions of pain (75). Interestingly, the positive results of this study were evident for both aerobic exercise and flexibility training, but not for resistance or balance training.

Effects of physical activity on depression and mood

In older adults, the prevalence of clinical depression has been reported as being anywhere from approximately 1% to 42%. The variability in prevalence is largely related to older adults' living status such that lower prevalence is evident among older adults living in private households (approximately 1%–9%) and higher prevalence is observed among older adults living in institutions (14%–42%) (24). The link between depression and physical activity is thought to work in both directions because people who are less physically active are at greater risk for depression and people who are more depressed tend to be less physically active. This link is supported by correlational studies (see Key Point 2-4) demonstrating an association between physical activity and depression (28, 29). However, there is also evidence from randomized controlled experimental studies (see Key Point 2-4), supporting that physical activity actually protects against depression. Recent meta-analytic reviews of studies testing the effects of physical activity on depression across age groups generally support that physical activity reduces both clinical depression and the experience of depressed mood (20, 53, 62, 66, 70, 78). For older adults, results from a meta-analysis that included only studies testing the effects of physical activity on clinical depression demonstrate that physical activity has large beneficial effects (66). Results with regard to the comparison of physical activity interventions with other interventions (psychological and pharmacological) have generally shown that physical activity is as beneficial as these other forms of treatment (53). When physical activity was examined in studies of clinically depressed older adults, it was found to be as effective as cognitive-behavioral therapy, psychoeducation, psychodynamic therapy, and cognitive therapy and had dropout rates that were generally comparable to (*i.e.*, not higher than) those observed for these forms of therapy (66). Thus, the existing research as a whole suggests that physical activity plays an antidepressant role in older adults.

KEY POINT 2-4

Correlational studies test relationships between variables (*e.g.*, physical activity levels and depression) in a group of people. Results from correlational studies cannot be used to draw conclusions regarding cause and effect because it is not possible to determine whether, for example, low physical activity causes depression or depression causes low physical activity.

Randomized controlled trials (experimental studies) are studies in which participants are randomly assigned to different conditions (*e.g.*, a treatment group, which is "given" the treatment, and a control group, which is not "given" the treatment), the treatment is manipulated (*e.g.*, physical activity participation), and the variable under study is measured (*e.g.*, depression). Results from these studies can be used to draw conclusions regarding cause and effect because the participants were essentially the same before their participation in the study. Therefore, differences at the end of the study can be attributed to the treatment that was manipulated.

Prospective studies are those in which similar participants are followed over a period of time. At the beginning and end of the period, data are collected on the variables of interest (*e.g.*, physical activity and depression). The goal (in this example) is to find out whether depression at the end of the period is predicted from the physical activity level at the beginning of the period.

Mood is defined as a transient and unfocused emotional experience that encompasses the concepts of depression, anxiety, vigor, and pleasantness. Although mood is a relatively unstable experience, physical activity is anticipated to increase positive mood and decrease negative mood in older adults. Results from a meta-analytic review of 32 studies (6) indicate that when older adults participate in physical activity, they tend to experience moderate improvements in mood and that these effects are equivalent for improvements in positive mood and decreases in negative mood. Surprisingly (because this is not consistent with findings for most other mental health outcomes), results of this review also suggest that resistance exercise results in larger effects than either combined aerobic and resistance exercise or aerobic exercise alone. Also of interest, positive effects can be observed after as few as 1 to 6 weeks of physical activity and do not appear to be dependent on a person's initial health and activity status.

Effects of physical activity on cognitive performance

Evidence suggests that cognitive performance, a person's ability to perform mentally demanding tasks, decreases with advancing age (72, 74). However, research also shows that there are lifestyle factors, including physical activity, that can reduce the risk of age-related cognitive decline (3). Although some prospective studies (Key Point 2-4) have not supported a beneficial effect of physical activity on cognitive performance (12, 23, 80, 88, 91, 95), the findings of most of these studies show that in a group of

Real Life Story 2-4   Sandy

As Sandy approaches her 60s, she is concerned because she is well aware that her own mother began to experience signs of dementia in her 60s, which ultimately culminated in Alzheimer disease. Because Sandy wants to do everything possible to ensure that she does not have a similar fate, she is pursuing life-style changes that could prevent cognitive decline. She quickly discovers evidence that being physically active can help, and immediately begins walking in her neighborhood in the evenings. She also starts doing little things to increase her strength, such as lifting canned goods repeatedly and using therabands to strengthen her legs. Although she has been exercising for only 6 months, she feels that she can already see improvements in her everyday abilities. For instance, her ability to navigate the grocery store when doing her shopping, to remember why she walked back into the bathroom when she was getting ready to leave the house, and to program her DVR to record television shows has benefited from her exercise.

older adults who have the same cognitive performance at baseline, those who are more physically active at baseline will perform better cognitively in future years than those who are less active at baseline (1, 3, 10, 45, 51, 52, 56, 58, 67, 71, 87, 90, 94, 96).

The effect of physical activity on the cognitive performance of older adults has also been tested in studies using experimental designs. When reviewed using meta-analytic techniques, the results of these studies show that physical activity has a moderate effect on cognitive performance (19). Importantly, meta-analyses also report that the size of the effect is dependent on the particular type of cognitive performance being measured. Unfortunately, the conclusions relative to the type of cognitive performance being measured are not consistent between the two meta-analyses testing its effects. Results from one meta-analysis (19) indicate that the larger effects occur for measures of executive function (tasks that require planning, the ability to inhibit a response, and working memory) than for controlled (tasks that require selections between stimuli), visuospatial (tasks that require mentally working with visual or spatial information), or speed tasks (tasks that require a quick simple response). Results from the other meta-analysis (5) indicated that the only significant positive effects were observed for speed tasks and visual attention (tasks that require attending to repetitive visual stimuli) and that the effects for executive function were negligible. These mixed results emphasize the importance of further study designed to expand our understanding of the specificity of the effects of physical activity on cognitive performance. Given the promising results for executive function reported by Colcombe and Kramer (19), future study should also consider examining different aspects of executive function to further delineate the extent to which physical activity impacts this particular category of cognitive performance (25).

With regard to specific recommendations regarding the type and volume of physical activity to participate in, evidence from the prospective studies suggests that even low-intensity activity (such as walking) can be protective (1, 94). Although there is no evidence from individual studies designed to directly test the relationship between the volume of physical activity and the cognitive benefits that accrue, summary data from a meta-analytic review (19) suggest that the largest benefits from initiating an exercise program occur when using a combined physical activity program that includes aerobic exercise and resistance training, and exercising for more than 6 months and for more than 30 minutes a session.

S U M M A R Y

A clear conclusion that can be drawn from the research on the effects of physical activity for physical and psychological health is that various types of moderate physical activity engaged in for a number of days each week have a positive effect on physical and psychological function in most older people. This is true for both men and women and for all ages of older adults. This is good news because engagement in moderate physical activity presents a minimal safety risk, requires a low financial cost, and can be done alone or with friends indoors or outdoors. Future research will help clarify the exact amount and type of physical activity necessary to obtain maximal benefits.

QUESTIONS FOR REFLECTION

1. What type of factors can be altered to positively impact or slow down the functional decline associated with increasing age?

2. Can exercise training increase aerobic capacity in older men and women, including those who are very old?

3. Over what period does an elderly person have to exercise regularly to lower resting and exercise heart rates?

4. Name the factors that dictate whether an older person can increase muscle strength?

5. What are some of the mechanisms that have been proposed to explain how exercise could have psychological benefits?

6. Evidence suggests that the effects of exercise on psychological outcomes differ depending on whether the exercise consists of aerobic, resistance, or flexibility training. Give specific examples to support this statement.

7. How do the results for exercise on clinical depression compare with the effects of other forms of therapy?

8. Describe how prospective studies on physical activity and cognitive performance are conducted and what the findings generally show.

REFERENCES

1. Abbott RD, White LR, Ross GW, Masaki KH, Curb JD, Petrovitch H. Walking and dementia in physically capable elderly men. *J Am Med Assoc.* 2004;292(12):1447–53.
2. Adams KJ, Swank AM, Berning JM, Sevene-Adams PG, Barnard KL, Shimp-Bowerman J. Progressive strength training in sedentary, older African American women. *Med Sci Sports Exerc.* 2001;33(9):1567–76.
3. Albert MS, Jones K, Savage CR, Berkman L, Seeman T, Blazer D, Rowe JW. Predictors of cognitive change in older persons: MacArthur studies of successful aging. *Psychol Aging.* 1995;10(4):578–89.
4. American College of Sports Medicine. In: Thompson WR, editor. *ACSM's Guidelines for Exercise Testing and Prescription.* 8th ed. Philadelphia (PA): Lippincott Williams & Wilkins; 2010. p. 2.
5. Angevaren M, Aufdemkampe G, Verhaar HJ, Aleman A, Vanhees L. Physical activity and enhanced fitness to improve cognitive function in older people without known cognitive impairment. *Cochrane Database Syst Rev.* 2008;(3):CD005381.
6. Arent SM, Landers DM, Etnier JL. The effects of exercise on mood in older adults: A meta-analytic review. *J Aging Phys Act.* 2000;8(4):407–30.
7. Arnold CM, Faulkner RA. The effect of aquatic exercise and education on lowering fall risk in older adults with hip osteoarthritis. *J Aging Phys Act.* 2010;18(3):245–60.
8. Asikainen TM, Kukkonen-Harjula K, Miilunpalo S. Exercise for health for early postmenopausal women: A systematic review of randomised controlled trials. *Sports Med.* 2004;34(11):753–78.
9. Bamman MM, Hill VJ, Adams GR, et al. Gender differences in resistance-training-induced myofiber hypertrophy among older adults. *J Gerontol A Biol Sci Med Sci.* 2003;58(2):108–16.
10. Barnes DE, Yaffe K, Satariano WA, Tager IB. A longitudinal study of cardiorespiratory fitness and cognitive function in healthy older adults. *J Am Geriatr Soc.* 2003;51(4):459–65.
11. Bea JW, Cussler EC, Going SB, Blew RM, Metcalfe LL, Lohman TG. Resistance training predicts 6-yr body composition change in postmenopausal women. *Med Sci Sports Exerc.* 2010;42(7):1286–95.
12. Broe GA, Creasey H, Jorm AF, et al. Health habits and risk of cognitive impairment and dementia in old age: A prospective study on the effects of exercise, smoking and alcohol consumption. *Aust N Z J Public Health.* 1998;22(5):621–3.
13. Campbell AJ, Robertson MC, Gardner MM, Norton RN, Buchner DM. Falls prevention over 2 years: A randomized controlled trial in women 80 years and older. *Age Ageing.* 1999;28(6):513–8.
14. Campbell AJ, Robertson MC, Gardner MM, Norton RN, Tilyard MW, Buchner DM. Randomised controlled trial of a general practice programme of home based exercise to prevent falls in elderly women. *Br Med J.* 1997;315(7115):1065–9.
15. Campbell PT, Gross MD, Potter JD, Schmitz KH, Duggan C, McTiernan A, Ulrich CM. Effect of exercise on oxidative stress: A 12-month randomized, controlled trial. *Med Sci Sports Exerc.* 2010;42(8):1448–53.
16. Carmeli E, Reznick AZ, Coleman R, Carmeli V. Muscle strength and mass of lower extremities in relation to functional abilities in elderly adults. *Gerontology.* 2000;46(5):249–57.
17. Chen TH, Li L, Kochen MM. A systematic review: How to choose appropriate health-related quality of life (HRQOL) measures in routine general practice? *J Zhejiang Univ Sci B.* 2005;6(9):936–40.
18. American College of Sports Medicine, Chodzko-Zajko WJ, Proctor DN, et al. American College of Sports Medicine position stand. Exercise and physical activity for older adults. *Med Sci Sports Exerc.* 2009;41(7):1510–30.
19. Colcombe S, Kramer AF. Fitness effects on the cognitive function of older adults: A meta-analytic study. *Psychol Sci.* 2003;14(2):125–30.
20. Conn VS. Depressive symptom outcomes of physical activity interventions: Meta-analysis findings. *Ann Behav Med.* 2010;39(2):128–38.
21. Conn VS, Hafdahl AR, Brown LM. Meta-analysis of quality-of-life outcomes from physical activity interventions. *Nurs Res.* 2009;58(3):175–83.
22. da Silva RB, Costa-Paiva L, Morais SS, Mezzalira R, Ferreira Nde O, Pinto-Neto AM. Predictors of falls in women with and without osteoporosis. *J Orthop Sports Phys Ther.* 2010;40(9):582–8.
23. Dik M, Deeg DJ, Visser M, Jonker C. Early life physical activity and cognition at old age. *J Clin Exp Neuropsychol.* 2003;25(5):643–53.

24. Djernes JK. Prevalence and predictors of depression in populations of elderly: A review. *Acta Psychiatr Scand.* 2006;113(5):372–87.

25. Etnier JL, Chang YK. The effect of physical activity on executive function: A brief commentary on definitions, measurement issues, and the current state of the literature. *J Sport Exerc Psychol.* 2009;31(4):469–83.

26. Ferketich AK, Kirby TE, Alway SE. Cardiovascular and muscular adaptations to combined endurance and strength training in elderly women. *Acta Physiol Scand.* 1998;164(3):259–67.

27. Frontera WR, Meredith CN, O'Reilly KP, Knuttgen HG, Evans WJ. Strength conditioning in older men: Skeletal muscle hypertrophy and improved function. *J Appl Physiol.* 1988;64(3):1038–44.

28. Galper DI, Trivedi MH, Barlow CE, Dunn AL, Kampert JB. Inverse association between physical inactivity and mental health in men and women. *Med Sci Sports Exerc.* 2006;38(1):173–8.

29. Goodwin RD. Association between physical activity and mental disorders among adults in the United States. *Prev Med.* 2003;36(6):698–703.

30. Grimby G, Aniansson A, Hedberg M, Henning GB, Grangard U, Kvist H. Training can improve muscle strength and endurance in 78- to 84-yr-old men. *J Appl Physiol.* 1992;73(6):2517–23.

31. Hagberg JM, Graves JE, Limacher M, et al. Cardiovascular responses of 70- to 79-yr-old men and women to exercise training. *J Appl Physiol.* 1989;66(6):2589–94.

32. Hakkinen K, Newton RU, Gordon SE, et al. Changes in muscle morphology, electromyographic activity, and force production characteristics during progressive strength training in young and older men. *J Gerontol A Biol Sci Med Sci.* 1998;53(6):B415–23.

33. Hirsch CH, Diehr P, Newman AB, Gerrior SA, Pratt C, Lebowitz MD, Jackson SA. Physical activity and years of healthy life in older adults: Results from the cardiovascular health study. *J Aging Phys Act.* 2010;18(3):313–34.

34. Huang G, Gibson CA, Tran ZV, Osness WH. Controlled endurance exercise training and VO2max changes in older adults: A meta-analysis. *Prev Cardiol.* 2005;8(4):217–25.

35. Hunter GR, Bryan DR, Wetzstein CJ, Zuckerman PA, Bamman MM. Resistance training and intra-abdominal adipose tissue in older men and women. *Med Sci Sports Exerc.* 2002;34(6):1023–8.

36. Hunter GR, McCarthy JP, Bamman MM. Effects of resistance training on older adults. *Sports Med.* 2004;34(5):329–48.

37. Hurley BF, Hagberg JM. Optimizing health in older persons: Aerobic or strength training? *Exerc Sport Sci Rev.* 1998;26:61–89.

38. Ibanez J, Izquierdo M, Arguelles I, et al. Twice-weekly progressive resistance training decreases abdominal fat and improves insulin sensitivity in older men with type 2 diabetes. *Diabetes Care.* 2005;28(3):662–7.

39. Ivey FM, Roth SM, Ferrell RE, et al. Effects of age, gender, and myostatin genotype on the hypertrophic response to heavy resistance strength training. *J Gerontol A Biol Sci Med Sci.* 2000;55(11):M641–8.

40. Izquierdo M, Hakkinen K, Ibanez J, et al. Effects of strength training on muscle power and serum hormones in middle-aged and older men. *J Appl Physiol.* 2001;90(4):1497–507.

41. Jacobs EJ, Newton CC, Wang Y, et al. Waist circumference and all-cause mortality in a large US cohort. *Arch Intern Med.* 2010;170(15):1293–301.

42. Joseph LJ, Davey SL, Evans WJ, Campbell WW. Differential effect of resistance training on the body composition and lipoprotein-lipid profile in older men and women. *Metabolism.* 1999;48(11):1474–80.

43. Jubrias SA, Esselman PC, Price LB, Cress ME, Conley KE. Large energetic adaptations of elderly muscle to resistance and endurance training. *J Appl Physiol.* 2001;90(5):1663–70.

44. Karavirta L, Tulppo MP, Laaksonen DE, et al. Heart rate dynamics after combined endurance and strength training in older men. *Med Sci Sports Exerc.* 2009;41(7):1436–43.

45. Karp A, Paillard-Borg S, Wang HX, Silverstein M, Winblad B, Fratiglioni L. Mental, physical and social components in leisure activities equally contribute to decrease dementia risk. *Dement Geriatr Cogn Disord.* 2006;21(2):65–73.

46. Kay SJ, Fiatarone Singh MA. The influence of physical activity on abdominal fat: A systematic review of the literature. *Obes Rev.* 2006;7(2):183–200.

47. Kelley GA. Exercise and regional bone mineral density in postmenopausal women: A meta-analytic review of randomized trials. *Am J Phys Med Rehabil.* 1998;77(1):76–87.

48. Kelley GA, Kelley KS, Tran ZV. Exercise and bone mineral density in men: A meta-analysis. *J Appl Physiol.* 2000;88(5):1730–6.

49. Kohrt WM, Bloomfield SA, Little KD, Nelson ME, Yingling VR, American College of Sports Medicine. American College of Sports Medicine Position Stand: Physical activity and bone health. *Med Sci Sports Exerc.* 2004;36(11):1985–96.

50. Konopack JF, Marquez DX, Hu L, Elavsky S, McAuley E, Kramer AF. Correlates of functional fitness in older adults. *Int J Behav Med.* 2008;15(4):311–8.

51. Larson EB, Wang L, Bowen JD, McCormick WC, Teri L, Crane P, Kulkull W. Exercise is associated with reduced risk for incident dementia among persons 65 years of age and older. *Ann Intern Med.* 2006;144(2):73–81.

52. Laurin D, Verreault R, Lindsay J, MacPherson K, Rockwood K. Physical activity and risk of cognitive impairment and dementia in elderly persons. *Arch Neurol.* 2001;58(3):498–504.

53. Lawlor DA, Hopker SW. The effectiveness of exercise as an intervention in the management of depression: Systematic review and meta-regression analysis of randomised controlled trials. *Br Med J.* 2001;322(7289):763–7.
54. Lexell J, Downham DY, Larsson Y, Bruhn E, Morsing B. Heavy-resistance training in older Scandinavian men and women: Short- and long-term effects on arm and leg muscles. *Scand J Med Sci Sports.* 1995;5(6):329–41.
55. Li F, Harmer P, Fisher KJ, McAuley E, Chaumeton N, Eckstrom E, Wilson NL. Tai Chi and fall reductions in older adults: A randomized controlled trial. *J Gerontol A Biol Sci Med Sci.* 2005;60(2):187–94.
56. Lindsay J, Laurin D, Verreault R, Hebert R, Helliwell B, Hill GB, McDowell I. Risk factors for Alzheimer's disease: A prospective analysis from the Canadian Study of Health and Aging. *Am J Epidemiol.* 2002;156(5):445–53.
57. Lovell DI, Cuneo R, Gass GC. Can aerobic training improve muscle strength and power in older men? *J Aging Phys Act.* 2010;18(1):14–26.
58. Lytle ME, Vander Bilt J, Pandav RS, Dodge HH, Ganguli M. Exercise level and cognitive decline: The MoVIES project. *Alzheimer Dis Assoc Disord.* 2004;18(2):57–64.
59. Malbut KE, Dinan S, Young A. Aerobic training in the "oldest old": The effect of 24 weeks of training. *Age Ageing.* 2002;31(4):255–60.
60. Marsh AP, Miller ME, Rejeski WJ, Hutton SL, Kritchevsky SB. Lower extremity muscle function after strength or power training in older adults. *J Aging Phys Act.* 2009;17(4):416–43.
61. Martin WH 3rd, Kohrt WM, Malley MT, Korte E, Stoltz S. Exercise training enhances leg vasodilatory capacity of 65-yr-old men and women. *J Appl Physiol.* 1990;69(5):1804–9.
62. Mead GE, Morley W, Campbell P, Greig CA, McMurdo M, Lawlor DA. Exercise for depression. *Cochrane Database Syst Rev.* 2009;(3):CD004366.
63. Netz Y, Wu MJ, Becker BJ, Tenenbaum G. Physical activity and psychological well-being in advanced age: A meta-analysis of intervention studies. *Psychol Aging.* 2005;20(2):272–84.
64. Newton RU, Hakkinen K, Hakkinen A, McCormick M, Volek J, Kraemer WJ. Mixed-methods resistance training increases power and strength of young and older men. *Med Sci Sports Exerc.* 2002;34(8):1367–75.
65. Norton R, Galgali G, Campbell AJ, Reid IR, Robinson E, Butler M, Gray H. Is physical activity protective against hip fracture in frail older people? *Age Ageing.* 2001;30(3):262–4.
66. Pinquart M, Duberstein PR, Lyness JM. Effects of psychotherapy and other behavioral interventions on clinically depressed older adults: A meta-analysis. *Aging Ment Health.* 2007;11(6):645–57.
67. Podewils LJ, Guallar E, Kuller LH, Fried LP, Lopez OL, Carlson M, Lyketsos CG. Physical activity, APOE genotype, and dementia risk: Findings from the cardiovascular health cognition study. *Am J Epidemiol.* 2005;161(7):639–51.
68. Rejeski WJ, Brawley LR, Shumaker SA. Physical activity and health-related quality of life. *Exerc Sport Sci Rev.* 1996;24:71–108.
69. Rejeski WJ, Mihalko SL. Physical activity and quality of life in older adults. *J Gerontol A Biol Sci Med Sci.* 2001;56 (Spec No 2):23–35.
70. Rethorst CD, Wipfli BM, Landers DM. The antidepressive effects of exercise: A meta-analysis of randomized trials. *Sports Med.* 2009;39(6):491–511.
71. Rovio S, Kareholt I, Helkala EL, et al. Leisure-time physical activity at midlife and the risk of dementia and Alzheimer's disease. *Lancet Neurol.* 2005;4(11):705–11.
72. Salthouse TA, Ferrer-Caja E. What needs to be explained to account for age-related effects on multiple cognitive variables? *Psychol Aging.* 2003;18(1):91–110.
73. Sawyer K, Castaneda-Sceppa C. Impact of aerobic physical activity on cardiovascular and noncardiovascular outcomes: Is anyone too old to exercise? *Aging Health.* 2010;6(2):251–60.
74. Schaie KW. The course of adult intellectual development. *Am Psychol.* 1994;49(4):304–13.
75. Schechtman KB, Ory MG. The effects of exercise on the quality of life of frail older adults: A preplanned meta-analysis of the FICSIT trials. *Ann Behav Med.* 2001;23(3):186–97.
76. Seals DR, Hagberg JM, Hurley BF, Ehsani AA, Holloszy JO. Endurance training in older men and women. I. Cardiovascular responses to exercise. *J Appl Physiol.* 1984;57(4):1024–9.
77. Spirduso WW, Francis KL, MacRae PG. *Physical Dimensions of Aging.* Champaign (IL): Human Kinetics; 2005.
78. Stathopoulou G, Powers MB, Berry AC, Smits JAJ, Otto MW. Exercise interventions for mental health: A quantitative and qualitative review. *Clin Psychol.* 2006;13(2):179–93.
79. Stephen WC, Janssen I. Influence of physical activity on age-related weight loss in the elderly. *J Phys Act Health.* 2010;7(1):78–86.
80. Sturman MT, Morris MC, Mendes de Leon CF, Bienias JL, Wilson RS, Evans DA. Physical activity, cognitive activity, and cognitive decline in a biracial community population. *Arch Neurol.* 2005;62(11):1750–4.
81. Tanaka H, Dinenno FA, Monahan KD, Clevenger CM, DeSouza CA, Seals DR. Aging, habitual exercise, and dynamic arterial compliance. *Circulation.* 2000;102(11):1270–5.
82. Taylor-Piliae RE, Newell KA, Cherin R, Lee MJ, King AC, Haskell WL. Effects of Tai Chi and Western exercise on physical and cognitive functioning in healthy community-dwelling older adults. *J Aging Phys Act.* 2010; 18(3):261–79.

83. Toth MJ, Beckett T, Poehlman ET. Physical activity and the progressive change in body composition with aging: Current evidence and research issues. *Med Sci Sports Exerc.* 1999;31(suppl 11):S590–6.

84. Treuth MS, Hunter GR, Kekes-Szabo T, Weinsier RL, Goran MI, Berland L. Reduction in intra-abdominal adipose tissue after strength training in older women. *J Appl Physiol.* 1995;78(4):1425–31.

85. Tricoci P, Allen JM, Kramer JM, Califf RM, Smith SC Jr. Scientific evidence underlying the ACC/AHA clinical practice guidelines. *JAMA.* 2009;301(8):831–41.

86. U.S. Department of Health and Human Services. *2008 Physical Activity Guidelines for Americans.* Rockville (MD): U.S. Department of Health and Human Services; 2008.

87. van Gelder BM, Tijhuis MA, Kalmijn S, Giampaoli S, Nissinen A, Kromhout D. Physical activity in relation to cognitive decline in elderly men: The FINE Study. *Neurology.* 2004;63(12):2316–21.

88. Verghese J, Lipton RB, Katz MJ, et al. Leisure activities and the risk of dementia in the elderly. *N Engl J Med.* 2003;348(25):2508–16.

89. Vincent KR, Braith RW, Feldman RA, et al. Resistance exercise and physical performance in adults aged 60 to 83. *J Am Geriatr Soc.* 2002;50(6):1100–7.

90. Weuve J, Kang JH, Manson JE, Breteler MM, Ware JH, Grodstein F. Physical activity, including walking, and cognitive function in older women. *J Am Med Assoc.* 2004;292(12):1454–61.

91. Wilson RS, Bennett DA, Bienias JL, et al. Cognitive activity and incident AD in a population-based sample of older persons. *Neurology.* 2002;59(12):1910–4.

92. Wolff I, van Croonenborg JJ, Kemper HC, Kostense PJ, Twisk JW. The effect of exercise training programs on bone mass: A meta-analysis of published controlled trials in pre- and postmenopausal women. *Osteoporos Int.* 1999;9(1):1–12.

93. Wray DW, Uberoi A, Lawrenson L, Richardson RS. Evidence of preserved endothelial function and vascular plasticity with age. *Am J Physiol Heart Circ Physiol.* 2006;290(3):H1271–7.

94. Yaffe K, Barnes D, Nevitt M, Lui LY, Covinsky K. A prospective study of physical activity and cognitive decline in elderly women — Women who walk. *Arch Intern Med.* 2001;161(14):1703–8.

95. Yamada M, Kasagi F, Sasaki H, Masunari N, Mimori Y, Suzuki G. Association between dementia and midlife risk factors: The Radiation Effects Research Foundation Adult Health Study. *J Am Geriatr Soc.* 2003;51(3):410–4.

96. Yoshitake T, Kiyohara Y, Kato I, et al. Incidence and risk factors of vascular dementia and Alzheimer's disease in a defined elderly Japanese population: The Hisayama Study. *Neurology.* 1995;45(6):1161–8.

CHAPTER 3

Active Living — Options and Benefits for Seniors

Scott J. Strath and Elizabeth EK. Lenz

▪▪▪ CHAPTER OUTLINE

- Introduction
- The concept of environmental and policy influences on physical activity
  - What are environmental variables
    - ▪ Concept of neighborhood and walkability
  - Assessing the environment
    - ▪ Perceived environmental assessment\
    - ▪ Measured environment assessment
  - What are policy variables
- Linking the environment to physical activity among seniors
  - Perceptions of the environment to promote senior physical activity
  - Environmental attributes and physical activity for seniors
- Linking the environment to health for seniors
  - The environmental impact on disability
  - The environmental impact on obesity
- Active living for seniors: a case study
- Summary

INTRODUCTION

There are few certainties in life, but an unmistakable one is that with each passing hour and each passing day, we are all getting chronologically older. Getting older, or aging, is accompanied by a slow deterioration of bodily systems. This rate of deterioration is affected by a constellation of factors such as genetic susceptibility, daily stressors, and the everyday choices of what we eat, where we go, and how we get there — whether by active means (such as walking) or by passive means (such as driving). All of our daily choices are affected by the broader environment that we interact with on a daily basis. The environment helps shape, or can even determine, the daily choices we make.

For decades, health professionals and researchers focused on the health and fitness benefits of exercise, primarily on leisure-time physical activity, typically engagement in sport-related activities. In such studies, exercise was usually performed in a vigorous fashion. From this work came traditional exercise guidelines that recommended that all adults should exercise three to five times a week for 20 to 60 minutes, at a vigorous (60%–90% heart rate maximum) intensity. Over the past 2 to 3 decades, this message has changed to also recognize that accumulating regular physical activity at a lower intensity than vigorous can also be health enhancing. Newer physical activity guidelines, now specific to older adults, recommend the accumulation of 30 minutes of moderate-intensity physical activity on 5 days each week, and that this moderate activity can be accumulated in bouts of 10 minutes or more (21). This recommendation supplements, but does not replace, traditional exercise guidelines.

KEY POINT 3-1

To promote and maintain health, older adults need moderate-intensity aerobic physical activity for a minimum of 30 minutes on 5 days each week or vigorous-intensity activity for a minimum of 20 minutes on 3 days each week. Combinations of moderate- and vigorous-intensity activity can be performed to meet this recommendation. Current guidelines recognize that increased amounts of physical activity are usually associated with increased health benefits.

It is important to define the two terms, *exercise* and *physical activity*. Exercise, or exercise training, pertains to something that is a planned, structured, and repetitive bodily movement done to improve or maintain one or more components of physical fitness (27). Physical activity pertains to any bodily movement that is produced by the contraction of skeletal muscle and that substantially increases energy expenditure (27). The importance in clearly distinguishing these terms is that there are different dimensions of physical activity. These different dimensions include (a) occupational activity, (b) transport-related activity, (c) domestic and incidental activity, and (d) structured activity/exercise. An increase in any of these dimensions would therefore count toward increasing overall physical activity and move someone closer to meeting health-enhancing physical activity recommendations. One such example would therefore include walking at a moderate intensity for a sufficient duration to meet current physical activity guidelines.

Physical activity has been shown to be effective in preventing and managing many health ailments in older adults. Regular physical activity has been shown to reduce coronary heart disease, Type 2 diabetes mellitus, obesity, hypertension, and some forms of cancer (9). Physical activity has also been shown to prevent functional limitations (20), prevent or delay cognitive impairment (1), and also improve the quality of sleep (10). The importance of engaging in regular physical activity is, therefore, essential to the health and well-being of an aging population.

During the time that important connections were being made between physical activity and health, societal and environmental changes were being made that have had major effects on our overall daily physical activity. The extraordinary fast pace of technological advancement has seen the creation of labor-saving devices at home, in our leisure time, and in our work. These changes have collectively made it possible, or even strongly encouraged, for people to live physically inactive and sedentary lives. In fact, at a time when total leisure-time physical activity has not changed much in our nation, sedentary behavior is likely to have increased, thereby actually decreasing our overall daily physical activity. Recent evidence suggests that older adults may spend as much as 9 hours a day engaging in sedentary activities (17).

In conjunction with technological advancement, many environmental and policy changes have come. The fast pace of our daily lives has impacted urban design catering more to the automobile, with the development of an extensive network of highways and roads, and a decreased emphasis on bicycling, walking, and public transportation. Or in other words, when designing or building a road or community, little thought was given to the person and to how physically active the environmental design would permit him or her to be. Building on our increased understanding of the connection between the environment and physical activity, a new area of scientific and public health emphasis has emerged — the impact of environment and policy change on physical activity. This important connection has led to the concept of **Active Living,** defined as a way of life that integrates physical activity into daily routines. The concept of Active Living is a fascinating one that involves many professions, such as urban planning, transportation, architecture, public health, and political offices, all working together in an interdisciplinary way, toward a common goal. The focus of this chapter will be to discuss the interplay between environmental and policy variables and physical activity, associations between the environment, physical activity, and health, and examples of Active Living for seniors.

KEY POINT 3-2

Active Living refers to a way of life that integrates physical activity into one's daily routines, such as walking to the store or biking to work. Active Living brings together many different professionals to work together to build and design places that encourage routine activity.

THE CONCEPT OF ENVIRONMENTAL AND POLICY INFLUENCES ON PHYSICAL ACTIVITY

The concept of environmental and policy factors being related to physical activity, and therefore public health, is still in its relative infancy, especially as they relate to an aging population. Much of our understanding of this relationship stems from studies

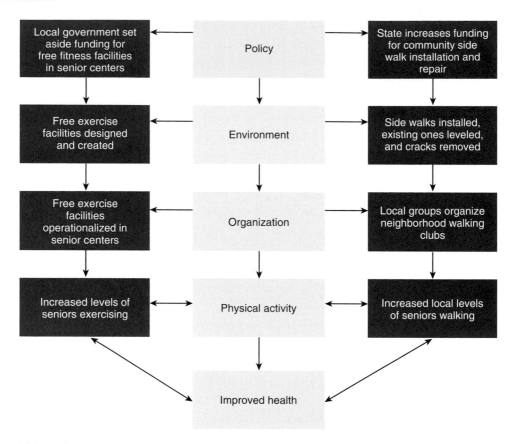

FIGURE 3-1 An example ecological framework for physical activity for seniors

that attempt to examine multiple levels of factors thought to influence physical activity. For such work, a social ecological perspective, or the ecological model, has been widely promoted and utilized (25). An ecological framework of how physical activity as a behavior is influenced by multiple levels is highlighted in Figure 3-1. Below we define and provide examples for both environmental and policy variables.

What are environmental variables?

Environmental variables include the social, economic, and physical environment. The social environment pertains to facets such as social relationships, the age of the neighborhood, social capital, and social isolation. It influences a person's desire for social participation. The economic environment pertains to factors such as socioeconomic status, educational level, and unemployment status. Physical environment features include both the built and the natural elements. The built environment includes roads, sidewalks, homes, stores, and the actual design and layout of our towns and cities. Thus, the built environment is subject to such things as urban design trends and zoning laws and practices. The natural environment includes elements such as the weather, length of day, and elevation of the land. There are clearly a large number of environmental variables that could be related to overall physical activity. Identifying them all is difficult because of the vast number of possibilities. In Table 3-1, we have listed some of the more widely studied environmental variables as they relate to different dimensions of physical activity behavior.

Concept of neighborhood and walkability

When considering the environment, environmental variables, and relationships with physical activity, the terms *neighborhood* and *walkability* often arise as important concepts. Both neighborhood and walkability are difficult to define. Neighborhood can pertain to a municipality, a region, or a vicinity surrounding a residential area. Neighborhoods can therefore be both formally or informally defined. Do you live in a good neighborhood? Is your neighborhood supportive of your physical activity? How you geographically define neighborhood therefore becomes critical. Neighborhood should have a sense of place, or a sense of community. Much of the research linking neighborhood attributes to physical activity has placed a distance or geographical boundary on the concept of neighborhood, for instance, within a 1 mile by 1 mile boundary, or within an 800-m or 400-m radius (sometimes referred to as a "buffer"),

Table 3-1   Examples of Environmental Characteristics Related to Physical Activity for Seniors

Environmental Variable	Brief Descriptor
Density	Compactness of land uses
Connectivity	Related to street level design, the directness between two points for travel
Mixed land use	Degree of integration within a given area for different land uses, *i.e.*, residential, commercial/retail, office, and public space
Distance to destinations	Related to density, the measured network distances between various destinations, such as residence to a local grocery store, park, or library
Sidewalks	Presence, or the actual number and condition, of sidewalks in a defined location
Traffic	Both the volume of traffic, traffic speed limits, and any traffic calming measures such as speed bumps
Parks, green spaces	The number of parks and open available green spaces within a defined location
Aesthetics	The overall visual appeal of an area, for instance, trees, tree canopy and flowers/plants, lack of graffiti
Safety	A feeling of safety, a lack of crime

> **Real Life Story 3-1   Betty — Neighborhood Change Has Helped**
>
> Betty lives in a community that has a small centralized area on one street for shopping and stores. Novelty stores, unique family-owned restaurants, boutiques, and so on line both sides of a street and off-streets for about one-third of a mile. Betty was always frustrated when she would visit this area because it was very popular and there was lots of traffic. Betty (and others) felt that the level of traffic and congestion made it almost impossible to cross the street. Three years ago, a group of community residents, and Betty, got together to lobby local government to help. After about 18 months, change happened. Traffic speed limits were decreased to 25 mph, and three traffic crossings were put in place with large yellow signs with flashing red perimeters on the signs. The result has Betty and others ecstatic. Considerably, more people are walking about the area; store and restaurant business is up; and because it is more difficult to drive through this area, traffic has elected to go around rather than through it. The end result was a major win for Betty and other residents. Simple neighborhood change seems to have increased local business, decreased traffic, and allowed more people to walk freely within the area.

of a person's residence. Placing such a boundary to the concept of neighborhood is important because to take advantage of neighborhood attributes supportive to physical activity, you have to be close to such attributes. The challenge is that one person's idea of "closeness" differs from another person's. Closeness also depends on perception and physiologic functioning of the person — critical when considering an aging population.

Walkability is another term that has become widely used and studied as it relates to connections between the environment, physical activity, and health. Although it may sound as if walkability refers to the presence of sidewalks and walking paths, it is much more than just that. A walkable neighborhood is a place where people are able to walk to useful destinations, such as a grocery store, retail shop, pharmacy, library, church, park, bank, and a friend's residence. A walkable neighborhood is a neighborhood that is visually or aesthetically appealing and is a safe and pleasant place. A walkable neighborhood is a neighborhood that is accessible to all populations, including seniors with all different levels of functional capabilities. A walkable neighborhood is therefore a place where walking is a convenient means of transit and is easier and preferred to personal motorized vehicle use. Certain terminology has arisen within the literature that makes intuitive sense. Saelens and colleagues (2003) described *high-walkable* neighborhoods as those neighborhoods with a high population density, a good mixture of land use, high connectivity, and good pedestrian/bicycling infrastructure, compared with *low-walkable* neighborhoods that displayed characteristics of low population density, segregated land use, low connectivity, and poor pedestrian/bicycling infrastructure (24). With this in mind, it becomes easy to conceptualize how a high-walkable neighborhood can promote Active Living for seniors, and vice versa, and how a low-walkable neighborhood can serve to deter Active Living for seniors Figure 3-2.

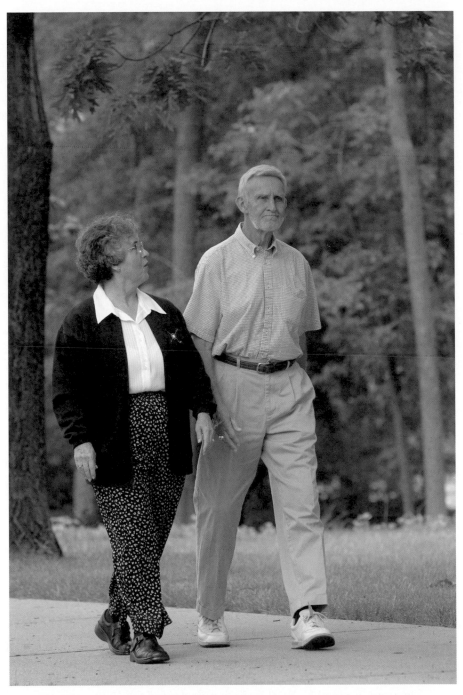

FIGURE 3-2   Seniors walking for health: It may only take a pair of walking shoes, but environmental support for such is critical

Assessing the environment

Measurement of environmental variables related to physical activity has come a long way in the past few years, with importance being paid to the development and testing of instruments and techniques able to reliably and validly measure environmental and neighborhood attributes as they relate to walkability. Enhancing to the field of environment and physical activity behavior inquiry has also been the increased use of geographical information systems (GIS). GIS is a software that has allowed for spatial connections to be drawn and made, overlaying environmental features on those of physically active behaviors. The actual measurement of environmental attributes can be broadly categorized as perceived measures versus objective or measured variables.

Perceived environmental assessment

Perceived environmental assessment refers to self-assessed questionnaire type instruments that are completed by an individual living within an area or neighborhood under study; for instance, the Neighborhood Environmental Walkability Scale (NEWS) is one such tool (23). Such an instrument would be administered to an adult living within a neighborhood that is under investigation to assess the linkage between the neighborhood attributes and the physical activity level of its residents. A set of questions are asked, and from the responses, an index is generated, with a higher score often associated with a neighborhood that is more conducive to walking, and therefore, being a more walkable neighborhood.

Measured environment assessment

The measured environment pertains to actual audits of environmental features and their qualities, typically carried out by trained professionals. There have been a number of such audit instruments created, and some specifically for older adults, such as the Senior Walking Environment Assessment Tool (19). Such audit tools typically consist of a long checklist containing a large number of environmental attributes, for instance, the presence, width, and condition of sidewalks in a given area. These checklists are often used by practitioners, community members, policy makers, and researchers to assess an environment.

What are policy variables?

Policy variables pertain to laws and regulations. These usually act in a top-down manner. For example, imagine that a new hypothetical Federal law states that all older adults who are physically active for 30 minutes a day will receive a twofold increase in monthly social security payouts, and for 60 minutes or more a day, a threefold increase in monthly social security payouts. Clearly, such a law would serve as an incentive for an older adult to increase his or her physical activity. Policy variables can also act to influence or change the environment. Consider a new urban planning policy that states that all roads must include a bike lane that is separated from the road by way of a raised grass median. Or, all cross-walks will now have a walk-cross time of 3 minutes minimum, giving more than ample time for a senior to cross the street. Such policies could reshape the environment, in a way that could promote biking and walking for seniors. Policy variables that could potentially influence physical activity are numerous. In Table 3-2, we give some basic examples of a few policy variables to promote Active Living and physical activity for seniors.

LINKING THE ENVIRONMENT TO PHYSICAL ACTIVITY AMONG SENIORS

Expert panels from the Transportation Research Board and Institute of Medicine (22), and the Task Force on Community Preventative Services (8) concluded, after reviewing available evidence, that investments are warranted and necessary to encourage the development of more walkable communities. Clear associations were found that suggest that the built environment can be supportive of physical activity. In this next section, we examine how perceptions of the environment can influence older adults' physical activity levels.

Table 3-2 Example Policy Variables Related to Physical Activity for Seniors

Policy Variable	Brief Descriptor
Senior Center/Church Other Organizational Approaches	
Incentivize	Take the stairs team and individual challenge with prizes Prizes for those who bike or walk to centers
Physical buildings	Provide showering facilities Highlight stairwells, provide music, decorations in stairwells, improve stairwell aesthetics
Access	Free access to supervised on-site physical activity/exercise facilities and classes Pay for transport to get to facilities if too far to walk/bike
Mass Media	
Promotional campaigns	Physical activity advertisements and associated benefits to air during primetime television and radio
State funding	Provide more funding for sidewalks/bike lanes, open green spaces/parks
Building/zoning policies	Require plans for all building projects to include large areas for green space, sidewalks, low traffic speeds, count-down timers on all crosswalks, and retail stores to be no more than 10 min from any one residence

Perceptions of the environment to promote senior physical activity

From interviews and focus groups carried out in both urban and suburban locations, across different ethnicities, we have learned that the physical environment is frequently cited as a factor that influences physical activity. African American and Hispanic women recently reported that a higher number and higher quality of parks, more sidewalks, and better maintained sidewalks, in conjunction with traffic calming measures, are possible changes to the environment that would increase their physical activity levels (13). Similar responses were also recently noted in a group of white men and women, who suggested that an enhanced infrastructure creating better sidewalks, traffic calming measures, and a greater separation between traffic and pedestrians and bicyclists would be supportive of higher levels of physical activity for seniors (26). This latter study also found that overall neighborhood aesthetics and aspects of the social environment were regarded as factors influencing physical activity. Many seniors report a strong interest in being active with others, rather than in isolation. Such findings support the importance of the built and social environment to physical activity levels for seniors.

Environmental attributes and physical activity for seniors

Studies have found positive relations between the built environment and walking. In a large study of 56 neighborhoods in Portland (Oregon, United States), neighborhood density, street connectivity, and open green spaces were all related to more walking among older adults (15). Other studies have reported similar findings using measures of pedestrian-friendly features, such as the presence of sidewalks, mixed land use, and higher street connectivity (12). Furthermore, others have reported that pedestrian infrastructure, such as crosswalks and curb cuts, is related to more walking for errands in older adults (11). Importantly, such findings

Real Life Story 3-2   Thomas and Ethel — Regular Users of Free Fitness Facilities in a Local Senior Center

Thomas and Ethel, a married couple for over 35 years, are both retired. Throughout their whole life, they have been fairly active, through work and play. When they retired, they noticed that they had more time, but less money. They both recognized the need to exercise, but could not afford any type of membership to exercise. A little over 10 years ago, a large Urban Midwestern University engaged in a partnership with the city's Department on Aging. The end result was to install fitness facilities into five local community senior centers that were free to any senior who wanted to use them. These fitness facilities are staffed by undergraduate University students in the health professions, and run by a joint academic-community partnership. The result: Thomas and Ethel have been regularly exercising in one of these free facilities (along with hundreds of others) for the past 10 years. When they were asked what they liked about it, they replied, "What's not to like? It's free, we have professional experts to help, the students are young and full of energy, and it gives us a place to go year-round — important with the long winters."

are consistent with perceptions of what older adults view as important built environmental features to increase their overall physical activity.

The social environmental has also emerged as an important factor influencing physical activity, albeit, not always consistently. Li and colleagues found that personal safety is related to physical activity levels (14). This finding has been confirmed by others who have shown that neighborhoods with high levels of vandalism and graffiti report lower levels of walking among older adults (18). However, others have suggested that the presence of vandalism and graffiti are not necessarily linked to unsafe neighborhoods, and because they are often found in urban locations with high population densities, the findings in this area are inconsistent (11).

It is worth mentioning that many of the environmental attributes related to higher physical activity levels for seniors are the same as those that have been found in the general adult literature. Further work is needed to understand whether there are environmental factors that serve as specific barriers or facilitators for older adults in particular.

> **KEY POINT 3-3**
> Neighborhood design — higher density, more places to walk to, greater land-use mix, and greater connectivity with more sidewalks — is positively related to older adult residents' physical activity levels and their health.

LINKING THE ENVIRONMENT TO HEALTH FOR SENIORS

Almost half of all older adults report functional disabilities, and this percentage increases with age to approximately three-quarters of adults older than 85 years reporting disabilities. Approximately two-thirds to three-quarters of older adults are overweight or obese, which is of concern given the linkage between obesity and coronary heart disease and other chronic conditions. The development of these conditions stems from a number of factors, predominately related to unhealthy behaviors (*i.e.*, smoking, poor diet, and being physically inactive), but such factors are also influenced by where one lives or one's surrounding environment.

The environmental impact on disability

Disability relates to having difficulties or depending on others to perform activities of daily living (ADLs). Mobility disability is often a precursor to the development of other disabilities and is defined as difficulty with functioning because of decreased walking ability, maneuverability, or speed. For the older adult population, disability begins with the development of chronic conditions, resulting in functional impairments and dependence on others. Therefore, if the demand of the environment is greater than an older adult's capacity to perform specific ADLs (*e.g.*, self-care activities or ambulation) or instrumental ADLs (IADLs; *e.g.*, cooking, housework, and shopping), that environment fosters dependence.

When various built environmental characteristics are examined, older adults living in environments that are not pedestrian friendly have a greater risk of developing disabilities. More older adults report physical disabilities and disabilities relating to going outside the home if they live in neighborhoods with fewer trees on the streets, less access to public transport, and less street connectivity (3). Overall incidence of functional loss and lower-extremity physical function decline is incrementally greater with deleterious environmental factors (*e.g.*, high traffic, low access to public transportation, and inadequate street lighting) (2). For older adult men, neighborhoods with higher street connectivity reduce the risk of reporting IADL difficulties (5). Such evidence supports the linkage between built neighborhood and disability in older adults.

Other social and economic environmental attributes have been shown to impact disability in older adults. For instance, older adults living in neighborhoods with high perceived social cohesion (*i.e.*, perceived strong social ties and mutual trust) are more likely to report going outside of their homes (3). Conceivably, improving the social climate of a neighborhood may be one way to encourage older adults to leave home and be more physically active. Data from the United States Health and Retirement Study show older adults living in economically advantaged neighborhoods have a lower risk of developing lower body limitations (5). Others have confirmed that men living in economically disadvantaged neighborhoods are at a higher risk for developing limitations with performing ADLs. This relationship is strongest for individuals living below the poverty line (4, 5). In summary, the built, social, and economic attributes of an environment appear to interact and be related to the development of the disablement process.

The environmental impact on obesity

The walkability of a neighborhood can have a positive influence on the amount of obesity observed among older adults. Neighborhoods that have higher street connectivity levels are associated with a decreased prevalence of women being overweight or obese (7). When land use includes a combination of residential, public, and commercial use, there is also a reported reduction in the prevalence of older adults being overweight or obese. However, if the neighborhood includes a large number of fast-food establishments, the prevalence of overweight and obesity increases (16).

Other social and economic environmental factors have been shown to impact obesity. Older adults living in neighborhoods with more social turmoil have higher body mass index levels than those living in neighborhoods with less turmoil, even after controlling for individual, diet, physical activity, and socioeconomic variables (6). When economic factors are examined, older adult men and women living in disadvantaged areas are more likely to be obese compared with those living in economically prosperous neighborhoods (7). As in the literature examining the relationship between the environment and the development of disability, the built, social, and economic environment in which older adults live can also impact the prevalence of obesity.

Having highlighted some of the available evidence linking environmental attributes to physical activity and health, in the next section, we draw attention to a case study that was effective at the community level to promote change to the environment in an effort to encourage Active Living for seniors.

ACTIVE LIVING FOR SENIORS: A CASE STUDY

In 2001, the Robert Wood Johnson Foundation launched a series of programs designed to facilitate change to the environment to promote Active Living. Programs ranged from the Active Living Research National Program, based at San Diego State University, to the Active for Life National Program, based at the Texas A&M University School of Rural Public Health, to the Active Living by Design (ALbD) National Program, based at the University of North Carolina School of Public Health. Specifically, the ALbD National Program was launched as a real world initiative with funding to support community-based innovations and applications to facilitate Active Living. The ALbD National Program Office funded 25 community initiatives, located all around the United States, employing ecological strategies to influence physical activity behavior. A supplement in the *American Journal of Preventive Medicine* (2009, S62) is dedicated to ALbD. The Get Active Orlando (GAO) is an excellent example of promoting ALbD.

Downtown Orlando is home to a large concentrated population of older adults. The neighborhood is bisected by two major highways, limiting resident mobility. A major GAO goal was to reduce community barriers to physical activity and to promote and create environments that support Active Living choices. Three activities were focused on: walking, bicycling, and community gardening. Initial marketing campaigns on the importance of Active Living were followed by forming public policy partnerships between such entities as the City of Orlando Planning Division, Transportation Department, and Families, Parks and Recreation Department; neighborhood associations; local hospitals; and bicycling associations. Influencing city policy was targeted for lasting, sustainable effects. Plans and policies around such things as downtown transportation plans, streetscape guidelines, growth management policies, a design standards checklist for new development, and a committee to serve the mayor and city council are just some areas that were targeted to great success.

Real Life Story 3-3   Margaret — Trees Make You Feel Better

Margaret has lived in the same house and in the same community for the past 39 years. The community is a nice one, with a lot of good neighbors and friends who look out for one another. Although the community was nice, there was not a lot of activity or a lot of people out and about. For an unknown reason about 8 years ago, the local area underwent a large tree, shrub, and flower planting endeavor throughout much of the community. The result is that the whole area is one of visual beauty for at least 6 months out of the year. Margaret and many of her neighborhood friends now take regular walks throughout the whole community admiring the scenery. When asked specifically what she likes, Margaret replied, "We all love seeing living color and trees, they make you feel better, it's just more pleasant to walk through."

Programs included such things as a senior walking program operated from a local park near a senior center, and biannual adult bicycle giveaways. Community gardens sprang up on previously abandoned land. Figure 3-3, the Parramore Community

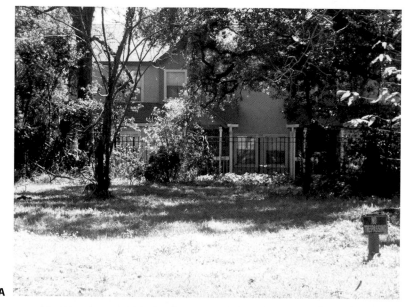

A

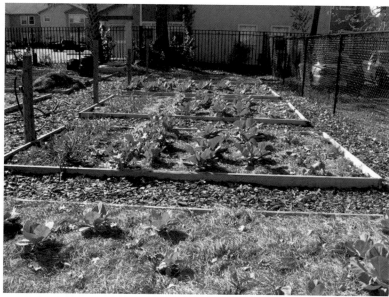

B

FIGURE 3-3   Get Active Orlando: Parramore Community Gardens, **(A)** before and **(B)** after pictures showcasing a successful environmental change to promote Active Living

> **Real Life Story 3-4   Fred — Things Change, but Not Always for the Best**
>
> Fred, a retired factory worker, reflects on how things have changed over the years. Fred recollects that when he was growing up, in a community not far from where he is living now, he was always walking everywhere. He could walk to school, walk to church, walk to the corner store, walk to the parks. Fred remembers that he could walk anywhere — and that was only 40 years ago. Now, you can't walk anywhere in this area; you have to get in your car to do anything or go anywhere. The biggest barrier to walk is that there is no purpose — if things are not close, you are not going to walk to them. His hope is that slowly people will realize that if you build it, and it is close, people will walk to it.

Gardens, shows a "before" and "after" look at what can be achieved through coordinated community effort. Gardens operate to enhance overall physical activity and Active Living, as well as to improve the visual landscape, while not forgetting the all-important yearly harvests of freshly grown fruits and vegetables. GAO is an example of success. By involving numerous community and local partners unified through a single message of encouraging Active Living, change to both policy and environment is possible.

S U M M A R Y

Historically, high numbers of seniors living within society, accompanied by high rates of chronic conditions and sedentary lifestyles, represent a major public health challenge for the 21st century and beyond. The paradigm of Active Living represents a fairly recent phenomenon, and through coordinated interdisciplinary efforts in the areas of research, policy, and practice, has been serving to slowly change the landscape in which we all live. Developing healthy, livable, and high-walkable communities for seniors is a challenge of unifying diverse disciplines, groups, and organizations toward a single goal. Examples, such as that of GAO, and others, showcase that successful partnerships can be fostered over time to implement sustainable Active Living approaches to enhance physical activity and ultimately health.

QUESTIONS FOR REFLECTION

1. What is the difference between physical activity and exercise?

2. What is Active Living?

3. On the basis of your understanding of policy and environmental variables, how do they relate to physical activity?

4. Describe how the walkability of a neighborhood can impact physical activity?

5. Can policy and environmental variables influence physical activity in seniors?

6. Can policy and environmental variables influence senior health?

7. Discuss ways in which you could modify the environment to promote senior physical activity and health.

REFERENCES

1. Abbott RD, White LR, Ross GW, Masaki KH, Curb JD, Petrovitch H. Walking and dementia in physically capable elderly men. *JAMA*. 2004;292:1447–53.
2. Balfour JL, Kaplan GA. Neighborhood environment and loss of physical function in older adults: Evidence from the Alameda County Study. *Am J Epidemiol*. 2002;155:507–15.
3. Beard J, Blaney S, Cerda M, et al. Neighborhood characteristics and disability in older adults. *J Gerontol: Soc Sci*. 2009;64B:252–7.
4. Clark C, Kawachi I, Ryan L, Ertel K, Fay M, Berkman L. Perceived neighborhood safety and incident mobility disability among elders: The hazards of poverty. *BMC Public Health*. 2009;9:162.
5. Freedman VA, Grafova IB, Schoeni RF, Rogowski J. Neighborhoods and disability in later life. *Soc Sci Med*. 2008;66:2253–67.
6. Glass TA, Rasmussen MD, Schwartz BS. Neighborhoods and obesity in older adults: The Baltimore Memory Study. *Am J Prev Med*. 2006;31:455–63.
7. Grafova IB, Freedman VA, Kumar R, Rogowski J. Neighborhoods and obesity in later life. *Am J Public Health*. 2008;98:2065–71.
8. Heath G, Brownson R, Kruger J, Miles R, Powell K, Ramsey L. TFoCP Services: The effectiveness of urban design and land use and transport policies and practices to increase physical activity: A systematic review. *J Phys Act Health*. 2006;3:S55–76.
9. Kesaniemi YK, Danforth E Jr, Jensen MD, Kopelman PG, Lefebvre P, Reeder BA. Dose–response issues concerning physical activity and health: An evidence-based symposium. *Med Sci Sports Exerc*. 2001;33:S351–8.
10. King AC, Oman RF, Brassington GS, Bliwise DL, Haskell WL. Moderate-intensity exercise and self-rated quality of sleep in older adults. A randomized controlled trial. *Jama*. 1997;277:32–7.
11. King, D. Neighborhood and individual factors in activity in older adults: Results from the neighborhood and senior health study. *J Aging Phys Act*. 2008;16:144–70.
12. King WC, Belle SH, Brach JS, Simkin-Silverman LR, Soska T, Kriska AM. Objective measures of neighborhood environment and physical activity in older women. *Am J Prev Med*. 2005;28:461–9.
13. Lees E, Taylor WC, Hepworth JT, Feliz K, Cassells A, Tobin JN. Environmental changes to increase physical activity: Perceptions of older urban ethnic-minority women. *J Aging Phys Act*. 2007;15:425–38.
14. Li F, Fisher KJ, Bauman A, et al. Neighborhood influences on physical activity in middle-aged and older adults: A multilevel perspective. *J Aging Phys Act*. 2005;13:87–114.
15. Li F, Fisher KJ, Brownson RC, Bosworth M. Multi-level modeling of built environment characteristics related to neighborhood walking activity in older adults. *J Epidemiol Commun Health*. 2005;59:558–64.
16. Li F, Harmer PA, Cardinal BJ, Bosworth M, Acock A, Johnson-Shelton D, Moore JM. Built environment, adiposity, and physical activity in adults aged 50–75. *Am J Prev Med*. 2008;35:38–46.
17. Matthews CE, Chen KY, Freedson PS, Buchowski MS, Beech BM, Pate RR, Troiano RP. Amount of time spent in sedentary behaviors in the United States, 2003–2004. *Am J Epidemiol*. 2008;167:875–81.
18. Michael Y, Beard T, Choi D, Farquhar S, Carlson N. Measuring the influence of built neighborhood environments on walking in older adults. *J Aging Phys Act*. 2006;14:302–12.
19. Michael YL, Keast EM, Chaudhury H, Day K, Mahmood A, Sarte AF. Revising the senior walking environmental assessment tool. *Prev Med*. 2009;48:247–9.
20. Nelson ME, Layne JE, Bernstein MJ, et al. The effects of multidimensional home-based exercise on functional performance in elderly people. *J Gerontol A Biol Sci Med Sci*. 2004;59:154–60.

21. Nelson ME, Rejeski WJ, Blair SN, et al. Physical activity and public health in older adults: Recommendation from the American College of Sports Medicine and the American Heart Association. *Circulation*. 2007;116:1094–105.

22. Transportation Research Board and Institute of Medicine. *Does the Built Environment Influence Physical Activity? Examining the Evidence* (Transportation Research Board Special Report 282). Washington (DC): Transportation Research Board; 2005.

23. Saelens BE, Sallis JF, Black JB, Chen D. Neighborhood-based differences in physical activity: An environment scale evaluation. *Am J Public Health*. 2003;93:1552–8.

24. Saelens BE, Sallis JF, Frank LD. Environmental correlates of walking and cycling: Findings from the transportation, urban design, and planning literatures. *Ann Behav Med*. 2003;25:80–91.

25. Sallis JF, Owen N. Ecological models of health behavior. In: Glanz K, Rimmer BK, Lewis FM, editors. *Health Behavior and Health Education: Theory, Research and Practice*. San Francisco (CA): Jossey-Bass; 2002. p. 462–84.

26. Strath S, Isaacs R, Greenwald MJ. Operationalizing environmental indicators for physical activity in older adults. *J Aging Phys Act*. 15:412–24, 2007.

27. U.S. Department of Health and Human Services. *Physical Activity and Health: A Report of the Surgeon General*. Atlanta (GA): U.S. Department of Health and Human Services, Centers for Disease Control and Prevention, National Center for Chronic Disease Prevention and Health Promotion; 1996.

CHAPTER 4

Motivating Older Adults to Initiate and Maintain a Physically Active Lifestyle

Diane Whaley and Agnes Schrider

●●● CHAPTER OUTLINE

INTRODUCTION

The two vignettes below describe real people with real issues. For example, both portray typical older adults — relatively healthy, but with some degree of medical issue that must be considered when designing an exercise program. In addition, they include information regarding potential motivators and barriers to their activity, such as lacking information or confidence, or enjoying solitary versus group activity. Finally, both have taken the initial step to be physically active, although they are in very different places. What they share is the need for a little assistance to exercise more efficiently, effectively, and over the long term. These are all aspects of *motivation,* the topic of this chapter. In pursuing the topic of motivation, we will take a *theory to practice approach.* We will begin by addressing the definition of motivation. After reviewing some descriptive research that focuses on barriers and determinants of exercise, we will describe three theoretical perspectives that have direct relevance for working with older adult exercisers. We will then put those theories to work, relating strategies health and fitness professionals actually used to motivate the individuals described in the vignettes to begin and maintain activity levels. Finally, we will use a case study approach to bring our concepts together, describing a "real-world" exercise story, so the reader can begin to imagine how he or she might work with an exerciser using the concepts that have been described. Through this process, you will learn to use theory and concepts to *inform* your practice. Along the way, we will share tips for working effectively with older adults based on our experience as a researcher (university professor) and a practitioner (physical therapist).

> **Real Life Story 4-1   Janet**
>
> Janet is a 79-year-old short, frail woman who lives alone and is seeking the services of a personal trainer to "increase my health and strength." She has never exercised before and reports feeling unsteady on her feet. She knows that she has to do something to maintain her independence but is very tentative and anxious about using "fancy machines." She purchased a 6-month fitness membership, but isn't sure how or where to start; however, she does share that she likes to be around other people.

> **Real Life Story 4-2   Bob**
>
> Bob is a 73-year-old overweight man who has a well-equipped home gym, yet has had several falls in the past year. Two falls have occurred in the gym while getting on and off equipment. He has knee arthritis and has had foot surgery. He states that he exercises daily and discusses the various exercises he does at home. He is vocal about how he has been exercising his whole life and that he has some medical training. When he sets up the stacked weights, he tries to lift the heaviest weight that he can, often with poor technique. He never asks anyone for help at the gym.

WHAT IS MOTIVATION?

Motivation focuses on "individuals' **choices** about which tasks to do, the **persistence** with which they pursue these tasks, the **intensity** of their engagement in these tasks, and their **perceptions** about their performance and their goals" (5, p. 1017). More simply, we can think of the study of motivation as answering two key questions: (1) What causes behavior (including reasons for initiation, persistence, and dropout)? and (2) Why does behavior vary in its intensity (both within the same individual over time and between individuals)? (24).

> **KEY POINT 4-1** Definition of Motivation:
> Motivation focuses on choices, persistence, intensity, and perceptions about an activity.

As implied in these definitions, motivation is particular to an individual and can change over time. In addition, it is different across individuals within the same target group (*e.g.*, older adults) and between target groups (*e.g.*, younger, middle, and older adults). From a lifespan development perspective, we would expect that older adults show more *interindividual differences* (differences between individuals) in their reasons for choosing to be active, motives for remaining active, and reasons for dropping out than younger adults. The reasons for this are complex, but related to the breadth of experiences older adults have been exposed to over their lifetimes (33). The end result is that a group of "similar" older adults are likely to have different reasons for exercising, as their needs, motives, and barriers are different. Next, we begin to unravel the complex reasons for older adult participation in exercise.

Motives for and barriers to participation in physical activity

A good deal of research has identified the reasons older adults cite for becoming active, that is, their *motives* for participation. Motives for older adults' participation in exercise include maintaining or improving fitness and health, enjoying the activity, releasing tension, improving joint mobility, improving appearance, and liking the company (13, 14, 18, 22, 32). However, many studies have found significant differences across individual difference variables. For example, women are more likely to cite social reasons or appearance for exercise (18, 22), whereas older adults with limited mobility are more likely to cite disease management (23). The take-home message here is that to promote sustained activity, that is, to motivate people over the long term, we must structure the exercise experience so that motives are likely to be achieved. However, keep in mind that these motives may change over time. This may seem relatively simple. For example, if older adults are motivated to increase health, fitness, and joint mobility, then exercise would appear to be an obvious way to meet those goals. The simple truth is that most older adults don't exercise enough to meet their health goals. In fact, about 46% of adults 65 to 74 years of age report being inactive, and 75% of individuals in this age group report no vigorous activity (29). Given the established connection between exercise and "living better rather than simply living longer," either older adults don't see themselves as capable of achieving these motives or something is getting in the way.

What gets in the way of achieving motives for participation? Barriers, or constraints to exercise, can be related to the person (time, health problems, fear of falling, or injury) or the environment (distance to or lack of an exercise facility, unsuitable environment) (e.g., 19, 23). In addition, the barriers present when one begins an exercise program may be quite different from those that present themselves a month, 6 months, or a year down the road. Barriers should not be viewed simply as excuses; whether individuals have a physical barrier to their participation (health condition, lack of access to an exercise facility) or *perceive* their situation as inhibiting or prohibiting their exercise (lack of time, don't feel capable), the end result can be the same. Grodesky and colleagues (7) noted that many barriers for older adults "reflected the value placed on the behavior" (p. 321). This provides an important clue regarding how we might help exercisers overcome perceived barriers; exercise needs to be viewed as relevant and important to the individual. For example, the trainer might say to the older client, "Using the leg press machine will strengthen your legs so that you can get out of a chair without struggling or get up from the ground while gardening." Any real or perceived barriers need to be acknowledged and addressed if we are to maximize the chance of older adults getting and remaining active, finding value in what they do, and feeling capable of achieving regular exercise.

KEY POINT 4-2 Summary of Motives and Barriers

Motives for older adult exercise: Maintaining/improving health, enjoying the activity, releasing tension, improving joint mobility, liking the company

Barriers to older adult exercise: Time, health problems, fear of injury, lack of access, distance to exercise facility, unsuitable environment

Addressing barriers gets to the heart of motivating individuals. Whether we are directly (as in the case of a group or individual exercise leader) or indirectly (as the manager or owner of a fitness club or community facility) involved with older adults and exercise, our goal should be to maximize the chance that barriers are perceived as a temporary setback that can be overcome. To do this, we move on to theories of motivation, which allow us to understand the process of exercise participation at a deeper level.

UNDERSTANDING THEORIES OF MOTIVATION

Recognizing the motives for and barriers against involvement in exercise is only part of the story. To create an atmosphere that motivates individuals to exercise, we need an understanding of how factors might come together to influence older adults' participation in exercise. A theory proposes relationships between and among variables that help us describe, explain, and predict behavior. Theories link together facts and findings from research, observation, and personal experiences in an effort to explain people's behaviors, attitudes, and beliefs (8). Theories give us the framework from which programs can be planned and interactions can be had effectively with exercisers. Although there are many theories that are relevant to the exercise context, we have chosen to focus on three that have practical application for someone working with older adult exercisers. The first theory we'll introduce describes how beliefs about one's ability to achieve a particular outcome influence behavior (self-efficacy theory; 1, 2). In the second, we turn our focus to the context in which learning takes place. This theory will show how to optimize the environment for teaching and learning skills (modeling or observational learning; 3, 21), including the important question of who might be the best choice to teach older adults new skills. In the third, we focus specifically on the self to examine how the way we see ourselves (our identity or self-definition) impacts our thoughts, feelings, and behaviors (11, 34). For each, there are practical applications of the theory to help us plan, execute, and evaluate programs so as to maximize the motivational content of our feedback and context.

Self-efficacy theory

According to self-efficacy theory, behavioral, physiologic, and cognitive factors, along with environmental influences, come together to influence *efficacy* and *outcome expectations* (2, 20). Efficacy expectations refer to a person's strength of conviction that he or she can do what it takes to successfully complete a task ("can I do this"), while outcome expectations refer to beliefs about the consequences of such an action ("will it work") (24). Albert Bandura uses the term *reciprocal determinism* to describe the interaction between the individual, the environment, and the behavior. What does this mean in practical terms? If we think back to the scenarios we opened the chapter with, Janet's poor balance (individual) contributes to her feeling tentative and anxious about exercise (behavior). The type of support and encouragement she gets in her exercise setting (environment) will likely impact her sense of confidence in her ability to be successful. With experience and increases in self-efficacy, she will start to see how exercise has positive outcomes (improved balance, more strength), which leads to greater confidence and more persistence. Thus, all three components continue to influence each other over time.

KEY POINT 4-3 Definition of Self-Efficacy

Self-efficacy is the strength of one's conviction that he or she can do what it takes to successfully complete a task.

How does an individual come to judge his or her efficacy for a particular task? According to the theory, efficacy expectations come from four primary sources: mastery experiences, vicarious experiences, verbal persuasion, and physiological states (2). Mastery experiences represent the strongest source of personal efficacy. Prior success in a task, in particular a task that was difficult but achievable, provides a strong source of efficacy information. We can think of this source as representing the phrase, "I did it before and I can do it again." However, in the case of an older adult exerciser, perhaps they *haven't* done it before (*e.g.*, used weight machines). That is when the second source, vicarious experiences, becomes important. Seeing someone else successfully complete a task can give you the confidence that you, too, can do it, but *only* if you can see yourself in the person modeling that behavior. We will talk more about who makes for a successful model a bit later in the chapter. For now, it is important to remember that vicarious experiences represent a source of information that translates to, "if he/she can do it, I can do it."

The third source of efficacy information is verbal or social persuasion, or the feedback an exerciser receives from others that supports the individual's belief that he or she can do it. Typical sources of verbal persuasion in older adults include the person's physician, family members, peers, or exercise instructor (27). Bandura (2) adds that it is critical that such feedback be realistic, as "unrealistic boosts in efficacy are quickly disconfirmed by disappointing results of one's efforts" (p. 72). Importantly then, for verbal persuasion to be a positive source of information, it needs to be from a credible source, realistic, and positive.

The fourth source of efficacy information is physiological and emotional states (2). These include fatigue, muscle tension, anxiety, or aches and pains. This source may be particularly important for older adult exercisers, for whom aches and pains before the exercise, coupled with soreness after, could easily be interpreted as a reason to discontinue exercise (4). In this case, it is the *interpretation* of the physiological state that could mean all the difference in the exercisers' subsequent behavior. An exercise leader or health care provider can help the exerciser see that soreness is a logical outcome of exercise in initial stages and will go away with time. This is particularly important with exercisers who have chronic conditions such as arthritis and may fear that exercise will increase their pain. It is vital that the fitness professional explain the difference between soreness that will go away and pain that may indicate injury. Now let's see how we might increase self-efficacy in an adult exerciser by using the four sources of information.

> **KEY POINT 4-4** The Four Sources of Efficacy Information
>
> Mastery experiences — having done something successfully before
>
> Vicarious experiences — seeing a similar other successfully complete the task
>
> Verbal persuasion — receiving realistic feedback from a credible source
>
> Physiological and emotional states — interpretation of states such as fatigue, muscle tension, aches and pains

Putting self-efficacy theory to work: The practitioner's perspective

In the case of Bob, his previous experience with exercise gave him mastery experiences and vicarious experiences, so he knew he could be successful with exercise. Before joining our facility, he had been coming to me once a year for personal training sessions to update his home exercise program. He was very detailed in recording every aspect of his exercise: date, repetitions, sets, and duration. However, Bob's perception of his abilities and his physical condition was altered by a series of falls. These falls in and around his home altered his confidence level and outcome expectations that he could achieve his goals without external support. He received verbal persuasion from his wife and physician to first seek physical therapy. He established a strong relationship with his physical therapist assistant, and after his course of physical therapy, he paid for personal training sessions for another month to focus on balance and agility activities. He regained confidence and mastered agility skills. The physical therapist assistant also offered verbal persuasion for him to exercise in a facility where his progress could be monitored and advanced appropriately. As for his physiological state, he was used to physical aches or pains when exercising, so he had no difficulty resuming an exercise program and feeling muscle soreness afterward.

In Janet's case, she had no mastery experience with exercise. However, through conversations with her peers who were exercising at our facility, she gained vicarious experiences and verbal encouragement to begin a program. When she joined the facility, she was very timid and shy. Gradually, as she watched her peers, her vicarious experiences observing others gave her the confidence to try new activities. Initially, she was sore after her workouts. Her program was adjusted, and she received instruction that her muscles and joints might feel that way when starting an exercise program. Our clients are questioned in-depth about the type of pain, so the therapists and trainers can differentiate between muscle aches from exercise or another type of physical ailment. Clients are then educated, so they differentiate between an acceptable ache and an abnormal pain that may need further evaluation. This type of regular communication fosters a trusting relationship between the trainer and the client and makes the client feel secure in the exercise environment.

Observational learning and modeling

Bandura is also responsible for the theory of observational learning through modeling, known as *social learning theory* (1, 3). This theory emphasizes the importance of observing and modeling the thoughts, actions, and attitudes of others as a way of guiding our own actions. Although learning can occur deliberately or inadvertently (3), we will focus on deliberate learning, as in the case of personal trainers and their clients. McCullagh and Weiss (21) describe Bandura's four essential components, or subprocesses of modeling: *attention, retention, motor production, and motivation*. Attention and retention deal with the acquisition of a behavior. The attention component refers to what is observed and extracted from an observed skill, as well as what is ignored. In this stage, focusing attention on the relative aspects of the skill, while avoiding the situation of the individual focusing on irrelevant components, is key. Talking clearly and directly to the exerciser and explaining the purpose of an action will help the exerciser attend to the task at hand. At the retention phase, information is coded into memory, organized, and rehearsed. To optimize this subprocess, the model should employ strategies that maximize the chance that information will be stored and organized; for example, asking the learner to repeat the steps in the process needed to use a given piece of equipment, or using terms that are easy to remember rather than technical.

Performance depends on the third and fourth components of modeling, motor production, and motivation. In motor production, mental conceptions of an action are translated into actual action (26). It is critical at this stage that participants have the necessary baseline skills to perform a given behavior. In the case of our older adults, even though they may watch someone model a skill (attending to the significant aspects and retaining that information in memory), they must have the necessary strength and flexibility to be able to successfully replicate the behavior. Finally, "people do not perform everything they learn" (3, p. 5514). They must be motivated to replicate the action of the model, which involves *wanting* to do the behavior. This implies valuing the activity, which is critical when we think of exercise. Some older adults don't see the purpose of structured exercise, whether it be on machines or in an exercise class; they prefer to do activity that, to them, contributes to the greater good (31). The job of the personal trainer or group exercise leader is to show older adults the value of exercise and to make it relevant to their daily functioning. For example, you could relate strength gains with measures of independence, such as getting out of a chair by themselves or carrying their own groceries. All together, the four components of modeling provide a template for structuring the exercise environment to maximize the chance that older adults will learn what they need to learn (attention), remember the important aspects (retention), be able to perform a given task (motor production), and be compelled to do so (motivation).

> **KEY POINT 4-5** The Four Subprocesses of Observational Learning
>
> Attention — attending to the relevant aspects of a skill while ignoring irrelevant components
>
> Retention — coding skill into memory; organizing and rehearsing information
>
> Motor production — mental action translated into physical action; must have requisite skill
>
> Motivation — individual must want to replicate skill

Does it matter who the model is?

Another aspect of modeling theory involves characteristics of the model (21). Research with children and adolescents suggests that *model similarity,* whether it be gender, age, or ability, can be important in helping individuals "see themselves" in the model. This brings us to the issue of the varying types of models and their effect on behavior. There are two basic types of models. In the first situation, the model knows considerably more than the observer. We call these models *mastery or correct models.* The second type of model involves individuals who may be learning right along with the observer; these models fall under the category of *learning or coping models* (21). Which type of model is best for teaching skills? This question is not as simple as it may seem. Although expert models may make sense in some situations, learning or coping models may be desirable in others. For example, expert models can motivate an individual to strive for higher levels of achievement, but only if the learner believes he can learn the skill. Coping models, on the other hand, show the learner the process of learning. This can be very helpful in situations where the learner is starting from scratch, or with a task that is perceived to be an optimal challenge. This could easily be the case for an older adult exerciser, who might have limited experience using exercise equipment. Little research has actually examined modeling in adult and older adult exercise contexts, so the best advice might be to use multiple models and ask questions throughout the demonstration.

Putting observational learning theory to work: The practitioner's perspective

In applying modeling theory to our case studies, Bob's case is more subtle than Janet's. He already had a long history of exercising independently and an education level that included basic anatomy and physiology. He felt that he knew more than his peers, and up to this year, he had been successful exercising on his own with annual sessions with his physical therapist/trainer. Although he was familiar with using stacked weight machines, he required individual sessions to perform the exercises with correct technique, proper foot position, and instruction in breathing. His attention and retention of the task had to be taught in such a manner that it didn't insult his level of education and demean his abilities. It was handled in a very tactful manner to advance his abilities and "fine tune" his performance. As with many older adults, retention in exercise takes repetition and more repetition. We use verbal cueing and frequent demonstration, and even Bob needed this to improve his program. Rehearsal of the exercise with positive verbal reinforcement worked well. When writing the client's exercise card, I often ask the client how he would like an exercise "named" or written on the card, so he will remember it better. Patience of the personal trainer is key in retention, as it often takes the older adult frequent attempts to learn to adjust exercise equipment (even starting a treadmill can be daunting). And the personal trainer must be sensitive that the older adult may be shy in asking for assistance, so it becomes necessary for the trainer to anticipate the client's needs and respond respectfully with instruction so as not to demean the older adult.

Bob easily approached exercise with the skills for motor production. He already knew that he was capable of exercising consistently; he just needed the correct program to reduce his falls. Preventing falls is his primary motivation for structured exercise, and he sees a direct correlation between exercise, agility, and balance activities and the reduction of falls. The role of the personal trainer/physical therapist as he continues to exercise is to challenge him with the appropriate activities that will hold his interest. I believe that Bob would have only accepted modeling the mastery or correct model — he wished to receive instruction only from the expert to help him attain a higher level of achievement because prior to his falls, he was very confident in his exercise skill set.

Unlike Bob, Janet's situation was perfect for observational learning. As you recall, she had no experience with exercise. For her, exercising was about learning not only new physical skills, but also a new language. Terms like *repetitions, sets, duration, exercise to fatigue, optimal heart rate, stretches, dumbbells, stacked weights, rows, curls,* and *lat pulls* were completely foreign to her. Acquiring her exercise skill set called for a lot of one-on-one attention from the trainer to teach her. She had to learn not only the exercises and stretches, but also to operate equipment such as the treadmill and stacked weight systems. To those of us for whom exercise has been an integral part of our lives, we are at ease entering a gym and operating equipment that we have never seen before. To an older adult, the multiple buttons, lights, and switches can be overwhelming. In fact, many of my clients who travel tell me that the reason they didn't exercise while they were on vacation was that the "machines were different." The older adult may have difficulty applying learned skills to different equipment. Over months of teaching with clear and gentle instruction, Janet became independent in her exercise program.

Considering the third and fourth components of modeling, motor production and motivation, respectively, Janet started at the beginner level. She is a petite and frail individual who did not possess a lot of strength. She did not have the motor production to perform exercises on any of the stacked weight systems or even with dumbbells. She started exercising with the weight of her own limbs, a few stretches, and a cardiovascular program using the Nustep machine. The duration of her program was limited, so she would not experience achiness after exercising. I wanted to reduce the barriers to exercise as much as possible. She started with exercises that she could perform well, so she could feel successful. Over the past 3 years, she has progressed to using the treadmill, stacked weights, and dumbbells. She appreciates where her starting point was and has experienced the improvement in her life. She gets sick less often than her peers, continues to live independently, and has more strength and energy. These factors motivate her to continue exercising in a structured manner because she feels the type of instruction and modeling received at our facility has been a key factor in her success.

Multiple models proved best for Janet's progression. The mastery or correct model was needed initially to teach her about exercise, but the learning or coping model was instrumental in her experience. Her peers acted as learning models; when she observed them performing an exercise that she wasn't doing, she asked them what they were doing and they would teach her the exercise. Her previous mastery of exercise gave her the confidence to try something new, and she began to challenge herself in various ways. Each time this happened, she felt more successful and has become one of our most loyal clients.

Theories of the self and identity

Self-efficacy and effective modeling, along with a host of other motivational constructs, have in common thoughts about the self (25). That is, we judge if we're capable of doing something, form ideas about who we are, and imagine what we might be able to do, based on how we see ourselves and our abilities. In this section, we will overview some key self-related concepts. In particular, we will focus on self-concept, defined as the different ways we describe ourselves (17, 30). From there, we will discuss two associated constructs, identity and self-definition (34, 11). These concepts will be explored with regard to how perceptions we have of ourselves guide our behavior, and importantly, how these perceptions can be shaped so as to maximize physical activity participation.

How do you describe yourself? Student, athlete, sibling, and close friend might be some of these descriptions. Together, these descriptors define who we are as individuals, as well as how we believe others see us, and perhaps who we would like to be (or avoid being) in the future. Our self-concept is formed from our experiences and reflections on those experiences (24). And, although we may not remember all the individual events that make up a particular part of ourselves (*e.g.*, "student"), we organize that information into knowledge structures that enable us to make sense of our life experiences (16). We call these knowledge structures identities (34), self-schemas (15), or self-descriptions (11). Thus, our self-concept is made up of domain-specific identities, each of which represents a different facet of our experience (as a student, an athlete, or a close friend). These identities are integrated into a "coherent, recognizable self-package" (6, p. xii) that continues to evolve over time. It makes sense that adults and older adults have multiple identities that accumulate over time, focusing on one's physical functioning, cognition, and social relationships (34). As we shall see, these identities can direct our behaviors, so they are critical for understanding our motivation. Once we understand the development and maintenance of identities, we can capitalize on these identities to encourage specific behaviors.

Identity is a powerful motivator. We do things that confirm our identities, and we avoid situations where our identities might be challenged (28). Research has shown us that our conceptions of our physical selves are particularly important. These include our physical appearance, our physical competence (defined as our ability to perform the tasks needed to get us through our daily activities), and our physical health (34). Kendzierski and her colleagues (11, 12) have developed a model of physical activity self-definition, which supplies us with a template for encouraging the development and nurturing of an identity for exercise. We turn next to that model and the factors proposed to contribute to an exerciser self-definition.

KEY POINT 4-6 Reasons to Help Exercisers Develop a Physical Activity Self-Definition

People who define themselves as "physically active" or "exercisers" exercise more frequently and for longer duration and are more likely to begin an exercise program than those who do not have such a self-definition.

The physical activity self-definition model

As indicated previously, people who define themselves in a particular way (*e.g.*, as an exerciser, runner, or tennis player) are more likely to participate in that activity. In addition, they are more likely to create plans to help them increase their activity and act on their intention to exercise, run, or play tennis (9, 10). Kendzierski and her colleagues (11, 12) developed the physical activity self-definition model in an attempt to discover how a specific (runner, tennis player) or general (exerciser, walker) identity might be formed and maintained. They based the components of the model on self-related theories, starting with the important premise that "self-definition is not simply a question of engagement in activity" (11, p. 177). An example illustrates this point. There are many people who run, but not everyone considers himself or herself a "runner." What is it that determines this status? Is it how often one runs? How far? How fast? Or is it something more complex — such as one's goals, attitude, or emotions associated with running? By examining a variety of theoretical perspectives, the researchers hypothesized that physical activity self-definitions would depend on three types of variables:

1. Perceptions about the behavior (effort extended, priority attributed to the behavior)
2. Motivation to engage in the behavior (perceived competence, perceived improvement, and perceived enjoyment of the activity)
3. The extent to which others in the person's social world acknowledge the self-definition

In a series of studies examining undergraduate exercisers and athletes (11), and adult runners and cyclists (12), a consistent pattern was found that best described a physical activity self-definition. Specifically, perceived *commitment* to the activity (defined as the importance of the behavior to the person) and perceived *competence* (defined as the person's perceptions of ability about the activity) directly affect self-definition. In turn, commitment is based on *wanting* to do the activity and *trying* to do the activity. Finally, *enjoying* the activity has been found to impact whether or not the person wants to do an activity.

What does this imply for motivating older adult exercisers? Undoubtedly, it is important to help exercisers foster an identity in the exercise context. Remember that physical self-definitions are related to activities that people voluntarily engage in (12); thus, if people feel as if they *have* to exercise, that is unlikely to result in an exerciser self-definition. Instead, you can help people see that exercise is something they *want* to do — for example, so they can be healthy and independent. Putting exercise in terms of a way to achieve goals is a sound strategy for motivating oneself and others. Second, physical activity self-definitions need to be triggered by something in the environment. You, as the exercise leader or facilitator, can and should be this trigger. Don't miss the opportunity to tell the person that he or she is a "dedicated exerciser" or that he or she is "really developing into a walker." Of course, make this feedback relevant to the person on the basis of facts. Third, let the person you are working with come up with their own term for their behavior. You may feel completely comfortable with the term *exerciser,* but an older adult might feel more comfortable using terms such as *healthy adult* or *active person* (32).

Once you have the person thinking about his or her identity, then it's your job to provide the means of confirming and building that self-definition. A good starting point is to make it enjoyable. Facilitating enjoyment, in turn, will help the person feel like this is something he or she wants to do rather than have to do, fostering commitment to the activity. Giving the exerciser opportunities to succeed at the task will help the exerciser know he or she is trying, helping to build perceptions of ability. Remember here to meet the person where they are; sometimes it is easy to either overestimate or underestimate an older adult's ability; keep in mind that everyone can get stronger, more fit, and more flexible. With support and encouragement, older adult exercisers can feel successful, show real improvement, and, when this is combined with commitment, build a strong physical activity self-definition.

Putting the self-definition model to work: The practitioner's perspective

As you may have guessed, Bob had a self-definition as an exerciser before joining our facility. He still works, so he also defines himself as a consultant and husband. However, his physical activity self-definition grew stronger and more specific during the year he joined our facility. He developed a renewed commitment and motivation to exercise under the guidance of a trainer/physical therapist assistant. Whereas before he exercised alone in his attic at home, he now enjoys his new exercise environment and the camaraderie with the trainer and other fitness members. He has become competent in using the exercise equipment properly and helps other members. He is engaging and social and stops in for a hug or to deliver a cookie for the staff. His self-definition of exerciser has changed from being a solo exerciser to being a fitness member. He feels a part of the exercise community at our facility, and we have helped to confirm his new identity through feedback and support.

In the first year of joining our facility, Janet did not define herself as an exerciser. Perhaps as a mother, widower, and friend would be how she defined herself. However, as her competence with learning new skills and enjoying increased function continued, she began to define herself as a regular exerciser and fitness member. She has experienced the connection between regular exercise and increased physical function, which has changed her perceptions about exercise ("it's too hard" or "it hurts" to "it's getting easier"), so she remains committed to her program. Her perceived competence has changed her entire outlook; she is more confident and is more outspoken in the gym. She takes it upon herself to update the staff on sick members in the community when she is at the gym or she calls our staff by phone. She has special staff whom she enjoys talking with when she exercises, and she makes it a point to work out when those staff members are working so that the experience is enjoyable.

It is important to note that in the case of both Bob and Janet, the gated community in which they live has an exercise facility that is free for their use. However, it is not staffed by any personnel, and they choose to drive 4 miles to our facility and pay our membership fees. As mentioned earlier, the trainers are the lead facilitators in developing and sustaining self-definition for their clients. The older adult enjoys verbal encouragement of some type on *each visit* to our facility. For example, staff notice where the client has improved and point that out to him or her. It is often hard for individuals to notice their own improvement. We often exercise with them, using that time to teach and engage with them in personal (yet professional) conversation. The relationship between trainer and client unfolds just as any close friendship would, and when the older adult sees value in you, the trainer, and in the facility, there is a great commitment and loyalty for the client to continue working with you. In this way, we work with what the client comes in with. We provide an enjoyable, comfortable, and supportive environment, so the client wants to do the activity, has plenty of opportunities to do activities, and thereby becomes competent and committed.

BRINGING THE KEY CONCEPTS TOGETHER: GERRI'S QUEST

The previous section showed how you might use three key concepts (self-efficacy, observational learning, and self-definition) to help exercisers become and stay motivated. We presented each theory and then showed how the concepts apply to two real-world cases. The next step in understanding a theory-to-practice perspective is to reverse the process. Instead of providing the theory and then fitting it to a case, we now present a case study of an older adult exerciser from one coauthor's physical therapy practice. Although the name has been changed, all the details are true. Remember, the idea here is to use the concepts and theories we reviewed previously to *inform* your practice. That is, for doctors, physical therapists, or personal trainers, it makes sense to use methods we can be confident lead to certain outcomes rather than "making it up as we go along," or even "using our gut." For example, we know that higher levels of self-efficacy lead to sustained effort and performance, and we judge our self-efficacy on the basis of four primary sources (mastery experiences, vicarious experiences, verbal persuasion, and physiological states). But how do we use the information we have about a client, patient, or participant to tailor our strategies in such a way as to maximize participation? This is the essence of a motivational plan. It is one thing to be able to list and define the four sources of efficacy information; it's quite another to fit it to the needs of an individual. Thus, in this final section, we will look inside a case study. After a few preliminary questions to consider, we will examine how we can use what we know about this person to create a motivational

---

Real Life Story 4-3   Gerri

Gerri is a 78-year-old woman who was diagnosed with osteopenia (a precursor to osteoporosis) in 2001. She has a family history of osteoporosis. She has additional medical complications such as cervical arthritis and adhesive capsulitis (a tightness in the shoulder capsule creating immobility in the shoulder). In 2001, it was recommended that she take medication to improve bone strength. She took the medication for 3 months and experienced side effects (malaise, stomach pain), so she stopped taking it and has gone without medication for her osteopenia. Around that time, she read an article that reported exercise was beneficial for osteoporosis and contacted a physical therapist (PT) for a consultation. In her discussion with Gerri, the PT learned that Gerri was very active as a child and adult. In high school, she walked 4 miles each way, and in college, she walked approximately 2 miles each direction to her classes. She also enjoyed hiking in her younger years. She states that what keeps her motivated "is keeping my bones strong." She also states, "My back begins to hurt" if she doesn't exercise and she wants to avoid shoulder pain.

plan to fit the individual's needs. We will include what worked, as well as some bumps that can (and did!) come up, so you can begin to plan for a real-life situation. As you read about Gerri, start to think about how her experiences, goals, and needs might influence how you would work with her.

Before beginning your motivational program, Gerri's trainer would need to carefully assess her readiness to exercise, as well as what type of exercise program would be appropriate. The following are some questions to consider:

1. What physical tests would you have Gerri perform to gain a baseline assessment of her strength? Her endurance? Her function?
2. What exercises/activities would you include in her exercise program considering her medical history?
3. Are there any exercises that you would avoid giving an individual who has a history of osteopenia?

Once we have the medical/physical issues addressed, it's time to move on to the motivational story. This begins by learning more about Gerri the person, rather than merely the patient. The following are some facts about Gerri that might impact her motivational status:

Gerri has been active her entire life. She considers herself self-motivated; the diagnosis of osteopenia elevated her motivation to do more to prevent the progression of the disease. She has a very no-nonsense type of personality; after she received the diagnosis of osteopenia, she read all the literature she could, and discovered that she needed strength and weight-bearing exercises. After feeling side effects from her medication, she made the decision to stop taking prescription medication for her osteopenia. She also shared that she expects to be a little sore after a "good workout."

KEY POINT 4-7 Creating a Motivational Plan — Questions to Pursue

What is the person's exercise history? Are they experienced or inexperienced? What does this suggest about sources of efficacy information?

Is the person eager and willing to learn, or tentative and anxious? What type of model might work best for this person? What can I do to maximize effective learning?

Does this person have components of a physical activity self-definition? What can I do to help this person form, confirm, or sustain such an identity?

What have we learned about Gerri so far and how does this help us?

- Self-efficacy: She has had previous mastery experiences for exercise and understands the difference between being sore and being hurt (physiological states). We can use these sources of information to continue to boost her levels of self-efficacy.
- Modeling: She is self-motivated and likes to learn — so she should respond well to information and explanations about activities you provide, and for you to be a

mastery model for the exercises you want her to do. Her desire to learn will help with attention and retention of information.

- Self-definition: We can expect that Gerri has an exerciser self-definition in place, since she seems committed and confident in her ability to exercise; she *wants* to exercise. However, she would benefit from feedback that helps her confirm that identity. In particular, helping her confirm her commitment to her program (through goal setting, for example) and building competence by having plenty of practice and instruction will help.

What happened at the clinic?

Gerri's physical therapist used lots of verbal persuasion in assuring her that she could be successful with exercise and proper nutrition ("you've done it before, and you can do it again"). When developing a program for her, we discussed what she liked to do (fostering enjoyment and commitment). She loved walking outdoors, taking in the beauty around her. Since walking is a weight-bearing exercise and appropriate for osteopenia, she was instructed in duration, frequency, and exercise heart rate goals (capitalizing on her desire for knowledge). On days of inclement weather, she could walk on the treadmill. Her gym program consisted of strength exercises for abdominals, back, hips, wrists, and shoulders, such as forward lunges, countertop push-ups, upper body dumbbells exercises, leg presses, and marching on the mini-trampoline. Gerri was very determined, but she required lots of modeling because she wanted to know all the nuances of each exercise to perform the technique perfectly. She was not timid in asking for assistance to acquire the skill and always demonstrated the exercise to be sure she had learned it properly.

Between 2003 and 2009, the bone mineral scans for Gerri showed an increase in bone mineral density: her bones were getting stronger. In fact, her "risk" for fracture improved from three to four times the risk to two times the risk. In addition, there was an improvement in her cholesterol levels because of regular exercise. She was ecstatic about the news and called me and brought in her test results for me to see. She continued to see me, her trainer/physical therapist playing a key role in her exercise program and the prevention against osteoporosis.

All goes well until . . .

Gerri and her husband spent their winters in Florida where they golfed and walked on the beach. In 2009–2010, the Florida winter was harsher than normal with frequent rainy and cloudy days. Gerri did not exercise regularly. She returned home with low back pain. Then she fell on some ice and fractured her left wrist. Her wrist was casted and immobile for 6 weeks, which limited the functional use of her left arm. She returned to physical therapy for her back and wrist discouraged about the way she was feeling physically. Unlike the first time, Gerri seemed unsure of her ability to exercise successfully, and her physiological and emotional states were altered. She questioned each new exercise that involved her left wrist, and each ache or pain left her wondering whether it was harming the healing process. She questioned why it was taking so long for the left wrist strength to improve.

What was going on with Gerri?

- Self-efficacy: Gerri had lost her previous confidence in her ability to be successful and didn't seem to see how exercise could get her back to her previous state (outcome expectation). Although she still had her mastery experiences, these were overshadowed by her focus on her back and wrist injuries and her perception of little to no progress. Gerri needs realistic feedback and support.
- Modeling: Gerri's model needs to be someone whom she sees as credible. This might take the form of a mastery *or* a learning model, but should definitely be accompanied by plenty of encouragement, information, and support. Her therapist/trainer will need to pay special attention to the motivation component of modeling — it seems she has moved from *wanting* to exercise to feeling she *has* to exercise.
- Self-definition: Gerri's exerciser self-definition seems to have slipped. Reminding her that she was such a successful exerciser previously and that she can regain her form and fitness with persistence and effort, and challenging her to commit to a new program (while providing support) are likely to help Gerri get back to where she was.

What happened at the clinic?

During her second round of PT, Gerri required more verbal persuasion to return to her previous program. With her left wrist in a cast, I encouraged her to focus on exercises for her back and right upper extremity. After three PT sessions, she no longer had back pain. At this stage, I was the only model she wanted; none of the other therapists, trainers, or coping models would suffice. She wanted a mastery model she trusted to transition her out of this uncertain phase. Gradually, the wrist and hand strength returned, and each week, she arrived with a new task that she was now able to accomplish at home, returning more to her old self. Gerri had seriously relapsed, but was well on the road to returning to her previous level of health and now had the confidence to continue on her own.

Questions to ponder:

1. How would Gerri's motivation to exercise have differed if she had not grown up accustomed to walking to school? What would you do differently?
2. What if Gerri had not gotten sick with the medication? What else could have been used to motivate her to begin exercise?

3. What impact did the Florida winter have on her self-efficacy and physiological response?

4. After the left wrist fracture and episode of low back pain, what positive mastery experiences did she learn about exercise that might help her down the road?

S U M M A R Y

In this chapter, we have provided a theory to practice approach to understanding motivation in older adult exercisers. It is important to note that older adults are perhaps the most diverse group of individuals; their varied histories and medical issues assure that no two people will react the same way, nor will the same techniques necessarily work across individuals. Although this may seem daunting, if we keep in mind that we can learn about an individual by listening and hearing their story, that will bring us a long way toward treating our clients, patients, or members with the respect and care they deserve. If we then plan our approach on the basis of the needs of the individual, keeping in mind concepts such as developing self-efficacy, demonstrating skills and techniques so as to optimize the learning experience, and fostering an exerciser self-definition, we will maximize the chance of the individual learning skills, feeling confident, enjoying the experience, and ultimately persisting at the activity. In turn, once a trusting relationship is formed between the older adult exerciser and the trainer, we have found that these older adults become very loyal and committed exercisers, creating a win-win situation for all involved. Motivating self and others is a skill that can be taught; it takes time and effort, but the rewards are plentiful.

 ## QUESTIONS FOR REFLECTION

1. What does it mean to take a "theory to practice approach" in solving problems related to exercise participation and adherence?

2. Why are older adults more varied in their motives for activity than younger adults are? What is the implication of this for designing programs?

3. What is the relationship between motivation and one's needs?

4. What sources of efficacy information did Janet use to become more confident in her ability to exercise regularly? How could you enhance these sources if you were her personal trainer?

5. If you were teaching Bob how to use a new piece of exercise equipment, how would you structure the learning environment to maximize a successful experience? Is it a problem if you were considerably younger and more skilled than he?

6. What is the difference between "running" and "being a runner"? Why is that distinction important?

7. Describe the factors that led to Gerri losing her confidence in her ability to exercise. How was the staff able to build her confidence back up?

8. What should a motivational plan include? Why is it important?

REFERENCES

1. Bandura A. *Social Foundations of Thought and Action: A Social Cognitive Theory.* Englewood Cliffs (NJ): Prentice-Hall; 1986.
2. Bandura A. Self-efficacy. In: Ramachaudran VS, editor. *Encyclopedia of Human Behavior.* Vol. 4. New York (NY): Academic Press; 1994. p. 71–81.
3. Bandura A. Social cognitive theory of human development. In: Husen T, Postlethwaite TN, editors. *International Encyclopedia of Education.* 2nd ed. Oxford, England: Pergamon Press; 1996. p. 5513–18.
4. Clark DO. Age, socioeconomic status, and exercise self-efficacy. *Gerontologist.* 1996;36:157–64.
5. Eccles JS, Wigfield A, Schiefele U. Motivation to succeed. In: Damon W, Lerner RM, Eisenberg N, editors. *Handbook of Child Psychology, Vol. 3: Social, Emotional, and Personality Development.* 5th ed. New York (NY): Wiley; 1998. p. 1017–95.
6. Fox KR. Let's get physical. In: Fox KR, editor. *The Physical Self: From Motivation to Well Being.* Champaign (IL): Human Kinetics; 1997. p. vii–xiii.
7. Grodesky JM, Kosma M, Solmon MA. Understanding older adults' physical activity behavior: A multi-theoretical approach. *Quest.* 2006;58:310–29.
8. Horn TS. Lifespan development in sport and exercise psychology: Theoretical perspectives. In: Weiss MR, editor. *Developmental Sport and Exercise Psychology: A Lifespan Perspective.* Morgantown (WV): Fitness Information Technology; 2004. p. 27–71.
9. Kendzierski D. Self-schemata and exercise. *Basic Appl Soc Psychol.* 1988;9:45–59.
10. Kendzierski D. Exercise self-schemata: Cognitive and behavioral correlates. *Health Psychol.* 1990;9:69–82.
11. Kendzierski D, Furr RM, Schiavoni J. Physical activity self-definitions: Correlates and perceived criteria. *J Sport Exer Psychol.* 1998;20:176–93.
12. Kendzierski D, Morganstein MS. Test, revision, and cross-validation of the physical activity self-definition model. *J Sport Exer Psychol.* 2009;31:484–504.
13. Kirkby R, Kolt G, Habel K, Adams J. Exercise in older women: Motives for participation. *Aust Psychol.* 1999;34(2):122–7. Available from: http://www.informaworld.com/smpp/title~db=all~content=g782655202. doi: 10.1080/00050069908257440
14. Kolt G, Driver R, Giles L. Why older Australians participate in exercise and sport. *J Aging Phys Act.* 2004;12(2):185–98.
15. Markus H. Self-schemata and processing information about the self. *J Personality Soc Psychol.* 1977;35(2):63–78.
16. Markus H, Cross S, Wurf E. The role of the self-system in competence. In: Sternberg RJ, Kolligan J Jr, editors. *Competence Considered.* New Haven (CT): Yale University Press; 1990. p. 205–25.
17. Markus HR, Herzog AR. The role of the self-concept in aging. In: Shaie KW, Lawton MP, editors. *Annual Review of Gerontology and Geriatrics.* Vol. 11. New York (NY): Springer; 1992. p. 110–43.
18. Martinez I, Kim K, Tanner E, Fried L, Seeman T. Ethnic and class variations in promoting social activities among older adults. *Act Adapt Aging.* 2009;33(2):96–119. Available from: http://www.informaworld.com/smpp/title~db=all~content=g912371905. doi: 10.1080/01924780902947082
19. Mathews AE, Laditka SB, Laditka JN, et al. Older adults' perceived physical activity enablers and barriers: A multicultural perspective. *J Aging Phys Act.* 2010;18(2):119–40.
20. McAuley E, Blissmer B. Self-efficacy determinants and consequences of physical activity. *Exer Sport Sci Rev.* 2000;28(2):85–8.
21. McCullagh P, Weiss MR. Observational learning: The forgotten method in sport psychology. In: Van Raalte JL, Brewer BW, editors. *Exploring Sport and Exercise Psychology.* Washington (DC): American Psychological Association; 2002. p. 131–49.

22. Mullen SP, Whaley DE. Age, gender, and fitness club membership: Factors related to initial involvement and sustained participation. *Int J Sport Exer Psychol.* 2010;8:24–35.

23. Rasinaho M, Hirvensalo M, Leinonen R, Lintunen T, Rantanen T. Motives for and barriers to physical activity among older adults with mobility limitations. *J Aging Phys Act.* 2007;15(1):90–102.

24. Reeve J. *Understanding Motivation and Emotion.* 4th ed. Hoboken (NJ): John Wiley & Sons; 2005.

25. Ruvolo AP, Markus HR. Possible selves and performance: The power of self-relevant imagery. *Social Cognition.* 1992;10(1):95–124.

26. Schunk DH. Teaching elementary students to self-regulate practice of mathematical skills with modeling. In: Schunk DH, Zimmerman BJ, editors. *Self-Regulated Learning: From Teaching to Self-Reflective Practice.* New York (NY): Guilford Press; 1998. p. 137–59.

27. Standage M, Duda JL. Motivational processes among older adults in sport and exercise settings. In: Weiss MR, editor. *Developmental Sport and Exercise Psychology: A Lifespan Perspective.* Morgantown (WV): Fitness Information Technology; 2004. p. 357–81.

28. Stets JE, Burke PJ. A sociological approach to self and identity. In: Leary MR, Tangney JP, editors. *Handbook of Self and Identity.* New York (NY): Guilford Press; 2003. p. 128–52.

29. U.S. Department of Health and Human Services. Summary Health Statistics for U.S. Adults: National Health Interview Survey. Centers for Disease Control and Prevention, National Center for Health Statistics; 2008. Washington (DC): U.S. Department of Health and Human Services; 2008. p. 76. Available from: http://www.cdc.gov/nchs/data/series/sr_10/sr10_242.pdf

30. Whaley DE. Seeing isn't always believing: Self-perceptions and physical activity behaviors in adults. In: Weiss MR, editor. *Developmental Sport and Exercise Psychology: A Lifespan Perspective.* Morgantown (WV): Fitness Information Technology; 2004. p. 289–311.

31. Whaley DE, Ebbeck V. Older adults' constraints to participation in structured exercise classes. *J Aging Phys Act.* 1997;5(3):190–212.

32. Whaley DE, Schrider A. The process of adult exercise adherence: Self-perceptions and competence. *Sport Psychol.* 2005;19(2):148–63.

33. Whitbourne SK. *Adult Development and Aging: Biopsychosocial Perspectives.* 3rd ed. Hoboken (NJ): Wiley; 2008.

34. Whitbourne SK, Collins KJ. Identity processes and perceptions of physical functioning in adults: Theoretical and clinical implications. *Psychotherapy.* 1998;35:519–30.

CHAPTER 5

Physical Activity Options for Healthy Older Adults

Mary Frances Visser and Pam MacFarlane

••• CHAPTER OUTLINE

INTRODUCTION

The intent of this chapter is to provide an overview of physical activity options available to normally healthy older adults. This includes men and women who are not regularly limited by acute or chronic disabilities, who have the capacity to perform a range of physical activities, and who would benefit from exercise regardless of age. Exercise for this segment of the population provides measurable improvements in physical fitness, but can serve as preventive and/or rehabilitative medicine in addition to enhancing the quality of life through social interaction engagement, a sense of accomplishment, and enhanced self-efficacy (18).

Although older adults may perform the same types of activities as younger adults, their reasons for adopting and maintaining an exercise routine may differ greatly (27). One type of exercise program does not suit everyone. Current recommendations for older adults suggest that effective programs should include a range of activities that enhance or maintain cardiorespiratory endurance, muscle function (strength, endurance, and power), balance and mobility (BAM), and flexibility (3). Given current knowledge of the benefits of physical activity for older adults, it appears that it is a key lifestyle factor that facilitates successful aging regardless of the age and prior experience.

One of the key recommendations from the most recent statement on physical activity and public health issued by the American College of Sports Medicine® (ACSM) and the American Heart Association (AHA) is that all older adults should have a workable plan that helps them to obtain a sufficient amount of physical activity in each of the recommended areas (21). It is hoped that the information contained in this chapter, as well as the text as a whole, will allow normally healthy older adults or the fitness professions they may work with to develop this type of plan. It is time that all adults, but especially older adults, create a personal health and wellness plan with a firm commitment to planning for regular physical activity in the same way that they approach planning for their retirement savings.

HISTORICAL PERSPECTIVES

It is important to acknowledge that older adults were not always encouraged to be physically active. Popular culture has traditionally viewed the path to old age as a steady reduction in activity leading to a prolonged time of leisure that was "earned" after years of work. Even medical professionals were slow to recognize the benefits of regular physical activity for older adults. Treatment of many illness and injuries included physical activity limitations and sometimes bed rest until researchers demonstrated that physical inactivity results in an accelerated loss of both bone mineral density and muscle tissue, which can actually compound health problems in this age group (6, 12). Recuperation strategies have evolved with this knowledge. In 2010, ACSM began its "Exercise is Medicine" campaign that pushes to the forefront the many health and wellness benefits of physical activity. This campaign, with resources targeted at individuals and the medical community, marks a milestone in the recognition and promotion of physical activity and exercise as integral parts of a health or wellness plan for all segments of the population including older adults.

The seeds of change in attitudes toward physical activity for adults in general were sown decades ago when the rates of heart attacks in British bus drivers and conductors were first traced. These data, published in 1953, indicated that conductors who climbed about 600 stairs a day had fewer than half the attacks of the drivers who sat for 90% of the day (19). Throughout the following decades, a number of research studies supported the beneficial effects of regular cardiovascular exercise in adults and older adults (5). Not only has the incidence of cardiovascular disease been reduced, but also standard treatment and management of the condition has evolved to incorporate regular exercise.

These successful outcomes encouraged examination of the effects of other types of exercise such as resistance and flexibility training on older men and women, as loss of muscular strength and range of motion (ROM) were recognized as contributing factors to loss of independent living skills and greater needs for higher levels of care (7). Concerns about the devastating outcomes of falls have spurred investigation of ways to prevent or decrease older adult BAM problems with targeted physical activities (4). This growing body of research on the effects of physical activity and exercise on older adults has provided overwhelming evidence that the training principle of specificity is as important for older exercisers as it is for younger exercisers.

In 1995, the Centers for Disease Control and Prevention (CDC) and ACSM released guidelines that recommended that all adults accumulate 30 minutes of moderate-intensity activity on all, if not most, days of the week (22). Experts soon concluded that the exercise needs of adults and older adults were qualitatively and quantitatively different. An ACSM position statement on physical activity for older adults was first published in 1998 (2) and was followed by periodic joint statements by professional organizations that updated and further clarified recommendations (4, 21, 23). The most recent and definitive position stand on exercise and physical activity for older adults was published in 2009. Recommendations from that document will shape the content of this chapter (3). The focus will be on those normally healthy older adults who are sedentary or less active and those who may wish to incorporate additional activity options to an existing program to align it with current recommendations. High-intensity recreational activity and sport is appropriate for older adults who have a good base of physical fitness; however, development and maintenance of this level of physical activity will not be specifically addressed in this chapter.

CONSIDERATIONS FOR ALL PHYSICAL ACTIVITY OPTIONS

Exercise participation is lowest for the older segments of the US population (10). Changing less healthy behaviors, especially when they have become habitual over time, is difficult, which makes it important to match older adults with exercise programs that meet their needs. To prevent dropout, a variety of options should be offered so that each may adopt an active lifestyle that they can adapt to and maintain.

An exercise session should include four basic components: a warm-up; a main conditioning session of endurance exercise, resistance training, neuromuscular exercises, or sports activities; a cool-down; and a flexibility session (1). ACSM guidelines suggest 5 to 10 minutes for the warm-up and cool-down, 20 to 60 minutes for the main conditioning, and 10 minutes of flexibility exercises. A somewhat longer warm-up period may be necessary to allow the older body to gradually adjust to changes in metabolic needs. A cool-down allows the body to readjust to normal conditions when the main bout of exercise has been completed. It is tempting to skip the warm-up, the cool-down, or the flexibility session when the exercise time is limited. All need to be included for a variety of reasons, including the safety and well-being of participants.

A successful main conditioning phase for older adults should include the same principles as for younger adults: frequency, intensity, time or duration, and type of exercise. Applying this "FITT" principle allows programs to be tailored to individual needs. ACSM guidelines provide clear direction for applying the FITT principles to exercises based on physical fitness classification *not* age (1). The FITT principles can be manipulated to increase the total *volume* of exercise in a safe and effective fashion. Some specific differences exist between application of these guidelines for younger and older exercisers. Initial exercise intensity and duration may need to be lower at the start of a program, and the progression of any of the FITT components also may need to be slower than for younger participants and specifically tailored to accommodate any chronic conditions that may impact their ability to perform certain tasks. If participants are unable to meet recommended amounts of activity because of their conditions, they should be encouraged to be as active as their limitations permit to avoid a sedentary lifestyle.

Maintaining an appropriate intensity is essential for the safety and well-being of all participants, but this is especially true for older exercisers. Managing intensity presents unique challenges for this population because of the number of commonly prescribed medications that may influence heart rate responses to exercise. ACSM guidelines recommend use of the Borg 1 to 10 rating of perceived exertion (RPE) scale, as it is easy to learn and can be used to monitor intensity across a number of types of exercise (1). Exertion refers to a subjective overall body sensation that takes into account personal fitness level, environmental conditions, and general fatigue. With this scale, 0 is equivalent to the exertion of sitting and 10 is equivalent to an all-out effort. Moderate-intensity exercise is defined as exertion level of 5 to 6, whereas vigorous-intensity is considered to be a level of 7 or higher (1). Participants should be taught or teach themselves to use this scale and be mindful of their intensity, especially when initiating a program. Exercising at the right intensity maximizes the benefits to be gained while reducing safety risks.

ENDURANCE EXERCISE OPTIONS

Figure 5-1 depicts the FITT framework for endurance exercise for older adults.

WHAT IS ENDURANCE EXERCISE?

ACSM has identified exercises that contribute to cardiovascular endurance as those that are rhythmic in nature, involve large muscle groups of the body, and are continuous (1). Endurance exercise is generally performed to promote cardiovascular health; however, it may also increase muscular strength and improve BAM in older adults, depending on its type and intensity (21, 23). As cardiovascular disease remains the primary cause of death in the United States, maintenance of heart health is an important goal of an exercise program.

Regular endurance exercise training (EET) can also reduce the risk of other common lifestyle diseases such as Type II diabetes and certain cancers. It is also recommended in the management of these and other common health conditions (1, 21, 23). Maintenance of aerobic fitness also contributes to performance of activities of daily life that are necessary for home and self-care. Declines in these abilities are major contributors to loss of independent living skills and increased dependence on others.

TYPES OF ENDURANCE EXERCISE

A wide range of activities from walking to recreational sports promote cardiovascular health. ACSM guidelines have partitioned various endurance activities into groups to facilitate appropriate choices for adults (1) (Table 5-1).

Frequency: For moderate-intensity activities, accumulate at least 30 or up to 60 (for greater benefit) minutes a day in bouts of at least 10 minutes each to total 150–300 minutes a week, at least 20–30 minutes a day or more of vigorous-intensity activities to total 75–150 minutes a week, an equivalent combination of moderate and vigorous activity.

Intensity: Between 5 to 6 for moderate intensity and 7 to 8 for vigorous intensity on an RPE scale of 0–10.

Time (Duration): For moderate intensity activities, accumulate at least 30 minutes a day in bouts of at least 10 minutes each or at least 20 minutes a day of continuous activity for vigorous-intensity activity.

Type: Any mode that does not impose excessive orthopedic stress; walking is the most common type of activity. Aquatic exercise and seated cycle or stepping exercise may be advantageous for those with limited tolerance for weight bearing activity.

FIGURE 5-1 The FITT framework for endurance exercise for older adults

Table 5-1 Aerobic (Cardiovascular Endurance) Exercise to Improve Physical Fitness

Exercise Group	Exercise Description	Recommended for	Examples
A	Endurance activities requiring minimal skill or physical fitness to perform	All adults	Walking, leisurely cycling, aqua aerobics, slow dancing
B	Vigorous-intensity endurance activities requiring minimal skill	Adults with a regular exercise program and/or at least average physical fitness	Jogging, running, rowing, aerobics, spinning, elliptical exercise, stepping exercise, fast dancing
C	Endurance activities requiring skill to perform	Adults with acquired skill and/or at least average physical fitness levels	Swimming, cross-country skiing, skating
D	Recreational sports	Adults with a regular exercise program and at least average physical fitness	Racquet sports, basketball, soccer, down-hill skiing, hiking

Reprinted with permission from American College of Sports Medicine. *ACSM's Guidelines for Exercise Testing and Prescription*, 8th ed. Philadelphia (PA): Lippincott Williams & Wilkins; 2010. 164 p.

Exercise Group A activities include types or modes of EET commonly performed by older adults such as walking. Cycling is an ideal choice for those who may have a lower tolerance for weight-bearing activities. Advantages include little training being needed for these activities and no special equipment being needed. More communities are providing safe and accessible indoor and outdoor sites, where people can walk and cycle to promote better health and well-being. The intensity of Group A activities can be more easily controlled than those requiring more skill, especially for novice exercisers. Maintaining an appropriate intensity is essential to the safety and effectiveness of an EET program, regardless of the level. This is especially true at the start and may become less of an issue, as individuals become more aerobically fit and understand the limits of their exercise capacity.

Aquatic (aqua) exercise has become a popular Group A option for many older adults who have access to aquatic facilities. Exercise in the water provides an excellent way for individuals who may have some mobility problems to remain active. The buoyancy of the water reduces the weight of the body and eliminates the risk of falling during activity. The warmth of the water can be soothing and can reduce discomfort associated with activity for many. Evidence suggests that aqua exercise can improve aerobic fitness and may also impact lower extremity muscular strength and ROM in individuals with osteoarthritis of the knee or hip (26).

Slow dance is also recommended as a Group A activity and may provide an interesting and enjoyable alternative to other forms of EET. A recent review of the physical benefits of dancing for healthy older adults revealed that improvements in endurance as well as lower body muscle function, flexibility, balance, gait, and agility can be gained from this type of activity (15).

Endurance exercises in Groups B to D are also appropriate for older adults, depending on health, fitness levels, skills, and interests. Individuals may choose to stay with one type of exercise or progress to more challenging kinds. When choosing a new type, it is important to monitor the intensity of activity regularly, as new activities can be more taxing until they are mastered. Increasing the complexity of movement may contribute to better balance and mobility, muscle function, or ROM. Physically conditioned older men and women may participate in vigorous-intensity EET and recreational sports well past the age where most adults have "retired" from those activities.

Endurance exercises to avoid are those that may impose excessive orthopedic stress that may injure bones or joints or those that put participants at heightened risk for falls or collision injuries (1). It is important to stress that the degree of limitation for participation depends entirely on exercise background and fitness level and not necessarily age.

STARTING AN ENDURANCE PROGRAM

Knowing how to safely start a program can be a barrier to older adult participation in EET. Figure 5-2 provides clear guidelines for determining a starting point within the FITT framework as suggested by ACSM guidelines. This information can be used by

Frequency: Train each muscle group (chest, shoulders, abdomen, back, hips, legs, and arms) at least 2 times a week with at least 48 hours between sessions. After a good resistance work out, the muscles need a day of recovery. This suggests working 2–3 days a week with a day between resistance workouts, or if daily exercise is preferred, split the resistance exercises so that each muscle group still gets a recovery day between workouts (e.g., M-W-F legs, and T-Th upper body).

Intensity: Between moderate (5–6) and vigorous (7–8) intensity on an RPE scale of 0–10. The correct resistance for this may take some time to determine, but participants can learn to use the scale and make appropriate adjustments. The aim is to complete 8–12 repetitions in a row at this intensity.

Type: Progressive weight training program or weight-bearing calisthenics (8–10 exercises involving major muscle groups) including stair climbing, and other strengthening activities.

Volume: The volume of work can be increased by adding sets (target 2–3 sets, increasing the resistance but still being able to complete 8–12 reps at a 7–8 RPE intensity), or adding an additional workout (still with a recovery day between workouts).

FIGURE 5-2   The FITT framework for resistance exercise for older adults

Table 5-2 Recommended FITT Framework for the Frequency, Intensity, and Time of Exercise

Habitual Physical Activity/Exercise Level	Frequency	Intensity	Time	
	Exercise (d.wk21)	RPE	Time (min.d^{-1})	Steps during Activity/Exercise Session
(1) Sedentary/no habitual activity/exercise/extremely deconditioned	3–5	Light to moderate (RPE 3–6)	20–30	3,000–3,500
(2) Minimal physical activity/no exercise/moderate to highly deconditioned	3–5	Light to moderate (RPE 3–6)	30–60	3,000–4,000
(3) Sporadic physical activity/ no or suboptimal exercise/ moderately to mildly deconditioned	3–5	Moderate to hard (RPE 6–8)	30–90	>3,000–4,000
(4) Habitual physical activity/regular moderate to vigorous-intensity exercise	3–5	Moderate to hard (RPE 6–8)	30–90	>3,000–4,000
(5) High amounts of habitual activity/regular vigorous-intensity exercise	3–5	Somewhat hard to hard	30–90	>3,000–4,000

Adapted with permission from American College of Sports Medicine. *ACSM's Guidelines for Exercise Testing and Prescription*, 8th ed. Philadelphia (PA): Lippincott Williams & Wilkins; 2010. 166–7 p.

participants themselves or the fitness professionals they work with. Once the entry point is established, the frequency, intensity, and time components can be adopted as appropriate for that level of habitual activity (Table 5-2).

Those beginning an EET program should start at the lower end of each of the FITT components that match their current level of activity. For example, someone who is doing minimal physical activity and who is moderately deconditioned (Category 2) might start with 3 days a week of 20 minutes of continuous endurance exercise at a light-to-moderate intensity. If completing 20 minutes of endurance activity at that intensity is initially too difficult, the target time might be 10 minutes. The 20 minutes may also be divided into two 10-minute segments each day, and this also provides health benefits. Additional minutes can be gradually added to increase total time per day from 20 to 30 minutes. Once the upper time limit has been attained, an additional day of activity can be added each week and the individual may choose to work out more at a moderate intensity rather than light. Generally, the *volume* of EET can be effectively managed by increasing one of the FITT components at a time. The key to maintaining a program is to keep it at a comfortable yet challenging level. Increasing more than one FITT component may push a participant too much and cause undue tiredness or muscle soreness.

Some individuals prefer to use a step counter to measure the "time" of their endurance exercise session. The goal is to complete a certain number of steps during a session, and the session ends when that goal is reached regardless of the time it takes. If a step counter is used, it must be secured to the body following the manufacturer's directions for the most accurate results. Most reputable companies provide clear direction for use and maintenance of their devices, including video clips on their Web sites as well as clear written directions. Many pedometers work effectively for years with routine battery replacements. Step counters can be a useful tool for many to quantify the amount of aerobic activity performed while walking, running, or dancing.

PROGRESSION FOR AN ENDURANCE PROGRAM

Variability among older adults due to interests, skills, and health will dictate the rate of progression toward meeting minimal recommendations of at least 30 minutes of moderate-intensity EET (a total of 150–300 min·wk^{-1}) or 20 to 30 minutes of vigorous activity (a total of 75–100 min·wk^{-1}) suggested by ACSM. No one best way to achieve either goal exists; however, both can be achieved through regular increases in the FITT components over time as suggested in Table 5-2. Meeting minimum goals provides numerous health and fitness benefits (1).

Moving beyond minimal goals may be recommended for older adults who have the time for additional aerobic exercise and want to continue to gain additional physiological benefits. A dose-benefit relationship appears to exist, but the exact nature of how much EET is enough for each individual remains to be determined (3). Older adults who are training for sporting events or who are used to regular exercise may safely push upper suggested limits. Although 30 minutes of moderate-intensity PA is associated with positive health benefits and is the amount recommended by governing bodies, individuals wishing to lose weight or to maintain weight loss may also choose to exercise for up to 60 minutes or more (1).

Resistance exercise options

Figure 5-2 depicts the FITT framework for resistance exercise for older adults.

WHAT IS RESISTANCE TRAINING?

Resistance exercise training (RET) refers to any exercise where the muscles exert a relatively large amount of force to move an object against a resistance, hold it in place, or control how quickly the object moves back to its original position. It is the most

Real Life Story 5-1   Richard

Richard (aged 76), an avid cyclist, works out in his basement during the Minnesota winters: "It's easier to maintain fitness than to get it back again."

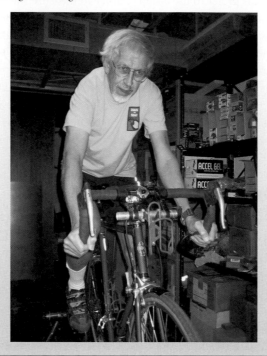

effective way to develop muscle endurance, strength, and power in adult populations (1). All three facets of muscle performance are essential for optimal functional performance and participation in many recreational activities. RET is an essential component of an exercise program for older adults because of systemic decrements that occur as muscle ages (3). To maintain mobility and function, it is recommended that RET include progressive weight training and weight-bearing calisthenics (21) (Table 5-3).

Strength and power, particularly in the lower body, tend to decline after age 40 with an accelerated loss after age 65 (3). This trend represents average data, and individuals can mitigate this decrease by including regular RET. Some loss of muscle function is inevitable as can be seen in the inability of senior elite athletes to maintain the same levels of performance regardless of continued high-intensity RET. Most age-related loss in muscle function in an average older adult seems to be a consequence of lowering levels of activity on account of injury, sickness, or adopting an inactive lifestyle. RET can be an effective mechanism to assist older adults in regaining muscle mass and,

	Table 5-3 Definitions and Examples of Different Aspects of Muscle Function	
Mode	**Definition and Assessments**	**Examples**
Muscle strength	Ability to exert high force a limited number of times. Strength is measured by the maximum amount of force that can be exerted 1–10 times.	Muscle strength will determine whether an object can be moved or lifted.
Muscle endurance	Ability of the muscles to exert force over a period. There are two types of muscle endurance: (a) holding a position for an extended time and (b) repeated bouts of lower strength to accomplish a task. Endurance is measured by determining how many times a weight can be lifted before fatigue.	Carrying a ladder requires a static contraction of the arm and back muscles for what can be an extended time, and climbing up the ladder requires repeated contractions of the leg muscles.
Muscle power	Ability to of the muscle to produce force quickly. Two factors that determine power are strength and the speed of muscle contraction. Power can have a speed or strength focus. Assessment of power is difficult due to the interaction of the speed and force involved. A weighted ball toss for distance, or speed to lift a submaximal weight are both measures of power.	Moving to hit a tennis ball or taking a quick step to prevent a fall depends very much on the speed the stepping leg can move the foot. Picking up a child and getting up from a chair without using arms requires use of a great deal of force but quickly.

more importantly, muscle strength even in very old frail people (11) or in people who have not previously been very active. Modest functional improvements in gait speed, time taken to stand from a chair, and walking endurance have also been a documented outcome of RET for this age group (16). Power training has been found more effective in improving performance on everyday tasks compared with strength training (20).

The combined loss of both strength and speed results in an even greater loss in power with aging (14). In a review comparing traditional RET with power RET, traditional training resulted in a greater increase in strength, whereas power training showed greater improvement in balance, chair rise time, and gait speed (20). These outcomes relate to the specificity of training where performance adaptations are greatest when resistances and speeds parallel those needed to function.

RET can focus specifically on developing any of these facets of muscle function, but many exercises and daily challenges to the musculoskeletal system are commonly a combination of the three facets. Some examples:

- Carrying a 40-pound suitcase is much more tiring (muscular endurance) if maximum lifting ability (strength) is only 60 pounds versus 80 pounds. Climbing a set of stairs is much easier (and safer) if legs have greater strength and can easily lift body weight. *As resistance increases, the maximum number of repetitions decreases and the time to fatigue shortens.*

- Using a hammer requires repetitive low levels of strength (muscle endurance), but the hammer needs to move quickly (power) to pound in the nails. *Swinging a heavy hammer will be more fatiguing because of the increased percentage of maximum strength needed for each hit.*
- Extending the arms and catching body weight when falling requires strong arm muscles (strength), but they must move quickly (power) to get in position and respond quickly to absorb the weight. *Quick moves can prevent injury but only if sufficient strength can be exerted when needed.*

TYPES OF RESISTANCE TRAINING EXERCISES

For effective RET, the muscle must work against some type of resistance. It makes no difference whether the resistance is supplied by lifting a weight, stretching a band, or moving the body. This fact helps increase the options available for RET so that individual preferences, functional levels, and budgets can be accommodated (Table 5-4).

Some fitness facilities may offer access to all types of RET, but in most cases, one or two are readily available. An effective and well-rounded program should train the

Table 5–4 Types of Resistance Training Including Advantages and Limitations

Option	Advantages	Limitations	Examples
Body weight	Always available for use in a variety of ways. Low cost. Exercises resemble activities of daily life with resistance relative to the individual.	Difficult to increase or decrease the resistance. Excess body weight or an injury can make the body's weight difficult. It may be challenging to find body weight exercises for all major muscle groups.	Chair raisers under control with limited arm use. Curl ups or push-ups. Side leg raises (standing or lying).
Weight machines	Motion is controlled. Weights cannot be dropped. A wide range of easily modified resistance. Exercises are easy to follow. Social interaction may be enhanced as machines are usually in a shared facility.	Instruction is recommended to start and modify a program. Expense may be an issue depending on access to a facility. Setting and machines can be intimidating initially. Not all machines are easily accessible or accommodate small changes in resistance. Most machines are designed for symmetrical exercise, and injuries may prohibit this.	Pneumatic resistance (*e.g.*, air or water pressure). Machines commonly available in fitness centers.

Option	Advantages	Limitations	Examples
Free weights	Many exercises mimic functional activities. Can be performed in many settings. Both seated and standing exercises are possible. Asymmetry of movement can be accommodated.	Instruction is needed to lift and return weights safely. Needing a range of resistance makes free weights a fairly expensive option. Gripping free weights may be a problem for those with low grip strength or injuries. Difficult to find exercises for all muscle groups that need training.	Dumbbells and barbells. Ankle and wrist weights. Household containers filled with water or sand.
Bands and tubes	Can be performed in many settings. Both seated and standing exercises are possible. Relatively low cost, but must be checked regularly for tears and material fatigue.	Monitoring resistance and improvement is difficult to measure. Tubing handles determine the resistance in several exercises because of the length of the tubing so a range of tubes is required. Wrist form and strain can be a concern.	Exercise bands with optional grip assists. Rubber tubing with handles. Tubing or bands attached to a solid structure.
Water	Recommended for those with certain painful conditions (arthritis or fibromyalgia). Social interaction is common in group. Stress on joints can be controlled by depth of water.	Intensity can depend on perceived exertion. Difficult to assess gains in strength. Difficulty in pool accessibility. Participant's discomfort in a bathing suit. Fear of water.	Foam floatation devices (weights, noodles). Leg and arm resistance.

major muscle groups of the body (chest, shoulders, abdomen, back, hips, legs, and arms) with other focal points as determined by individual needs (1).

STARTING OR RESUMING A RET PROGRAM

Individual goals and objectives as well as exercise history and the current level of activity will determine the focus for the RET, including the type of resistance chosen and the number and type of exercises performed. Regardless of the starting point, certain principles remain consistent across all types of training. The initial sessions of RET programs should focus on learning and performing safe techniques that allow the body to adapt to the activity. During this time, resistance should be kept low and the exercises should be performed in a manner that the body can easily control to minimize risk of injury or residual stiffness or soreness.

ACSM guidelines suggest that 8 to 10 exercises be included that are multi-joint or compound exercise and target more than one muscle or joint (1). Novice exercisers may start with four to six exercises with a minimal resistance and increase resistance as confidence and the ability to correctly perform the exercises improves. Many avenues exist for determining correct form for the exercises, including mimicking pictures or videos from reputable sources, practicing in front of a mirror, or consulting a fitness professional for advice and information. Excellent resources to guide resistance exercises are available (see resources at the end of this chapter).

PROGRESSION FOR A RESISTANCE TRAINING PROGRAM

When good form and skill have been developed, the quantity of work should be increased until ACSM guidelines of RET at a moderate (5–6) or vigorous (7–8) intensity for 8 to 12 repetitions for two to four sets are met (1). Intermediary steps toward the target could be performing one set of 10 to 15 repetitions at a comfortable weight, then performing one set of the same repetitions at the target intensity, and then adding the additional sets. This may allow an easy transition to the recommended volume of RET. Sets may be performed back-to-back with 3 minutes of rest between each or in a circuit where sets of different exercise (*e.g.,* arms and legs) may be alternated. In this way, transition between exercises can provide rest for muscles worked. Each muscle group should be trained two to three times a week to gain maximal benefits. The muscle groups need at least a day of rest to allow for muscle development between strength workouts if training is at the recommended intensity. This is an important aspect of RET that should be continually adhered to.

The speed of lifting the weight, or stretching the band or tube, can be increased to develop power once good form and strength have been developed. High-speed RET, where the shortening phase is as fast as possible or less than 1 second using a low resistance, is more effective in improving functional tasks such as standing up from a chair than using higher resistance but at a slower speed (20). Increasing the speed of muscle shortening using light, moderate, or even high intensities (if appropriate) appears to be closely related to dynamic activities of daily living and preventing falls in older adults (9, 23). Regardless of the shortening speed adopted, the lengthening phase of the exercise, as happens when lowering the weight or allowing the band or tube to return to a resting length, should be under control without dropping the weight or allowing a band or tube to spring back to its resting length. Taking 2 to 4 seconds for this phase of the movement increases the total muscle work performed and can protect the joints from injury.

When a given set of an exercise can be completed at an RPE of lower than the recommended 5 to 8, the resistance should be increased. This may mean returning to one set of the exercise until it is possible to complete more sets at that resistance. This type of progressive increase in RET can be most easily met through the use of free weights and/or machines (21).

When strength goals have been reached, the RET program can be maintained without increasing the resistance or it can be modified. ACSM guidelines suggest that a given level of muscular strength, power, and/or endurance can be maintained with one training day a week if the intensity remains at the goal level (1). Participants can determine whether that point has been reached either by the amount of resistance used or more simply by noting that their daily activities can now be easily performed. All muscles of the body may not progress at the same rate, so the RET program should be modified on an exercise-by-exercise basis. Stopping a program will result in a steady loss of strength, endurance, or power, so it is important to continue a maintenance RET program over time. When returning to an RET program after time away, resuming with a lower resistance may best accommodate any losses in muscle function.

Real Life Story 5-2   Grace

Grace (aged 73), a recent convert to resistance training: "When I was making cookies, I used to have to stop stirring because I'd get so tired. Now, I can stir!"

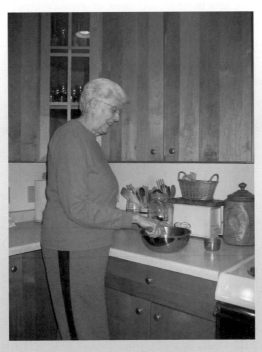

Balance and fall prevention options

Figure 5-3 depicts the FITT framework for balance exercise for older adults.

WHAT IS BALANCE TRAINING?

Balance is defined as the ability to maintain control of the body movements whether in an attempt to remain stationary or to move in a controlled fashion. To accomplish this, good sensory information about the position must be quickly integrated with the intent to move. Balance requires good anticipatory and reactive control of body movement (24). Anticipatory responses are those that occur or can be planned before movement. Reactive control of balance is needed when balance is disturbed and a rapid correction is required. Examples of this include stepping quickly after catching a foot on the carpet or grabbing a railing while sliding on front porch ice. The benefits of including balance training in all exercise programs for older adults are to build a reserve of anticipatory and reactive control through exercise that challenges each in a safe and systematic manner.

Good balance is often taken for granted until it becomes impaired or fails, and then the consequences can be dire. Balance may be impaired because of many clinical conditions such as Parkinson disease, hypotension, vestibular disturbances, or, occasionally, a side effect of some medications. Typical age-related changes that contribute to balance loss include decreases in sensory input, motor ability, and cognitive changes that alter biomechanics of sitting, standing, and locomotion.

Frequency: 2–3 days a week in a program; however, individual balance exercises can be done as often as the individual likes (NIA, 2010).

Intensity: There are no specific recommendations. If the individual is at the appropriate intensity for a balance challenge, any increase in difficulty would cause a loss of balance and the need to step or use support. The challenge is insufficient if the participant can easily maintain stability. Examples of intensity differences for one-foot support are: (a) touch the wall and barely raise one foot for a short time, (b) stand steadily with hands across chest, and (c) stand on one leg and move a medicine ball from left to right of the body.

Type: Various challenges are needed that include (a) progressively difficult postures that gradually reduce the base of support, (b) dynamic movements that perturb the center of gravity, (c) stressing postural muscle groups, and (d) reducing sensory input.

Caution: Care must be taken that the participants can self-monitor and remain safe if they are working in a group without one-on-one support from an experienced activity leader. For safety in group settings, each individual should understand his or her appropriate challenge level and not proceed to a higher level until having mastered the lower level. Safety requires having a sturdy support (chair, counter, or stable person) to give support whenever needed.

FIGURE 5-3   The FITT framework for balance exercise for older adults

These together with environmental constraints can adversely affect BAM and lead toward having difficulty in staying stationary, moving around in the environment, and recognizing appropriate levels of environmental challenges (3). Experts now recommend balance exercise for individuals who are frequent fallers or those with mobility problems and for all older adults who are experiencing a decline in function (3, 4, 23).

HOW DOES BALANCE TRAINING RELATE TO FALL PREVENTION?

The two strongest predictors of a fall are muscle weakness and having had a previous fall (4). The fear of falling, a common consequence of having fallen (although it can be present without having fallen), is an additional risk factor for falling. This is mediated through a decrease in activity, triggering further declines in strength and balance and a cascading deterioration in mobility (8). It appears prudent to include strength, balance, gait, and stability challenges in all physical activity programs for older adults to maintain their function and to prevent a fall.

Mobility is a combination of many aspects of physical functioning including balance that allows the older adult to lead an active independent life. The mobility needs vary by individual and include transfers (getting in and out of bed, using an escalator, climbing into the back seat of a car), moving about the environment (walking, climbing stairs, or bleachers), and being able to pursue activities such as travel, gardening, and playing with children. Mobility clearly relies on all modes of activity, including balance, muscular strength endurance and power, flexibility, and cardiovascular endurance. BAM exercises become more important components of a physical activity program for older adults as the individuals' level of functioning declines and their risk of falling increases (21).

TYPES OF BALANCE EXERCISES

Distinct types of balance exercises have been identified and categorized (3). Researchers have not identified particular types of balance exercise as being "best" for all older adults. Currently, recommendations suggest including a range of exercises each performed at a level that challenges the individual and makes them feel somewhat off-balance or wobbly, but still able to remain under control. Table 5-5 identifies the focus of balance challenge, general categories of balance exercises, examples of individual challenges in each, and how each exercise may relate to actual environmental challenges.

Some evidence suggests that tai chi styles that involve slow and continuous variations of head and neck rotations, weight shifting with different arm movements, following hand moves with the eyes, and changes from double to single limb support improve balance (17). As with other facets of physical fitness, the intensity or level of difficulty of each exercise must be progressed to maintain improvement. Simple

Table 5-5   Balance Exercises and How Each May Relate to Environmental Challenges

Focus of Challenge	Balance Exercise Challenges and Progressions	Relationship to Balance and Function	Examples of Environmental Challenges
Progressively difficult postures that gradually reduce the base of support.	Two-legged stand with feet shoulder width apart, stand with feet together, stand on one leg. Semi-tandem stand (big toe touching inside of contralateral back heel), full-tandem stand (feet directly in line with each other), walk on a line on the floor or a balance beam.	Inactive older adults find it difficult to keep the center of gravity over a small base of support.	Walk with big steps that include a heel strike, step up and down a curb or over a crack in the sidewalk (requires time with weight supported on one foot).
Dynamic movements that perturb the center of gravity (COG).	Walk, stop, continue walking. Walk, stop, back step, walk. Diagonal step, swing arms out and up, return to start. Catch and throw a medicine or other ball.	Moving about freely requires automatic corrections without concentration.	Maneuver around and between people and avoid others. Bend over to retrieve a dropped object.
Stressing postural muscle groups.	Heel stands, toe stands. Lean forward, back, to each side without moving feet. Rotate a ball in a big *figure 8* across the front of the body.	All muscle groups need to coordinate automatically to maintain balance.	Lean forward to pick up a heavy object. Stretch up on toes to reach something from a high shelf.
Reducing input from the senses that contribute to balance.	Decrease touch while challenging balance. Progression: Start with a good grip on something stable, loosen the grip, move to one hand touching, decrease touch to fingertips, hover hands over the surface.	Touch gives very strong input.	Walk without use of handrails or assistive device.
	Decrease vision while challenging balance. Keep head steady and shift focus from side to side of room, focus on something that is moving. Progress to closing eyes.	Focusing on a stable object is often the most used sense to keep balanced.	Scan as you walk or make eye contact with others.
	Decrease vestibular input by maintaining focus on something stable while moving the head. Look up at the ceiling.	Moving the head or being dizzy decreases vestibular input.	Look up, down, left, and right.
	Decrease sensory input from ankles and feet. Stand on a foam cushion, half round roller, rocker board, or inflated disc. Walk on an exercise mat.	Foot position is detected by the sensory input from the lower leg.	Walk on grass or a rocky surface or walk-up a ramp.

Adapted with permission from American College of Sports Medicine. *ACSM's Guidelines for Exercise Testing and Prescription*, 8th ed. Philadelphia (PA): Lippincott Williams & Wilkins; 2010. 193–4 p.

repetition of the same types of movement activities may not provide that stimulus and either the exercise or level of challenge needs to be modified (23).

STARTING A BALANCE AND MOBILITY PROGRAM

BAM exercises can be easily incorporated into an existing exercise program regardless of its primary focus. Because these exercises require focus and concentration, it is important to include them at a point in the session when a participant is not overly fatigued or tired. A session of stepping exercises may be performed toward the end of the warm-up, extending it slightly longer than general recommendation. They may also be included during the main portion of activity at a point that blends well with other movements. The tempo of BAM exercises should be less than that of endurance or strength exercises. Care *must* be taken to perform them slowly and with control to gain maximal benefit. A constant safety precaution is to have a firmly grounded object or stable exercise partner nearby to serve as a support if needed.

Stationary (static) and moving (dynamic) balance challenges each have a place in programs. Static postures are used initially by older adults with poor balance, as it is easier to use good support when staying in the same position. Examples are practicing toe stands, and one-foot balance at a counter or holding on to the back of a stable chair. Dynamic challenges, such as walking across an exercise mat or walking in full tandem, are needed to adapt the systems while moving around. A combination of static and dynamic moves requires good control of both types of balance. Walking and stopping quickly on one foot or walking and stepping over imaginary boxes with a stationary balance posture while the leg is lifted is a combination challenge. Table 5-6 presents ideas for incorporating BAM exercises into an existing endurance or resistance training program.

HOW DOES THIS INFORMATION RELATE TO FALL PREVENTION?

Preventing falls is a complex social and health problem. The age-related increased risk for falls is part of an ongoing process that is more like a chronic disease that must be managed, rather than a unique incident that presents with the first fall. Good evidence exists for including fall prevention exercise programs for non- or prefrail individuals living in the community (4). In community living, nonfrail populations exercise in the form of strength, balance, gait and coordination training should be included as part of all interventions and available to all older adults who are at risk for falling. For those who are frequent fallers or have mobility problems, an individually tailored mobility program is recommended. Depending on the awareness of the individual, it might be necessary to practice balance exercises only with a trained assistant who is able to provide support when needed. In all cases, care must be taken to provide appropriate support during challenges that are within the safe capabilities of each individual (4).

Table 5-6 Examples of BAM Activities That Can Be Incorporated into Existing Endurance and Resistance Programs	
Primary Focus	**Suggested BAM Exercises**
Endurance training	
Walking	Walk on toes, take slow steps as if stepping over a series of boxes, walk heel-toe, walk and look from side to side with each step, walk on grass, rocks, or an exercise mat.
Dancing and aerobics	Combine slow and quick, short and long steps, include weight shifts in all directions with arm movements, include turns, pivots, forward and backward steps.
Seated exercise	Shift weight from side to side, maintain stability with one foot on the ground, sit on an inflated cushion, move head from side to side, change visual focus from one stationary object to another, track moving objects with head and eyes moving.
Resistance training	
Body weight and calisthenics	Large step with lowering body down and minimizing support, shift weight from foot to foot progressing to a bounce, maintain balance while walking on toes or heels, balance on an exercise ball while doing bridges, push-ups, and curls.
Free weights, bands, or tubes	Stand up for upper body exercises, or sit on an exercise ball, perform upper body exercises one side at a time.
Medicine ball	Toss and catch a medicine ball using a variety of tosses, perform large ROM medicine ball movements while walking.

Flexibility exercise options

Figure 5-4 depicts the FITT framework for flexibility exercise for older adults.

WHAT IS FLEXIBILITY EXERCISE?

Regular flexibility exercise training (FET) or stretching is recommended for all adults, including older adults, as part of a well-rounded exercise program to maintain or increase ROM at targeted joints (1). Flexibility exercises are specific body positions or poses that stretch muscles and tendons around a joint. It is recommended that the stretch for each position be moved to the point of moderate discomfort, not pain, and held for a specific time before being released. If increased ROM is desired at a specific joint, exercises that target that joint must be performed.

General recommendations for inclusion of FET in exercise programs have not changed substantially, but statements about its efficacy have (1). It is important to note that less research has been conducted on the effects of stretching on older men and women. Some evidence exists to suggest that ROM can be improved in older adults (3), and consequently, recommendations for improving this facet of physical fitness

Real Life Story 5-3   Ann

Ann, aged 80, a local community volunteer of the year who never misses her exercise session: "My balance is so much better now, I know it has allowed me to be busier now in retirement than I ever thought possible."

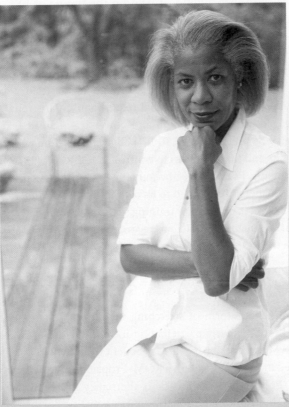

Frequency: At least 2 days a week.

Intensity: Between 5 and 6 for moderate intensity on an RPE scale of 0–10.

Time (Duration): Static stretches should be held for 15–60 seconds and repeated at least 4 times a session for a total of approximately 10 minutes a session.

Type: Any activities that maintain or increase flexibility using sustained stretches for each major muscle and static rather than ballistic movements.

FIGURE 5-4   The FITT framework for flexibility exercise for older adults

have been extrapolated from results based primarily on outcomes from younger populations. Long-held beliefs that increased ROM reduces the chance for injury during exercise or reduces muscle soreness after exercise have not been supported by research findings (1, 23).

Research has also shed additional light on the timing of FET within an overall training session. It has been commonly accepted that stretching is more effective when muscles to be stretched are warm. ACSM guidelines suggest that FET may be performed after a warm-up period of 5 to 10 minutes or after a cool-down of about the same length of time (1) when the muscles are sufficiently warm so that maximal benefits can be obtained if exercises are performed correctly. For those who participate regularly in recreational activities that require muscular strength and/or power, or who are engaged in regular strength and power training, FET after the primary training bout may be preferred (1, 13). It is advised to begin a FET with slow controlled movements and then progress to controlled full ROM (23). Owing to injuries or other impairments, ROM at specific joints may not be the same on both sides of the body and each should be worked to its own individual limits. Advising inclusion of stretching at a point in an exercise training session where it makes sense and where muscles are warm remains a judicious recommendation, especially for those who wish to increase the ROM about any or all joints.

TYPES OF FLEXIBILITY EXERCISES

The most recommended form of stretching for older adults is sustained or static stretching (1). Those regularly participating in more vigorous-intensity endurance, strength, and BAM exercises or sports may benefit from dynamic stretching that consists of controlled movement through a ROM. Proprioceptive neuromuscular facilitation stretching (PNF), where the muscle is alternately stretched and contracted, can also be effective. It requires additional training, assistive devices, and/or the aid of another individual. This makes it a less attractive option for many although a benefit is that some level of strength may be developed, especially in weaker participants.

Different types of static stretches can be performed to increase ROM at selected joints. ACSM guidelines suggest focusing on the major muscle groups of the body such as the neck, shoulders, upper and lower back, pelvis, hips, and legs (1). The choice of which stretch is best for a given area of the body depends on a number of factors, including the habitual physical activity level and ROM at each joint. Stretches can be performed standing, sitting in a chair or on the ground, and lying on a table or the ground. Personal preferences and the ability to comfortably get on the ground and get up again may limit the range of choices.

Readily available resources provide examples of the types of FET that can be safely performed by older adults. Safe and effective stretches may also be learned and practiced by following video or CD-based programs that are designed specifically for older adults. Care should be taken to purchase these types of products from reputable sources and to ensure that they adhere to recognized guidelines for older adult exercise.

Some individuals have turned to yoga and tai chi programs to enhance flexibility. Many fitness facilities and community recreation programs offer classes from certified instructors to allow people to learn and practice these activities. Although the programs have become popular options, less is known about their effects on older populations than other forms of FET (3, 21, 23). A recent study evaluated the effects of a year-long tai chi program versus a traditional FET on several physical measures including ROM. Results indicated that both groups improved upper and lower body flexibility; however, individuals who practiced traditional FET had greater improvements in upper body flexibility than the tai chi group (25).

STARTING A FLEXIBILITY PROGRAM

Each flexibility exercise should be performed a minimum of 2 days a week up to a maximum of 7 days a week. A basic FET portion of an exercise session should last approximately 10 minutes (1). It is also recommended that each flexibility exercise should be performed or held for 15 to 60 seconds and repeated up to four times. Exercises that target major joints used in the primary modes of endurance and strengthening exercises should be used as the core of the 10-minute program.

With minimal planning, flexibility exercises for all major joints of the body may be performed on alternate days with each joint targeted 2 to 3 days a week. Standalone FET programs should always begin with a warm-up session to allow muscles to become warm for comfort and optimal outcomes. As a note of caution, many group exercise programs for older adults spend a large time on flexibility at the expense of other modes of exercise that might be more beneficial to the participants (23). It is recommended that ROM activities be included in a well-rounded program but not be the primary activity.

PROGRESSION FOR FLEXIBILITY EXERCISES

Flexibility exercises can be progressed in different ways. The same exercises performed correctly over time should permit a greater ROM or stretch to be held up to a point of natural stoppage due to the limit of the joint or the anatomy of the individual. It is a reasonable goal to simply maintain an optimal ROM once that point has been reached for each exercise.

Additional and possibly more complex exercises can be substituted for those that have been mastered. An example might be when a chair-based hamstring stretch evolves over time into a floor-based hamstring stretch as an individual gains greater ROM in the hip and lower back. Another example of progression may be to incorporate stretching into a different section of an overall program. This could be inclusion

Real Life Story 5-4   Rosemary

Rosemary, aged 93, started a formal exercise program at 89: "I have always been flexible, but now I have power and balance to go along with it."

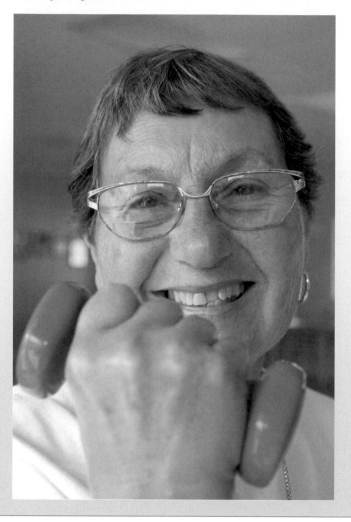

of a variety of yoga-type poses or full ROM movements in tai chi moves that might be in a balance, warm-up, or cool-down segment.

"All in one" exercise programs

Previous sections of this chapter have dealt with specifics of programs for endurance, resistance training, flexibility, and BAM. As emphasized in each segment, normally healthy older adults need to regularly perform exercises in each area to achieve and maintain optimal benefits. "All in one" (AIO) programs incorporate all recommended components of fitness in an efficient program that is usually group based. These programs are specifically designed to be attractive to independent older adults who can make decisions about the appropriate levels of exercise intensity for themselves. Fitness professionals with training in group exercise and with experience in working with older adults can create and lead effective AIO programs at a variety of locations. Most include a warm-up, endurance, BAM, strengthening, cool-down, and flexibility segments. An example of a format for an AIO program is contained in Table 5-7.

Several organizations have created AIO programs that combine exercise components in this fashion. These programs are offered at easily accessible sites in many communities, with some sponsored by Health Maintenance Organizations for their members who can attend the programs free of charge or at limited costs. The standard group exercise sessions are generally 1 hour in duration and held 3 days a week or every other day and include periodic assessments. These programs are led by fitness leaders who have been trained to understand unique considerations associated with older adult exercise and who possess basic first-aid/CPR skills. An instructor-to-participant ratio is maintained, which provides a safe and welcoming situation for many.

Advantages of AIO programs are that all components of physical fitness are addressed in a systematic fashion and that an exercise leader may provide guidance for correct performance of exercises and prompt exercisers to maintain an appropriate intensity. The group exercise setting can provide a venue where participants may find company, friendship, and additional encouragement to become and remain active. Disadvantages may include the issue that the intensity of the activity selected by the leader to meet the needs of the majority of the group may not be optimal for individual participants. Some participants could benefit from additional focus on a particular component of fitness rather than the combination provided. In addition, this type of group program may not be attractive to those who wish to exercise on their own.

Table 5-7   Example of an "AIO" Program

	Duration (min)	Sample Exercises/Activity
Warm-up	10	ROM, seated low-intensity aerobics
Endurance	10	Standing calisthenics/aerobic exercises and walking patterns
Balance and mobility	10	Specific balance challenges
Resistance exercise	10	Exercise band or wrist or free weight routine
Cool-down	10	Slow tai chi–like movements
Flexibility	10	Full body stretching

Real Life Story 5-5   Frank

Frank, aged 83, joined an AIO program with his wife's encouragement: "I have lost weight, I am stronger, and I know this program has helped me prevent falls. I can do so much more."

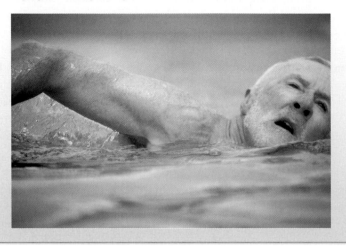

AIO programs can provide a viable option for older adults to become and remain more physically active. Participants should examine the program, its individual components, the leader, and the site where it is held to determine whether it is suitable for them. Many have successfully adopted an exercise program by attending group sessions such as these and then have continued a program on their own once they are confident in their ability to do so.

S U M M A R Y

It is generally recognized that physical activity or exercise is of benefit to all adults regardless of age, gender, or previous experience. Regular participation can improve functional performance and general quality of life over time. This chapter identified a range of endurance, resistance, BAM, and flexibility activities that can be safely performed by normally healthy older adults who conform to the most current professional recommendations. A variety of information was provided so that individuals can determine appropriate levels to initiate or continue physical activities that improve or maintain fitness in each area. This information can also be used by fitness professionals to guide and assist older adults in making safe and effective exercise choices.

QUESTIONS FOR REFLECTION

1. What are important milestones in the development of the current exercise recommendations for older adults?

2. Identify and describe the ACSM-recommended format for a well-rounded exercise session for older adults.

3. What are the exercise options that should be included in a well-rounded exercise program for normally healthy older adults? What benefit does each type provide for this age group?

4. How does the ACSM "FITT" framework apply to each of the exercise options?

5. What are two to three kinds of physical activities or exercises that can be performed to increase physical performance capacities with each exercise option?

6. What are the advantages and disadvantages of "AIO" exercise programs?

7. Think of four adults older than 65 years whom you know well. What component of exercise may be the most important for each of them individually to include in their exercise plan to bring them into compliance with current exercise recommendations?

RESOURCES TO GUIDE EXERCISE PROGRAMMING

Resource	Content and Location
CDC/NCIPC	Downloadable Manual: Preventing Falls: How to develop community-based Fall Prevention Programs for Older Adults. Atlanta, GA: Centers for Disease control and Prevention 2008. www.cdc.gov/ncip/preventingfall/CDC_Guide.pdf
Exercise and Wellness strategies for Older Adults (2nd ed.)	2010 Textbook by Van Norman. Practical programming and exercise guidance. Available from Human Kinetics Publishers.
AHA and ACSM	Exercise is Medicine. Web site with resources for health care providers, health and fitness professionals and the public. www.exerciseismedicine.org
Health and Human Services	Be Active Your Way. A guide to help older adults prepare to be active. www.health.gov/paguidelines/pdf/adultguide.pdf

Idaho Health and Welfare	Downloadable manual: Fit and Fall Proof Class Leader Manual. Good diagrams of exercises for an AIO program. Available from prevention resources on www.healthandwelfare.idaho.gov
International Council on Active Aging	Media and consumer links from the Web site include extensive content related to programming issues. www.icaa.cc
Journal of Aging and Physical Activity	Professional journal that publishes current research on aging and physical activity. Human Kinetics Publisher. www.humankinetcs.com
National Council on Aging	Web site with extensive resources on physical activity. www.agingblueprint.org
National Institute on Aging	Exercise and Physical Activity. Detailed guide including many exercises to be used as a guide for older adults as they become more active. http://www.nia.nih.gov/HealthInformation/Publications
	Web site with resources to order. Go4life. http://go4life.niapublications.org

REFERENCES

1. American College of Sports Medicine. *ACSM's Guidelines for Exercise Testing and Prescription.* 8th ed. Philadelphia (PA): Wolters Kluwer/Lippincott Williams & Wilkins; 2010. 380 p.
2. American College of Sport Medicine Position Stand. Exercise and physical activity for older adults. *Med Sci Sports Exerc.*1998;30(6):992–1008.
3. American College of Sports Medicine, Chodzko-Zajko WJ, Proctor DN, et al. American College of Sport Medicine Position Stand: Exercise and physical activity for older adults. *Med Sci Sports Exerc.* 2009;41(2):1510–30.
4. AGS/BGS Clinical Practice Guideline: 2010; Prevention of falls in older persons. [cited 2010 December 15]. Available from: http://www.americangeriatrics.org/files/documents/health_care_pros/Falls.Summary.Guide.pdf
5. Blair SN, Kampert JB, Kohl HW 3rd, Barlow CE, Macera CA, Paffenbarger RS Jr, Gibbons LW. Influences of cardio-respiratory fitness and other precursors on cardiovascular disease and all-cause mortality in men and women. *JAMA.* 1996;276:205–10.
6. Bloomfield S. Changes in muscle structure and function with prolonged bed rest. *Med Sci Sports Exerc.* 1997;29(2):197–206.
7. Chandler JM, Duncan PW, Kochersberger G, Studenski S. Is lower extremity strength gain associated with improvement in physical performance and disability in frail, community-dwelling elders? *Arch Phys Med Rehabil.* 1998;79:24–30.
8. Delbaere K, Crombez G, Vanderstraeten G, Willems T, Cambier D. Fear-related avoidance of activities, falls and physical frailty. A prospective community-based cohort study. *Age Ageing.* 2004;33(4):368–73.
9. deVos NJ, Singh NA, Ross DA, Stavrinos TM, Orr R, Fiatarone-Singh MA. Optimal load for increasing muscle power during explosive resistance training in older adults. *J Gerontol A Biol Sci Med Sci.* 2005;60:638–47.
10. Federal Interagency Forum on Ageing-related Statistics. *Older Americans 2004: Key Indicators of Well-Being.* Washington (DC): U.S. Government Printing Office; 2004.
11. Fiatarone MA, Marks EC, Ryan ND, Meredith CN, Lipsitz LA, Evans WJ. High-intensity strength training in nonagenarians: Effects on skeletal muscle. *JAMA.* 1990;263:3029–34.
12. Guadalupe-Grau A, Fuentes T, Guerra B, Calbet JAL. Exercise and bone mass in adults. *Sports Med.* 2009;39(6):439–68.
13. Gurjao ALD, Goncalves R, De Moura RF, Gobbi S. Acute effect of static stretching on rate of force development and maximal voluntary contractions in older women. *J Strength Cond Res.* 2009;23(7):214–9.
14. Hazell T, Kenno K, Jakobi J. Functional benefit of power training for older adults. *J Aging Phys Act.* 2007;15:349–59.
15. Keogh JWL, Kilding A, Pidgeon P, Ashley L, Gillis D. Physical benefits of dancing for health older adults: A review. *J Aging Phys Act.* 2009;17(4):479–500.
16. Latham NK, Bennett DA, Stretton CM, Anderson CS. Systematic review of progressive resistance training in older adults. *J Gerontol A Biol Sci Med Sci.* 2004;59:48–61.

17. Li F, Harmer P, Fisher KJ, McAuley E, Chaumeton N, Eckstrom E, Wilson NL. Tai chi and fall reductions in older adults: A randomized controlled trial. *J Gerontol A Biol Sci Med Sci.* 2005;60:187–94.
18. McAuley E, Blissmer B, Marquez DX, Jerome GJ, Kramer AF, Katula J. Social relations, physical activity, and well-being in older adults. *Prev Med.* 2000;31(5):608–17.
19. Morris JN, Heady JA, Raffle PAB, Roberts CG, Parks JW. Coronary artery disease and physical activity of work. *Lancet.* 1953;262(6795):1053–7.
20. Miszko TA, Cress ME, Slade JM, Covey CJ, Agrawal SK, Doer CE. Effect of strength and power training on physical function in community-dwelling older adults. *J Gerontol A Biol Sci Med Sci.* 2003;58A:171–5.
21. Nelson ME, Rejeski WJ, Blair SN, et al. Physical activity and public health in older adults: Recommendation from the American College of Sports Medicine and the American Heart Association. *Med Sci Sports Exerc.* 2007;39(8):1435–45.
22. Pate R, Pratt M, Blair S, et al. Physical activity and public health. A recommendation from the Centers for Disease Control and Prevention and the American College of Sports Medicine. *JAMA.* 1995;273:402–7.
23. Paterson DH, Jones GR, Rice CL. Ageing and physical activity: Evidence to develop exercise recommendations for older adults. *Appl Physiolo Nutr Metab.* 2007;32:S69–108.
24. Rose DJ. *Fallproof! A Comprehensive Balance and Mobility Training Program.* 2nd ed. Champaign (IL): Human Kinetics; 2010. 313 p.
25. Tailor-Piliae RE, Newall KA, Cherin R, Lee MJ, King AC, Haskell WL. Effects of Tai Chi and western exercise on physical and cognitive function in healthy, community-dwelling, older adults. *J Aging Phys Act.* 2010;18:261–79.
26. Wang TJ, Belza B, Thompson EF, Whitney JD, Bennett K. Effects of aquatic exercise on flexibility, strength, and aerobic fitness in adults with osteoarthritis of the hip or knee. *J Adv Nurs.* 2007;57(2):141–52.
27. Ziggelmann JP, Lippke S, Schwarzer R. Adoption and maintenance of physical activity: Planning interventions in young, middle-aged, and older adult. *Psychol Health.* 2006;21(2):145–63.

CHAPTER 6

Active Options for Older Adults with Special Issues and Concerns

Bo Fernhall, Abbi Lane, and Huimin Yan

●●● **CHAPTER OUTLINE**

INTRODUCTION

Although there are many health issues and concerns for older individuals, three specific but common conditions will be discussed in this chapter: (a) cardiovascular disease (CVD), (b) diabetes, and (c) cognitive impairment. All of these conditions share certain common features. The prevalence of each condition is fairly high, each condition can be very limiting and produce concomitant health concerns not directly attributable to the specific condition, and each condition is usually associated with reduced levels of activity and independence. However, there is considerable evidence that increased levels of physical activity or more organized exercise programs can have beneficial physical, physiological, and psychological effects for individuals with these conditions. Consequently, exercise and physical activity are usually recommended for individuals with CVD, diabetes, or cognitive impairment.

CARDIOVASCULAR DISEASE AND EXERCISE

Introduction to cardiovascular disease and exercise

The term *cardiovascular disease* refers to the broad category of diseases involving the heart and circulatory system. This includes coronary artery disease, heart failure (HF), stroke, myocardial infarction, hypertension (HT), and peripheral arterial disease (PAD). CVD is the major cause of mortality in many countries. According to the 2009 cardiovascular and stroke statistical update from the American Heart Association (AHA), about 73% of adults older than 60 years have been diagnosed with CVD, making it a major health care expense and a larger mortality threat than cancer, Alzheimer disease, or accidents. Exercise, and associated increases in fitness level, can help prevent or decrease the risk of developing CVD and reduce CVD mortality (11). The incorporation of exercise into a prevention or maintenance plan of moderate- to high-risk patients is strongly recommended (19).

Individuals with CVD may face challenges when exercising, depending on the severity of the disease. Because exercise is characterized by increased metabolism, more blood must be delivered to the working muscles. The cardiovascular system makes many physiological changes during exercise to accommodate the increased demand by active tissues. For instance, individuals who have had a heart attack or who have HF may experience difficulties in pumping blood from the heart, adapting to the increased pressure in the arteries, or expanding the peripheral arteries to allow for increased blood flow. Fortunately, exercise training can stimulate improvement in all of these areas. Thus, exercise and physical activity have a large role in improving physical and psychological function in people with CVD (35).

Issues associated with cardiovascular disease

CVD is an umbrella term referring to a constellation of diseases, many of which become more prominent with aging. It is beyond the scope of this chapter to provide a detailed overview of all types of CVD. Some common CVDs include HT, coronary heart disease including myocardial infarction, HF, and PAD. Each of these conditions has associated symptoms and considerations for exercise. A well-planned exercise intervention will need to consider both severity and type of CVD.

Hypertension

Essential hypertension (HT), or high blood pressure, has no known cause, but is associated with arterial stiffness, high peripheral resistance, and augmented sympathetic tone. This is problematic because stiffer arteries result in increased pressure throughout the arterial system. This can lead to capillary damage, which in turn can increase the risk of end-organ (eye, kidney, brain) damage. Stiffer arteries offer more resistance against the flow of blood from the heart. This increased workload on the heart can lead to enlargement of the heart muscle. The heart and arteries themselves become structurally or physiologically altered in response to this stress.

HT is the most common CVD in the United States, and many individuals are on treatments to assist in the lowering of blood pressure. Medication status may affect exercise tolerance. Some medications are associated with increased arterial dilation, making light-headedness a possibility. Individuals on these medications may wish to emphasize a warm-up and increase effort gradually to avoid complications. β-Blockers also lower heart rate; consequently, if target heart rates are used to monitor exercise intensity, it may be necessary to modify exercise heart rates to adjust for these factors.

Coronary heart disease

It is a condition where plaque is formed in the walls of the coronary arteries, decreasing the size of the artery and thus limiting blood flow. This can cause angina (classic "chest pain" or other associated discomfort). A myocardial infarction is almost always caused by a ruptured plaque coupled with the formation of a blood clot. This prevents blood flow to the area of the heart downstream from the plaque rupture and causes oxygen deprivation and eventually cell death. Thus, a heart attack usually results in cell death in parts of the heart muscle, which may, in turn, affect the heart's ability to pump blood.

Peripheral arterial disease

Peripheral arterial disease (PAD) occurs when plaque is formed in the peripheral arteries of the arms or legs (the legs are more frequently affected). The plaque buildup makes the arteries unable to dilate enough to supply the musculature with adequate oxygenated blood during exercise. This disease is characterized by intermittent claudication, or painful tightness and squeezing in the legs on exertion. Because blood flow is restricted, other symptoms may include cold or numbness and lack of sensitivity in the legs and feet.

CVD risk factors

Much of the benefit of regular exercise in CVD disease modification stems from its ability to favorably impact risk factors (12, 28). Exercise can help manage body weight, and a regular exercise routine can also lead to improvements in glucose control, blood pressure, and lipid levels. Indeed, the combined effect of exercise on multiple CVD risk factors makes it more effective and less complicated than any drug for reducing CVD risk.

Exercise guidelines

High-risk patients should consider attending cardiac rehabilitation programs, where they can be closely supervised by trained personnel. In these programs, the patients are often continuously ECG monitored for additional safety. Other CVD patients

---

Real Life Story 6-1   Jones

Jones, a 65-year-old retired librarian, moved to New York from Tennessee 2 years ago to be close to his elder son. He has had mild HT for 10 years, but surprisingly, he was recently told by his doctor that his blood glucose was a little high, too. Jones also noticed that he gained 20 pounds after moving to New York. He enjoyed gardening in the past in Tennessee. He used to spend at least 5 hours in his garden every day. He found it difficult to develop a garden in his apartment in New York, so he stopped gardening. Jones's doctor suggested that he get back to regular daily physical activity. Jones took this advice and joined a fitness program near his apartment. He now made friends with the people in his gym and really enjoyed going there. A follow-up checkup with his doctor showed that his weight had decreased 10 pounds and that his blood sugar was now close to normal.

who are at lower risk can exercise on their own following their physicians' or exercise professionals' recommendations. Since almost all patients with CVD can benefit from resistance exercise training, weight training is now recommended for most people with CVD (12, 24, 28). Thus, an appropriate exercise program consists of both aerobic and resistance exercise training.

The AHA and the American College of Sports Medicine® (ACSM) have set guidelines for exercise specifically for both older adults and people with CVD (12, 24, 28). In Chapters 2, 3, 5, and 9 specific guidelines and recommendations regarding the quantity and quality of physical activity needed to ensure significant outcomes are discussed in detail.

Exercise sessions should include a warm-up and a cool-down. The warm-up should begin slowly at a very comfortable and "easy" effort level. Intensity should gradually increase until the desired effort level for the workout is reached. At the end of the exercise session, this pattern should be reversed, with intensity gradually decreasing until the individual is recovered. The cool-down is especially important in persons with CVD, as most complications that are associated with exercise occur after exercise (28).

Resistance training is extremely important for people with CVD. Because CVD is often associated with poor peripheral circulation, muscle catabolism (breakdown) is common. This can greatly affect functional and performance-related abilities. Even normal, nonclinical aging is characterized by a significant and progressive loss of muscle each year after age 30 (12). Because of this, body mass index may stay relatively stable, masking the onset of obesity because loss of muscle exceeds gain of fat mass. Balance exercise is also recommended, particularly for those at a heightened risk for falling. Currently, there are no specific guidelines, but the ACSM suggests incorporating one of the following techniques: postures that gradually reduce the base of support, such as a one-legged stand; perturbing the body's center of gravity while performing dynamic movements; using postural muscle groups (heel stands, toe stands); or reducing visual input (standing with eyes closed).

Real Life Story 6-2   Carol

Carol's physician told her at her last physical examination that her blood pressure was too high (148/88), as was her cholesterol (210 mg·dL^{-1} total). With medication, her blood pressure and cholesterol levels were reduced, but not to the extent recommended by her doctor. Carol was interested in learning more about controlling her blood pressure cholesterol without increasing her dosage of medications. She began walking 3 days a week and has recently incorporated some calisthenics and balance activities into her weekly routine. Since beginning exercise, Carol has maintained a healthy blood pressure and cholesterol level without increasing her dosage of medicine. She also finds it easier to complete her daily activities.

Contraindications to exercise

- Unstable angina
- Resting BP >180/110 or exercise BP >240/110
- Orthostatic intolerance or a BP drop of >20 mm Hg during or immediately after exercise
- Unpredictable ventricular or atrial arrhythmias
- Uncompensated HF
- Uncontrolled diabetes
- Orthopedic issues that prevent proper movement patterns
- Fever or severe illness
- Severe muscle soreness or pain that restricts activities of daily living

Observing these symptoms before, during, or after exercise is cause for concern, and exercise should be stopped (or not initiated). Consult a physician before continuation of exercise if any of the aforementioned symptoms occur.

Expected benefits of exercise in cardiovascular disease

Much of the benefit of regular exercise is due to reduction in CVD risk factors. For example, regular exercise can reduce body fat percentage, body weight, BP, blood glucose levels, and total and LDL cholesterol while increasing HDL cholesterol (12, 28, 40). Regular exercise can improve fitness level, which is strongly correlated with reduced mortality in people with CVD (2).

Exercise has also been consistently shown to improve quality of life and reduce effort required to complete activities of daily living (12). Indeed, regular exercise helps reduce heart rate and blood pressure at given, submaximal exertion levels. Patients with HF have recorded improvements in aerobic fitness between 12% and 31%. Other clinical groups, such as individuals with PAD, have been able to double their tolerable walking distances after exercise training (1). This has important implications regarding ability to return to work or comfortably complete tasks associated with daily living.

Including resistance training can help counteract not only disease-related weakness, but also the decline in muscle strength and muscle mass that occurs with aging. Increased muscle mass and strength makes it easier to perform daily activities, increases metabolism, and helps with glucose tolerance (12).

Exercise is important for everyone, but those with CVD have much to gain from an exercise regime. Although beginning an exercise program can seem daunting, communication with exercise professionals and following the advice provided in the chapters of this book can help a person with CVD develop a structured plan. The use of exercise as medicine can improve functional ability, fitness, strength, and flexibility, as well as survival in individuals with CVD (11).

DIABETES

Introduction to Type 2 diabetes mellitus

According to the American Diabetes Association (ADA), in 2007, 12.2 million or 23.1% of people 60 years or older have diabetes. Type 2 diabetes mellitus (T2DM) is a metabolic disorder resulting in high blood glucose even in the presence of adequate or high levels of insulin, and accounts for 90% to 95% of all diagnosed cases of diabetes in adults. Long-term complications for high blood glucose and poor blood glucose control can cause an increased risk of heart attacks, strokes, HT, amputation, and kidney failure.

People with diabetes are encouraged to exercise regularly for better glucose control and to reduce the risk of CVDs. Exercise can acutely lower blood glucose by using glucose as fuel. Long-term exercise training can also be used as weight management and increase muscle mass. Insulin action becomes more effective with less fat mass and increased muscle mass. Other health benefits associated with exercise include better management of blood lipids and blood pressure and reduced severity of diabetes complications.

Issues associated with Type 2 diabetes

Older adults with T2DM may be more likely to be in an advanced stage of diabetes than younger people, simply because of a longer duration of disease and progression of pancreatic β-cell failure. Potential health conditions (not necessarily related to T2DM) may contraindicate specific exercises. Specific T2DM conditions that should be considered before adopting an exercise program include inability to bear weight, peripheral vascular disease, retinopathy, nephropathy, and autonomic neuropathy.

Blood glucose control

T2DM is characterized by poor control of blood glucose level. Blood glucose level increases shortly after eating, temporarily rising to 180 mg·dL^{-1} (10 mmol·L^{-1}) or greater. Generally, hyperglycemia (high blood glucose level) does not affect participation in physical activities. People should be cautious about engaging in strenuous exercises if they have an elevated blood glucose level of 300 mg·dL^{-1} (16.7 mmol·L^{-1}) or above. In general, individuals with T2DM should be active, provided they feel well and are adequately hydrated (14, 15, 41).

Hypoglycemia (low blood glucose level) should not affect T2DM exercisers being treated exclusively with lifestyle modifications, but it may become an issue in exercisers who are insulin users. It is far more dangerous to have too little glucose in the blood than too much, at least temporarily. Brain cells use blood glucose for fuel; thus, hypoglycemia during exercise is accompanied by both physical and cognitive symptoms such as fatigue, mental confusion, or even unconsciousness. Symptoms of hypoglycemia start to appear with blood glucose levels lower than 70 mg·dL^{-1} (3.9 mmol·L^{-1}). Both exercise and insulin may decrease blood glucose, and therefore it is important to monitor the magnitude of their effects on blood glucose during and after exercise. Those who take insulin should monitor their blood glucose before, immediately after, and several hours after completing a session of physical activity. Several strategies can be used if blood glucose levels tend to drop during or after exercise: (a) doses of insulin can be reduced before sessions of physical activity, (b) extra carbohydrate can be consumed before or during physical activity, or (c) both strategies can be implemented (38).

Diabetic neuropathic foot ulcers

Diabetic neuropathic foot ulcers are a frequent complication in diabetes. Nerve damage due to diabetes causes altered or complete loss of sensation in the foot and/or leg and changes to foot structure. Limited joint mobility and pressure on the bottom of the foot (called plantar pressure) may contribute to neuropathic foot ulcers (32). Therefore, reducing the central and inner forefoot plantar pressures by wearing proper shoes should be considered for both prevention and treatment purposes. People with active ulcers or who are at high risk may consider partial or non–weight-bearing exercises. If active ulcers are an issue, aquatic exercise should be eliminated because of the increased risk of bacterial infections (3). Once ulcers have developed, the cause should be determined. Neuropathic ulcers must be protected from further injury until they heal, and strenuous efforts should be avoided. Prevention of the development of another ulcer can be accomplished by wearing well-fitting shoes and conducting frequent skin examinations.

Peripheral arterial disease

The prevalence of PAD is higher in diabetic than in nondiabetic patients. However, only one-half of elderly persons with documented PAD are symptomatic. PAD may cause intermittent claudication (pain or weakness with walking) that is relieved with rest. For exercise guidelines, please see section on CVD.

Retinopathy

With appropriate precautions and monitoring, diabetic patients with retinopathy are capable of undertaking an exercise program inclusive of both aerobic and resistance training portions. In a well-supervised environment, a low-intensity aerobic exercise program can be performed. This program should take the following precautions: ensure that systolic blood pressure does not exceed 20 to 30 mm Hg above baseline and that activities do not involve head-down or arms overhead positions, and avoid exercise with excessive jarring (38). However, with proliferative or severe nonproliferative diabetic retinopathy, vigorous exercise may produce vitreous hemorrhage or retinal detachment and should be avoided. To mitigate unsafe spikes in blood pressure, it is important that patients employ appropriate breathing techniques during lifting. Although it is ultimately the responsibility of the patient to conduct the lift correctly, the technician must carefully monitor and assist the patient with this technique. Yoga and tai chi offer the benefit of lower increases in blood pressure and postural options. When the patient has more advanced disease, consultation with an ophthalmologist can provide individualized recommendations.

Autonomic neuropathy

Autonomic neuropathy (damage to nerves that regulate blood pressure, heart rate, bowel and bladder emptying, digestion, and other body functions) can increase the risk of exercise-induced injury by decreasing cardiac responsiveness to exercise. Using the Borg RPE scale to qualitatively describe effort may be more appropriate than heart rate guidelines for prescribing intensity in patients with autonomic neuropathy. Patients with severe autonomic neuropathy may be best served by emphasizing functional activities of daily living, yoga, or tai chi. To decrease the risk of dehydration, appropriate rest and water breaks should be built into the protocol. Individuals with diabetic autonomic neuropathy should undergo a medical checkup before beginning physical activity more intense than that to which they are accustomed.

Microalbuminuria and nephropathy

Nephropathy is a pathological condition resulting from disrupted kidney function. Microalbuminuria is the presence of a small amount of protein in the urine and is the earliest clinical evidence of nephropathy. Physical activity can acutely increase urinary protein excretion. The magnitude of this increase rises in proportion to the acute increase in blood pressure. It is recommended that people with diabetic kidney disease perform only light or moderate exercise so that blood pressure during exercise does not exceed 200 mm Hg. However, the improvements in blood glucose control and blood pressure from heavy exercise may outweigh the impairment in kidney function. There is no current evidence demonstrating that vigorous exercise increases the rate of progression of diabetic kidney disease.

Evaluation for exercise

Evaluation for participating in physical activities can be complicated by the presence of diabetes-related complications such as CVD, HT, or microvascular changes. Previous physical activity level should also be considered. Low-intensity exercise, such as walking or typical daily activities, does not require exercise capacity tests other than general health care. Graded exercise tests (stress test) are recommended in older people with diabetes who are sedentary but want to engage in moderate to vigorous exercise, other than brisk walking.

Exercise program guidelines

The exercise program for older people with diabetes should be individualized to accommodate previous physical activity and fitness levels, medication schedule, presence and severity of diabetic complications, and expected benefits of the exercise program. Older people with T2DM may have difficulties meeting the current recommendations for structured physical activity. However, individual accommodations should be made with a goal of increasing the total volume of physical activity. The recommendations for structured physical activities are as follows:

Frequency. Regular physical activity is of primary importance in the exercise prescription for T2DM. The acute effects of a single bout of exercise on blood glucose are maintained for 24 to 72 hours. Therefore, it is imperative to increase exercise frequency to more than 3 days a week to optimize its benefits, with the goal being 5 or more days a week. Resistance exercise can be performed less frequently. It is recommended that resistance exercise be performed at least twice weekly on nonconsecutive days (37).

Intensity. The goal should be to perform moderate-intensity aerobic exercise. Brisk walking may be a very appropriate exercise for older individuals with diabetes. Moderate- to high-intensity exercises are encouraged because of the greater benefit associated with this intensity of exercise in controlling blood glucose. Evaluations of the intensity can be made using the RPE scale. Light (1–2 on the RPE scale) to somewhat hard (7–8) exercise is also recommended. Additional information about setting the intensity of exercise is included in Chapters 2, 3, 5, and 9 of this book.

Duration. Physical activity recommendations for T2DM and the general population closely align. Patients should strive to achieve 150 minutes of moderate- to high-intensity aerobic exercise each week. Cardiovascular benefits associated with this volume of activity are well documented in the literature (13, 36), even for diabetics (7, 26).

Mode. Any form of exercise using large muscle groups is recommended, such as brisk walking, yoga, biking, and swimming. Exercise programs combining aerobic, resistance, flexibility, and lifestyle activities tailored to the patient's preference are recommended to maximize success. Brisk walking is the most common exercise for T2DM.

Non–weight-bearing activities may need to be considered because of the progression of diabetic symptoms.

Tips for exercising safely in older individuals with T2DM include the following:

- Keep a source of rapidly acting carbohydrate, such as fruits, fruit juice, or granola bars, available during exercise.

- Consume adequate fluids before, during, and after exercise.
- Prepare for optimal foot care by wearing proper shoes and cotton socks, and inspect feet both before and after exercise.
- Carry medical identifications.

Exercise contraindications

- Fatigue, light-headed, or dizziness
- Pain or blisters on the feet
- Blood glucose level <70 mg·dL^{-1} (3.9 mmol·L^{-1}) or >300 mg·dL^{-1} (16.7 mmol·L^{-1})
- Blurred vision
- The presence of ketone bodies or protein in the urine

Expected benefits/outcomes

Exercise is especially important for individuals with diabetes. It improves blood glucose control by allowing muscles to use insulin more effectively, by maintaining or reducing body weight, and by increasing muscle to promote glucose use. This may decrease the amount of insulin or oral hypoglycemic medication needed.

Exercise helps control T2DM by

- improving insulin sensitivity and insulin handling;
- reducing excess body fat, thus helping to decrease and control weight (decreased body fat results in improved insulin sensitivity);
- improving muscle strength;
- increasing bone density and strength;
- lowering blood pressure;
- helping to protect against heart and blood vessel disease by lowering LDL cholesterol and increasing HDL cholesterol;
- improving peripheral circulation;
- increasing energy level and enhancing work capacity;
- reducing stress, promoting relaxation, and releasing tension and anxiety;
- improving quality of life.

FRAILTY

Introduction to frailty

Although there are many definitions of frailty, most geriatricians agree that it describes an elderly person facing some sort of functional disability (17). However, frailty is not synonymous with disability. Frailty can be thought of as deterioration of various body systems, creating instability and the risk of loss of function (8, 17). Frailty can also be thought of as a biologic syndrome, involving decreased physiological and psychological reserves, which lead to decreased resistance to various stressors

(23). Thus, there are various types of frailty, including functional, medical, mental/psychological, and physical frailty. Recently, frailty has been described as a phenotype, which can be measured in five areas: unintentional weight loss, exhaustion, low energy expenditure, slowness, and weakness (5, 23). A person would be considered frail in the presence of three of the five criteria. Using this definition, 7% of the population older than 65 years met the criteria of frailty (23). Exercise and physical activity are associated with improvements in function that may prevent and/or improve frailty in older individuals (17, 29, 31).

Issues and concerns

Frail individuals are much more vulnerable to untoward exercise-related difficulties and complications than nonfrail persons are. Frail individuals often have one or more disabilities (*e.g.*, both hearing and vision disabilities), which impact their ability to perform activities of daily living. Considering that the fastest-growing segment of the population is the oldest old, it is very likely that a significant number of these individuals will also be frail, and this is likely to become a more prominent problem in the future. Thus, it is imperative for exercise professionals to be aware of and consider conditions that increase the vulnerability of frail older adults. Although it is not possible to list all such conditions, the following are well documented and likely to be encountered:

- Presence of other medical conditions that may impact the ability to exercise.
- It is likely that the person will experience fatigue and weakness.
- The risk of falls and fractures is high in this population as balance is often compromised.
- The person may be easily confused or agitated.
- It is likely that an older frail person will be on multiple medications. These medications may alter heart rate and blood pressure response during exercise or postural change.
- Mobility and motor coordination are usually limited, and this impacts the ability of the person to perform exercise.
- Many, if not most, of the above conditions may coexist. This forms a challenging set of conditions to consider when developing exercise programming for old and frail individuals.

Exercise evaluation

Before evaluating a person with frailty for exercise participation, a thorough medical history should be obtained. This is best accomplished through medical checkup by the personal physician, but could also be done by a trained medical professional. Information on chronic diseases and medication use is especially important. The information obtained will then guide the selection of tests for the exercise evaluation. In addition, evaluation of performance in areas deemed important for activities of daily living or an identified individual weakness should also be conducted. Depending on the overall condition of the frail individual, some or all of the following tests may be valuable:

- Body weight — present weight and annual history of body weight.
- Muscle strength: Handgrip dynamometry is most usually assessed. However, it may also be useful to also evaluate muscle strength in other muscle groups.
- Muscle endurance: Self-report of exhaustion; timed walk test; 400-m walk test.
- Activities of daily living: Timed get-up-and-go test, timed chair stands test, and activities of daily living questionnaire.
- Slowness: Timed walk.
- Physical activity: Questionnaire to evaluate weekly caloric expenditure through physical activity.
- Balance: One-legged stance and/or eight-step tandem gait tests.
- Flexibility: Sit and reach.

In addition to these tests, standard clinical exercise testing using either a treadmill or a cycle ergometer with ECG and blood pressure measurements may be warranted, depending on the individual.

Exercise prescription/programming

The exercise prescription for an old frail person should be based on individual ability and preference. The three main goals of exercise prescription for frail older adults are to increase muscle strength, increase cardiovascular endurance, and increase overall physical activity levels and energy expenditure. In addition, it may also be helpful to provide specific exercise programming for improving activities of daily living and balance. Finally, it is helpful to provide a nutrition intervention to prevent/offset weight loss. In general, exercise programs for frail individuals should be supervised

---

Real Life Story 6-3   Debbie

Debbie is a 74-year-old woman who has never been very physically active. Recently, she noticed that she had lost some of her appetite and that she has trouble getting out of her comfortable TV chair. Her children also complain that she has become very forgetful, but she does not believe this to be the case. She scheduled a doctor's visit for a regular checkup, and her physician suggested she should join an exercise group. After doing some research, she found a walking program for older adults sponsored by the local Y, and she joined the program. The program met 3 times a week for 90 minutes and actually included both walking and theraband resistance exercises. Debbie really enjoyed the social aspects of the program, as most of the members were older women. When she started, she could only walk for 10 to 15 minutes without resting. However, after 2 months in the program, she had no trouble walking at a comfortable pace for 45 to 60 minutes. She commented to her children how much she enjoyed the program and how she had regained her appetite, and even gained some weight. Her friends noticed a remarkable change in her attitude, and she seemed less forgetful. She had definitely improved her energy level. Debbie also thought that the best part was she no longer had any difficulty getting out of her comfortable TV chair!

Table 6-1 Exercise prescription guidelines for frail individuals

Targeted area	Goal	Exercise Prescription
Muscle strength	• Increase upper and lower body muscle strength • Increase or prevent loss of lean body mass • Decrease risk of falling • Increase balance • Improve activities of daily living	• Use weight machines, therabands, or body weight • 3 d · wk^{-1} • Sets of 12–15 reps for each muscle group • 1 set progressing to 2 sets • Start with low resistance eventually progressing to 12–15 RM • Tai chi type exercises
Endurance	• Increase endurance and functional capacity • Improve activities of daily living	• Use large muscle exercise modes such as walking, cycling, swimming, etc. • 3–5 d · wk^{-1} • 30–60 min session^{-1} — smaller increments of 5 min can be used to accumulate 30–60 min • Start at low intensity to ensure exercise is comfortable and well tolerated. Progress to moderate intensity using rating of perceived exertion
Physical activity	• Increase energy expenditure • Improve activities of daily living	• Any activity that keeps the person moving and is enjoyable • Every day of the week if possible • Low to moderate intensity — intensity should not be a focus
Activities of daily living	• Increase the ability to perform activities of daily living • Improve quality of life	• Practice activities such as chair rises (with and without hand support), stair climbing, and moving objects of various sizes • 3–5 d · wk^{-1}. • Start with activities the person can do at least once, and increase number and difficulty of activities progressively as improvement is observed
Balance	• Improve balance • Decrease risk of falling • Improve quality of life	• Balance type activities, such as heel-to-toe walk, one-legged stands, walk straight line, forward, backward, and sideward • 3–5 d · wk^{-1}

to ensure safety and appropriateness of the exercise prescription. Guidelines for exercise prescription in each of the areas identified are presented in Table 6-1.

Expected outcomes

A well-designed exercise program targeted at improving conditions associated with frailty may result in the following outcomes (9, 17, 18):

1. Improved muscle strength. This may also be accompanied by increased lean body mass, or at least prevention of the loss of lean body mass.
2. Improved endurance. This may or may not be accompanied by improvements in aerobic capacity, depending on the intensity of the exercise prescription.

3. Increases in physical activity energy expenditure. This will also help alleviate the feeling of exhaustion and improve quality of life.
4. Improved ability to perform activities of daily living. Activities of daily living will be easier to perform and will result in fewer limitations for the individual.
5. Balance may improve and may be associated with a reduced fear of falling.

INTELLECTUAL DISABILITY AND AGE-RELATED COGNITIVE IMPAIRMENT

Introduction

Intellectual disability (ID) and cognitive impairment refer to two distinctly different conditions with some common features, such as reduced cognitive function. ID is a developmental disorder defined as significantly below average intelligence (2 standard deviations below the mean or an IQ <70 for mild ID, <35 for severe/profound ID). This has to be coupled with limitations in two or more adaptive skills areas such as communication, self-care, home living, social skills, community use, self-direction, health and safety, functional academics, leisure and work, and the level of care the individual requires (20), and must be evident before the age of 18 years. ID is the most common developmental disorder in the United States with a prevalence rate of approximately 3% (4). Life expectancy is slightly lower in persons with ID than in the general population, the gap has narrowed in recent years, and the difference is no longer large. An exception to this is individuals with Down syndrome, with a life expectancy of around 60 years (25, 34). A key difference between ID and age-related cognitive impairment is that ID is a life-long condition, usually diagnosed in early childhood, whereas age-related cognitive impairment is an acquired condition with an age-related onset (27). Age-related cognitive impairment is also usually progressive and thus becomes more accentuated with age, whereas cognitive function per se is not altered with age in ID, unless ID is also coupled with age-related cognitive impairment.

Age-related cognitive impairment includes a constellation of syndromes and diseases, ranging from mild cognitive impairment to severe dementia and Alzheimer disease. The prevalence of dementia is around 14% among persons 71 years of age or older, and there are an additional 10% with Alzheimer disease (33). However, these rates are age dependent, as dementia prevalence increases from 5% at age 71 to 79 to over 37% at age 90 or above (33). These rates are expected to increase as our aging population grows, and a larger proportion of Americans are older than 70 years. Thus, current estimates of over 10 million older people with either ID or age-related cognitive impairment are expected to grow substantially over the next 30 years.

Issues and concerns

A common feature in both ID and age-related cognitive impairment is a sedentary lifestyle, with little physical activity (16, 22). Not surprisingly, physical fitness levels are also often low. This includes very low levels of both cardiovascular fitness and muscle strength. In individuals with ID, obesity may also be common, particularly in persons with Down syndrome. Persons with Down syndrome usually have extremely low levels of cardiovascular fitness and muscle strength, regardless of age (6). Individuals with Down syndrome also have very low maximal heart rates (30 beats below expected levels), which may be a factor in their low cardiovascular fitness (21). Down syndrome is also associated with unstable joints at the base of the spine known as atlantoaxial instability, which can lead to an increased risk of spinal fracture. Consequently, if a person is diagnosed with atlantoaxial instability, any activity that can cause severe jarring or excessive neck motion is discouraged.

Many individuals with age-related cognitive impairment are also frail and thus subject to the limitations associated with frailty (see section on frailty above). Many older individuals with ID and age-related cognitive impairment will be on multiple medications, which may affect the exercise response, and some may also experience side effects associated with the medications they are taking.

Exercise evaluation

It is important for individuals with ID and age-related cognitive impairment to undergo a thorough medical evaluation before starting an exercise program. This is especially important for persons with ID, who often do not receive adequate preventive annual care (34). Considering that both individuals with ID and age-related cognitive impairment have low levels of cardiovascular fitness and muscle strength, both groups often experience problems with activities of daily living and many may be frail. Therefore, the exercise evaluation recommended for frailty will also apply for these populations (see above).

Exercise prescription/programming

The exercise evaluation will provide the information necessary to individualize the exercise prescription. However, the focus should almost always be on improving cardiovascular fitness and muscle strength, coupled with targeted increases in physical activity and activities of daily living. Consequently, the exercise prescription guidelines provided above for frailty also apply to both individuals with ID and those with age-related cognitive impairment. However, it is important to remember that the use of RPE may be problematic in these populations, and heart rate prescriptions should never be based on age-predicted heart rate, especially not in persons with Down syndrome. Consequently, exercise intensity during cardiovascular activities become more difficult to assess. Thus, close supervision coupled with subjective clues is recommended. A simple clue is the talk test — if the person can comfortably carry on a conversation, the exercise intensity is likely not excessive.

It is important to help an individual with ID or age-related cognitive impairment to become familiar and comfortable with an exercise routine. This can be accomplished by demonstration and explanation, coupled with extensive practice. This is especially important for resistance exercise training, where proper technique is important to maximize improvements and avoid injury. Thus, several weeks may need to be dedicated to familiarization and practice before the person is able to perform the prescribed exercise adequately.

Expected outcomes

Since the exercise program for people with ID and age-related cognitive impairment is essentially the same as that for frail individuals, the outcomes of the program will also be similar (see above). Although there is some information in the literature that individuals with Down syndrome seldom improve aerobic capacity with endurance training (30), they still improve work capacity. Newer information also suggests that endurance training in older individuals with Down syndrome improves not only aerobic capacity, but also muscle strength (10). For individuals with age-related cognitive impairment, small improvements in cognitive performance can sometimes occur (39). However, the larger impact of exercise and physical activity on age-related cognitive impairment is through prevention. Several studies show that physical exercise at midlife reduces the likelihood of dementia and cognitive impairment in older adulthood (16). Thus, the greater impact of exercise and physical activity is in prevention, not in treatment of age-related cognitive impairment.

S U M M A R Y

It is clear that planned exercise programs or increased physical activity is beneficial for individuals with CVD, diabetes, or cognitive impairment. Although exercise and physical activity are beneficial, it is important to remember that there are few direct effects on the disease or condition. The major effects appear to be a reduction in risk factors associated with the disease/condition, thus potentially slowing or preventing progression of the disease/condition. Importantly, although exercise is often used in rehabilitation for persons with these conditions, it is likely that exercise and physical activity are more effective for prevention than for rehabilitation; thus, lifelong exercise or physical activity habits are essential. Nevertheless, beneficial outcomes such as improved fitness, increased muscle strength, decreased body fat, improved glucose tolerance, reduced risk factors, improved quality of life, and increased independence provide the opportunity for a healthier and happier life for individuals with CVD, diabetes, or cognitive impairment. Therefore, carefully planned exercise rehabilitation interventions are recommended for most individuals with these conditions.

QUESTIONS FOR REFLECTION

1. What are some different types of CVD?

2. How does the cardiovascular system adapt to the stress of an acute bout of exercise?

3. What are some adaptations made by the cardiovascular system in response to long-term, consistent exercise training?

4. What challenges are associated with exercise in CVD?

5. How does progression of exercise duration and intensity differ between an apparently healthy older adult and one with diagnosed CVD?

6. What are the warning signs of potential danger in exercising older adults with known CVD.

7. Discuss the precautions for exercise in older people with diabetes.

8. How do the major complications of diabetes limit the mode of exercise people can perform?

9. Why should we make individualized exercise programs for older people with diabetes? What are the key aspects we should consider when we design the program?

10. What are the benefits associated with weightlifting and aerobic exercise in older adults with Type 2 diabetes?

11. Is exercise beneficial for older people with Type 1 diabetes? How?

12. What is frailty?

13. What are some of the concerns regarding exercise for a frail person?

14. What can exercise training do for a frail person?

15. How is the exercise prescription altered for a frail person compared with an older person without frailty?

16. What are the main exercise concerns for individuals with cognitive decline and/ or ID?

17. Can exercise training "cure" cognitive decline and/or ID?

18. What type of exercise would be most beneficial for a person with cognitive decline and/or ID?

REFERENCES

1. Antignani PL. Treatment of chronic peripheral arterial disease. *Curr Vasc Pharmacol*. 2003;1:205–16.

2. Arena R, Myers J, Abella J, Peberdy MA, Bensimhon D, Chase P, Guazzi M. Prognostic characteristics of cardiopulmonary exercise testing in caucasian and African American patients with heart failure. *Congest Heart Fail*. 2008;14:310–5.

3. Aronow WS. Peripheral arterial disease in the elderly. *Clin Interv Aging*. 2007;2:645–54.

4. Auxter D, Pfyfer J, Huettig C. *Principles and Methods of Adapted Physical Education and Recreation*. New York (NY): McGraw-Hill Companies; 2001.

5. Bandeen-Roche K, Xue QL, Ferrucci L, et al. Phenotype of frailty: Characterization in the women's health and aging studies. *J Gerontol A Biol Sci Med Sci*. 2006;61:262–6.

6. Baynard T, Pitetti KH, Guerra M, Unnithan VB, Fernhall B. Age-related changes in aerobic capacity in individuals with mental retardation: A 20-yr review. *Med Sci Sports Exerc*. 2008;40:1984–9.

7. Black LE, Swan PD, Alvar BA. Effects of intensity and volume on insulin sensitivity during acute bouts of resistance training. *J Strength Cond Res*. 24:1109–16.

8. Bortz WM 2nd. A conceptual framework of frailty: A review. *J Gerontol A Biol Sci Med Sci*. 2002;57:M283–8.

9. Campbell AJ, Robertson MC, Gardner MM, Norton RN, Buchner DM. Falls prevention over 2 years: A randomized controlled trial in women 80 years and older. *Age Ageing*. 1999;28:513–8.

10. Carmeli E, Kessel S, Coleman R, Ayalon M. Effects of a treadmill walking program on muscle strength and balance in elderly people with Down syndrome. *J Gerontol A Biol Sci Med Sci*. 2002;57:M106–10.

11. Carnethon MR, Gulati M, Greenland P. Prevalence and cardiovascular disease correlates of low cardiorespiratory fitness in adolescents and adults. *JAMA*. 2005;294:2981–8.

12. American College of Sports Medicine, Chodzko-Zajko WJ, Proctor DN, et al. American College of Sports Medicine position stand. Exercise and physical activity for older adults. *Med Sci Sports Exerc*. 2009;41:1510–30.

13. Church TS, Earnest CP, Skinner JS, Blair SN. Effects of different doses of physical activity on cardiorespiratory fitness among sedentary, overweight or obese postmenopausal women with elevated blood pressure: A randomized controlled trial. *JAMA*. 2007;297:2081–91.

14. Coyle EF. Fluid and fuel intake during exercise. *J Sports Sci*. 2004;22:39–55.

15. Coyle EF, Montain SJ. Benefits of fluid replacement with carbohydrate during exercise. *Med Sci Sports Exerc*. 1992;24:S324–30.

16. Deslandes A, Moraes H, Ferreira C, et al. Exercise and mental health: Many reasons to move. *Neuropsychobiology*. 2009;59:191–8.

17. Faber MJ, Bosscher RJ, Chin APMJ, van Wieringen PC. Effects of exercise programs on falls and mobility in frail and pre-frail older adults: A multicenter randomized controlled trial. *Arch Phys Med Rehabil*. 2006;87:885–96.

18. Fairhall N, Aggar C, Kurrle SE, et al. Frailty Intervention Trial (FIT). *BMC Geriatr*. 2008;8:27.

19. Fang J, Wylie-Rosett J, Alderman MH. Exercise and cardiovascular outcomes by hypertensive status: NHANES I epidemiological follow-up study, 1971–1992. *Am J Hypertens*. 2005;18:751–8.

20. Fernhall B. Mental retardation. In: Durstine J, Moore G. editors. *ACSM's Exercise Management for Persons with Chronic Diseases and Disabilities*. Champaign (IL): Human Kinetics; 2003. p. 304–10.

21. Fernhall B, McCubbin J, Pitetti K, Rintala P, Rimmer J, Millar AL, de Silva A. Prediction of maximal heart rate in individuals with mental retardation. *Med Sci Sports Exer*. 2001;33:1655–60.

22. Fernhall B, Pitetti K, Rimmer JH, et al. Cardiorespiratory capacity of individuals with mental retardation including Down syndrome. *Med Sci Sports Exer*. 1996;28:366–71.

23. Fried LP, Tangen CM, Walston J, et al. Frailty in older adults: Evidence for a phenotype. *J Gerontol A Biol Sci Med Sci*. 2001;56:M146–56.

24. Gordon NF, Gulanick M, Costa F, Fletcher G, Franklin BA, Roth EJ, Shephard T. Physical activity and exercise recommendations for stroke survivors: An American Heart Association scientific statement from the Council on Clinical Cardiology, Subcommittee on Exercise, Cardiac Rehabilitation, and Prevention; the Council on Cardiovascular Nursing; the Council on Nutrition, Physical Activity, and Metabolism; and the Stroke Council. *Circulation*. 2004;109:2031–41.

25. Hayden MF. Mortality among people with mental retardation living in the United States: Research review and policy application. *Ment Retard*. 1998;36:345–59.

26. Houmard JA, Tanner CJ, Slentz CA, Duscha BD, McCartney JS, Kraus WE. Effect of the volume and intensity of exercise training on insulin sensitivity. *J Appl Physiol*. 2004;96:101–6.

27. Jedrziewski MK, Ewbank DC, Wang H, Trojanowski JQ. Exercise and cognition: Results from the National Long Term Care Survey. *Alzheimers Dement*. 2010;6:448–55.

28. Leon AS, Franklin BA, Costa F, et al. Cardiac rehabilitation and secondary prevention of coronary heart disease: An American Heart Association scientific statement from the Council on Clinical Cardiology (Subcommittee on Exercise, Cardiac Rehabilitation, and Prevention) and the Council on Nutrition, Physical Activity, and Metabolism

(Subcommittee on Physical Activity), in collaboration with the American Association of Cardiovascular and Pulmonary Rehabilitation. *Circulation.* 2005;111:369–76.

29. Manini TM, Everhart JE, Patel KV, et al. Activity energy expenditure and mobility limitation in older adults: Differential associations by sex. *Am J Epidemiol.* 2009;169:1507–16.

30. Millar AL, Fernhall B, Burkett LN. Effects of aerobic training in adolescents with Down syndrome. *Med Sci Sports Exerc.* 1993;25:270–4.

31. Newman AB, Simonsick EM, Naydeck BL, et al. Association of long-distance corridor walk performance with mortality, cardiovascular disease, mobility limitation, and disability. *JAMA.* 2006;295:2018–26.

32. Piaggesi A, Viacava P, Rizzo L, et al. Semiquantitative analysis of the histopathological features of the neuropathic foot ulcer: Effects of pressure relief. *Diabetes Care.* 2003;26:3123–8.

33. Plassman BL, Langa KM, Fisher GG, et al. Prevalence of dementia in the United States: The aging, demographics, and memory study. *Neuroepidemiology.* 2007;29:125–32.

34. Roizen NJ, Patterson D. Down's syndrome. *Lancet.* 2003;361:1281–9.

35. Seals DR, Desouza CA, Donato AJ, Tanaka H. Habitual exercise and arterial aging. *J Appl Physiol.* 2008;105:1323–32.

36. Sesso HD, Paffenbarger RS Jr, Lee IM. Physical activity and coronary heart disease in men: The Harvard Alumni Health Study. *Circulation.* 2000;102:975–80.

37. Sigal RJ, Kenny GP, Wasserman DH, Castaneda-Sceppa C. Physical activity/exercise and type 2 diabetes. *Diabetes Care.* 2004;27:2518–39.

38. Sigal RJ, Kenny GP, Wasserman DH, Castaneda-Sceppa C, White RD. Physical activity/exercise and type 2 diabetes: A consensus statement from the American Diabetes Association. *Diabetes Care.* 2006;29:1433–8.

39. Teri L, Logsdon RG, McCurry SM. Exercise interventions for dementia and cognitive impairment: The Seattle Protocols. *J Nutr Health Aging.* 2008;12:391–4.

40. Thompson PD, Buchner D, Pina IL, et al. Exercise and physical activity in the prevention and treatment of atherosclerotic cardiovascular disease: A statement from the Council on Clinical Cardiology (Subcommittee on Exercise, Rehabilitation, and Prevention) and the Council on Nutrition, Physical Activity, and Metabolism (Subcommittee on Physical Activity). *Circulation.* 2003;107:3109–16.

41. Zinman B, Ruderman N, Campaigne BN, Devlin JT, Schneider SH, American Diabetes Association. Physical activity/exercise and diabetes mellitus. *Diabetes Care.* 2003;26(suppl 1):S73–7.

CHAPTER 7

Assessing Physical Activity, Fitness, and Progress in Older Adults

Jakob L. Vingren, Anne-Lorraine T. Woolsey,
and James R. Morrow, Jr.

●●● CHAPTER OUTLINE

INTRODUCTION

In previous chapters, you have learned why older adults should engage in physical activity and have been given options for implementation and maintenance of physical activity programs for the older adult population. In this chapter, you will learn the importance of assessing current levels of fitness and tracking for progress. In addition, you will learn to differentiate between types of fitness testing, which will assist you in developing and interpreting assessments so that you can create appropriate individualized physical activity programs.

The body of evidence continues to mount on the relationship between physical activity behavior and the prevention of chronic disease and functional loss. It is imperative that older adults understand how assessment identifies their current states of fitness and allows them to monitor how they are progressing toward the long-term goal of sustained independence and health. Regardless of the participant's age, their current physical activity status and fitness level should be determined as part of the initial needs assessment. Although physical activity assessments should be completed for all ages, it does not mean that *all* assessments are appropriate across *all* ages and fitness levels. It is, therefore, important that health/fitness professionals know how to individualize assessment on the basis of the needs of the older adult they are working with and that they understand how to accurately interpret and use the results from these assessments.

Tracking Our Progress 7-1

My husband (age 67) and I (age 68) engage in physical activity every day. Although he is retired and I am still working, we go to the local YMCA every morning for about 60 minutes. Assessment has played an important part in what we do every day. When we joined "The Y" 2 years ago, we met with a certified personal trainer and completed fitness assessments that included tests for cardiorespiratory endurance, muscle strength, and balance. We then created a fitness program on the basis of these baseline data and our history of physical activity, current medical conditions, and goals. I actually track my progress more often than my husband. I keep a notebook/log of my workouts that I update each day. We talk every day about how that day's workout was easier, more difficult, or simply different from previous workouts. We also purchased pedometers and use them to track our walking and physical activity each week. We keep logs of our steps taken and have developed goals of walking the distance equivalent to crossing the state and ultimately the nation. Assessment was important for us when we initially adopted a physically active lifestyle as we approached retirement, and it continues to influence our physical activity decisions today.

ASSESSMENT IN OUR LIVES

Assessment is important in all areas of life, and we make daily decisions based on of the data that we collect (*e.g.*, determining whether the baking is done and whether you need gasoline for your car). Similarly, it is important to collect data (assess) regarding the fitness level of your older adult clients to make good decisions about physical activity program prescription and their progress. Although we might not always enjoy being tested, testing serves important roles in our everyday lives. Height, weight, temperature, and blood pressure are often recorded when visiting a personal physician. These indices provide information about your current state of health, your progress, and your response to treatment. Similarly, ongoing assessment of your physical fitness level can provide insight into the effects of aging, intervention, and tracking of important health, performance, and functional outcomes.

Of primary importance to older adults is maintenance of health and fitness sufficient to sustain quality of life and independence. Generally, fitness levels decline with age. However, physically active people have declines in fitness parameters that are slower than those who are physically inactive (see Figure 7-1).

The importance of assessing older adults for the health/fitness professional

There are two primary reasons why physical fitness should be assessed for older adults. First, assessment establishes the current performance status of the participant, and second, it allows for evaluation of the participant's progress over time. Assessment also allows you to answer questions such as How should the workout be designed? Are the levels of physical activity and/or physical fitness sufficient to maintain independent living, to obtain/maintain good health, or to perform desired physical activities? Even though the participant might not be interested in his or her current performance results or even progression of physical capability, initial and regular fitness assessments are important aspects of any physical activity program. If you do not assess fitness, you are acting "blindly" and simply guessing when you design and implement physical activity programs. This is a particular concern when working with older adults because improper physical activity program design or implementation can result in serious health/life-threatening outcomes.

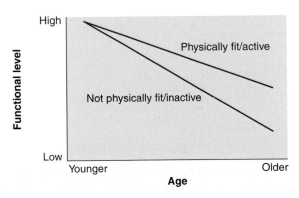

FIGURE 7-1   Relative decline in function between fit and unfit individuals across age

Why assess current performance status?

Physical fitness (biological/physiological age) can vary drastically among older adults even when the adults are of the same chronological age. It is, therefore, imperative for the health/fitness professional to know the participant's current performance status to design a safe and scientifically sound physical activity program, including selecting among the acute program variables such as exercise mode, intensity, and volume (see Chapters 5 and 9 for details on program design). In fact, to select appropriate and safe tests for older adults, a preliminary evaluation should be conducted before designing the physical fitness evaluation. Finally, the results from the initial fitness assessments allow for comparisons with norm- and criterion-referenced data (how does the participant compare with others and with health standards: more detail on this important concept is presented later in this chapter).

Why assess performance progression?

When performance is measured at two or, ideally, more points across time (*e.g.*, quarterly), progress in physical fitness can be determined. There are several reasons why fitness progression should be monitored: (a) to ensure that the physical activity program tailored for the older adult achieves the desired outcomes, (b) to aid the health/fitness professional in determining appropriate program modification including the progression of the acute program variables, and (c) to provide motivation for the participant to continue the program (motivation is covered in detail in Chapter 4). From the health/fitness professional's perspective, showing participants that they have improved or maintained fitness validates the prescribed physical activity program and helps justify the expense of the trainer and thus ultimately results in client retention.)

KEY POINT 7-1 Reasons for Assessing Older Adults' Physical Fitness Levels

Know current level

Identify strengths

Diagnose weaknesses

Help set goals

See progress toward goals

Motivate

Monitor program

Important assessment concepts and considerations

Before we discuss the specifics of fitness testing, it is important that you understand the fundamental concepts involved in assessments. This understanding is needed to make assessment results accurate, interpretable, and thus ultimately valuable.

Fundamental assessment concepts

Reliability is consistency of measurement — if a test is reliable, the participant will obtain a score with little variability when tested several times within a short time span.

Objectivity is a special case of reliability — test scores reflect objectivity if similar results are obtained regardless of who administers the test; that is, there is little variability in results when different test administrators are used.

Relevance is whether the test is related to the construct/concept being measured. For example, a skinfold test is relevant to body composition assessment because it measures subcutaneous fat.

Validity is the most important concern when testing. Validity is the ability of the test to measure what it reports to measure. That is, does the test truthfully measure what it is supposed to measure? Validity is a function of test reliability and relevance. A test can be valid only if it is both reliable (consistent) and relevant.

Generalizability is the degree to which a test can be administered to a variety of individuals, that is, across ages, genders, cultures, and physical activity levels. Generally, one should *not* assume that test items or test batteries generalize from one population to another. Evidence should be available that the test under consideration is appropriate for the specific population with which you are working. Remember that there are many different subpopulations in the general category of older adults.

Error is common to all measurements. It is important to realize that all measures contain some amount of measurement error. Reporting results should always be done with the caveat that the assessment results are an estimate of the true ability or skill and thus contain some error. The actual error is reflected in the reliability and validity of the measures taken. Greater reliability and validity result in less error.

Norm-referenced measurement is a way of interpreting test results. With norm-referenced testing, participants' test results are compared with their peers (generally, age and gender) to see how well they compare. Are they near the top, the middle, or the bottom of performers of their age and gender? Norm-referenced evaluation results are often reported in percentiles. Percentiles indicate the percentage of people who have achieved at the specific level or below. It is important to remember that norms do not tell you whether the fitness test score obtained is good or bad. Someone in the 50th percentile for body composition in the United States might still be overweight or obese.

Criterion-referenced measurement is distinguished from norm-referenced measurement. With criterion-referenced measurement, one is not concerned with how others have performed. Rather, having achieved a criterion or met a minimal standard is the goal. For example, a person wants to achieve an aerobic endurance level sufficient to indicate that he or she has achieved health benefits, is at reduced risk for disease or mortality, or can complete a certain task. The values for a healthy blood pressure (<130 mm Hg) or total cholesterol (<200 mg·dL^{-1}) are other examples of criteria.

Formative and summative evaluations are considered together. Formative evaluation processes involve the ongoing assessment of achievement during the process of learning. This is distinguished from summative evaluation, which is the assessment of achievement at the end of an intervention or process. Essentially, formative evaluation processes let you determine ongoing progress and success, whereas summative evaluation investigates the total progress at the end of a period of training/intervention.

KEY POINT 7-2 Important Testing Considerations

Reliability
Objectivity
Relevance
Validity
Generalizability
Error

Evaluation types
Norm-referenced
Criterion-referenced
Formative evaluation
Summative evaluation

Testing considerations

Purpose: The initial question you should ask yourself is "Why am I testing this participant?" The purpose of the assessment should be the primary guide in the selection of the specific tests to be used. There is no standard test or selection of tests that is appropriate or meaningful for *all* older adults (see Assessing Fitness later in this chapter for more details).

Preparation: As a health/fitness professional, you should take the following steps to prepare for testing:

- Familiarize yourself with each test and ensure that you can administer it validly.
- Ensure that all equipment is available and functioning properly.
- Prepare the testing area so that it is safe and ready for testing.
- Describe each test to your clients and obtain their signed consent to perform the test. This is similar to what is required by law before conducting testing for

a research study. This signed form indicates that the participant understands the stresses required and potential risks associated with the specific fitness testing you have selected for them.

- Lead your clients in sufficient warm-up.
- Familiarize your clients with the procedures of each test (preferably days in advance of the actual test day).

Preliminary Approval and Evaluation: Given that you are working with older adults, it is essential that you obtain written medical clearance from the participant's personal physician before you conduct any physical fitness testing. Often the physician's examination will include a monitored vigorous exercise test involving an ECG, also called a "stress test." You should also conduct a preliminary health and fitness evaluation, and the findings should direct your selection of tests. For example, for individuals with a herniated disc, you should avoid testing that involves loading the spine (*e.g.*, squats), or for individuals with hypertension, you should avoid tests that could substantially increase their blood pressure (*e.g.*, isometric muscle actions of long duration). The preliminary evaluation will also determine whether a physician should be present during testing (see Table 7-1). At a minimum, you should obtain the following preliminary information before the evaluation:

- Participant health history, including significant injury, illness, and treatment
- Family history of significant injury, illness, and treatment
- Risk factor appraisal
- Current medications (prescription and over-the-counter)
- Current and history of lifestyle behaviors, including physical activity, weight loss/gain, smoking

---

KEY POINT 7-3 Physical Activity Readiness Questionnaire

YES	NO		
☐	☐	1.	Has your doctor ever said that you have a heart condition <u>and</u> that you should only do physical activity recommended by a doctor?
☐	☐	2.	Do you feel pain in your chest when you do physical activity?
☐	☐	3.	In the past month, have you had chest pain when you were not doing physical activity?
☐	☐	4	Do you lose your balance because of dizziness or do you ever lose consciousness?
☐	☐	5.	Do you have a bone or joint problem that could be made worse by a change in your physical activity?
☐	☐	6.	Is your doctor currently prescribing drugs (for example, water pills) for your blood pressure or heart condition?
☐	☐	7.	Do you know of *any other reason* why you should not do physical activity?

Table 7-1 ACSM Guidelines for Physician Presence During Exercise Testing		
	Submaximal Testing	**Maximal Testing**
Asymptomatic, no risk factor other than age ($\geq$45 yr for men and $\geq$55 yr for women)	MD supervision not recommended	MD supervision not recommended
Asymptomatic, $\geq$1 risk factor other than age	MD supervision not required	MD supervision recommended
Symptomatic or known cardiovascular, metabolic, or pulmonary disease	MD supervision recommended	MD supervision recommended

KEY POINT 7-4 Considerations When Testing Fitness in Older Adults

Is it necessary for a physician to be close to the area during testing (see Table 7-1)? In most cases, you should not conduct maximal aerobic tests without a physician present.

Ambulation ability: Do they have difficulties maintaining good balance?

Hydration: Older adults are often dehydrated.

KEY POINT 7-5 Safety Precautions When Testing Older Adults

Discuss items with the participant and obtain consent.

Get physician's approval for exercise participation (note any exceptions).

Ensure availability of emergency contact.

Make sure testing site and personnel are well prepared.

Establish emergency procedures (plan) (including access to phone).

Ensure availability of automated external defibrillator (AED).

Ensure availability of personnel trained in emergency procedures, including CPR and use of AED.

Current physical activity performance considerations

Physical activity behavior assessment

The focus of this chapter is on fitness assessment, but recent research and national guidelines have illustrated the importance of assessing physical activity behaviors. There are a variety of methods used to assess physical activity, including self-report, accelerometers, and pedometers. Self-reports are the most widely used, but are subject to bias (also called social desirability). Accelerometers can be rather expensive. Pedometers are widely used, but do not differentiate between intensities of physical activity and cannot measure strengthening activities. Nevertheless, having clients wear pedometers can help you learn about daily physical activity behaviors. As illustrated in Figure 7-2, older adults are generally less physically active than younger adults (2).

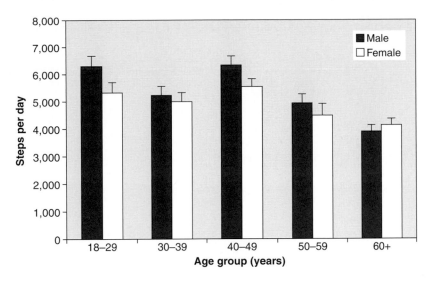

FIGURE 7-2   Steps per day by age categories

Assessment during physical activity training sessions (in-session monitoring)

Just as it is important to conduct assessments over time to evaluate and modify the training program, it is important to continuously conduct minor assessments throughout each physical activity training session. The selected acute program variables (*e.g.*, intensity and volume) should be monitored to ensure that they meet the trainer's prescription. This in-session monitoring can be done informally by observing the client's physical response to the exercise and/or by asking the clients how they are feeling/doing, or more formally using assessment tools such as rating of perceived exertion (RPE) or measurement of heart rate.

Several RPE scales exist, but the most commonly used are the 6- to 20-point "Borg Scale" (6) and the 0- to 10-point Category Ratio Scale (CR-10) (15) (see Key Points 7-6 and 7-7). Heart rate is a good indicator of the physiological demand of the exercise, especially for endurance exercises, and can be used to prescribe exercise intensity. Maximal heart rate declines with age, and can be estimated as 220 – age (in years). However, there is a great variation in maximal heart rate among individuals of the same age, so it is important to remember that although this equation can be used to estimate maximal heart rate, many older clients will have a substantially lower or higher maximal heart rate. Heart rate, therefore, should only be used as one of several means of in-session monitoring of intensity, especially if the true maximal heart rate is not known.

KEY POINT 7-6 6 to 20 Point Borg Scale — Rating of Perceived Exertion

6	
7	Very, very light
8	
9	Very light — gentle walking
10	
11	Fairly light
12	
13	Somewhat hard — steady pace
14	
15	Hard
16	
17	Very hard
18	
19	Very, very hard
20	

KEY POINT 7-7 CR-10 Scale of Perceived Exertion

0	Nothing at all
0.5	Very, very weak (just noticeable)
1	Very weak
2	Weak (light)
3	Moderate
4	Somewhat strong
5	Strong (heavy)
6	
7	Very strong
8	
9	
10	Very, very strong (almost max)
•	Maximal

Assessing fitness

So far, in this chapter, you have learned the importance of fitness assessment for the older adult population and important assessment concepts and considerations. You have also learned how to conduct a preliminary evaluation for use in your assessment selection for each client. In the following section, you will learn about how to assess the three general fitness domains (functional, health-related, and performance) for older adults. Although there are overlapping characteristics among these domains, there are important distinctions and tests assessing specific aspects of one or more of these domains. As you will learn, assessment of *all* three fitness domains is not appropriate for *all* older adults.

KEY POINT 7-8 Types of Fitness Tests

Functional
    Cardiorespiratory fitness
    Musculoskeletal fitness
    Balance/gait
    Flexibility
    Motor agility
    Body composition
Health-related
    Cardiorespiratory fitness
    Musculoskeletal fitness
    Body composition
Performance
    Cardiorespiratory fitness
    Musculoskeletal fitness
    Body composition
    Speed/agility
    Power

Functional fitness testing for older adults

For older adults, the passage of time shifts life's priorities from establishing career and domestic aspirations to maintaining the functional independence implicit in former years, but not freely extended in later years. Hence, running a marathon, bench pressing 200 lb, or hitting a home run becomes less of a motivation than the desire to maintain functional independence for as long as possible. This ability to maintain independence is vulnerable to the effects of the normal increase in sedentary behavior during the later stages of life. Increased sedentary behavior coupled with the effects of natural biological aging creates a progressive path from physiologic impairment to functional limitation to disability and premature death. Functional fitness tests can serve as a guide for the health/fitness professional in identifying where the older adult is located within this progression of functionality. Once the complete picture of functionality is identified, the health/fitness professional can more accurately implement physical activity programs that target physiological impairments, delay the onset of functional limitations, and prevent the premature progression into disability.

Functional fitness assessment consists of tests related to conducting activities of daily living (ADL), instrumental activities of daily living (IADL), and balance. The ability to conduct ADLs and IADLs is vital to take care of oneself and to live independently (see Key Point 7-9), but is not a good measure of aerobic endurance or neuromuscular strength in most physically active older adults. Therefore, functional fitness tests are mainly appropriate for older adults who have been largely sedentary throughout life as well as the frail and senior elderly (older than 85 yr). For the latter populations especially, functional fitness testing can provide objective data on their ability to perform ADL and IADL and thus their capability for independent living. Two test batteries are identified specifically for the older adult. The Groningen Fitness Test for the Elderly (12) consists of grip strength, leg extension, sit-and-reach, circumduction, balance board, block transfer, reaction time, and a walking endurance test. The Senior Fitness Test (19) is widely reported. We will expand our discussion of the Senior Fitness Test battery below.

KEY POINT 7-9 Activities of Daily Living (ADL) and Instrumental Activities of Daily Living (IADL)

ADLs — Self-care

Personal hygiene (bathing, grooming)

Toileting (restroom use, continence)

Dressing oneself

Feeding oneself

Transferring from position to position (bed to standing, standing to sitting, sitting to standing)

IADLs — Help one to live independently

Using personal and community resources (telephone, appointments)

Travel (driving or arranging)

Kitchen tasks (preparing meals, opening containers, using equipment)

Shopping (getting around, carrying)

Household chores (laundry, light cleaning)

Managing self-treatment (medications)

Managing finances (budgeting, paying bills)

Senior Fitness Test battery for assessing functional fitness in older adults. Rikli and Jones (17, 18) recognized the accelerated progression toward disability in older adults and developed a test battery that specifically and comprehensively evaluates areas of functional fitness in older adults (19). These areas consist of cardiorespiratory endurance, muscular strength and endurance, balance/gait, flexibility, agility, and body composition. An overview of equipment and objective and physical fitness parameters for each item in the Senior Fitness Test is provided in Table 7-2. For complete instructions on how to administer this battery of tests, please refer to the *Senior Fitness Test Manual* (19). There are many additional functional fitness tests that are not included in the Senior Fitness Test; however, because this test battery evaluates across functional fitness areas and requires minimal equipment and space, it is probably the most widely used test battery by health/fitness professionals for older adult health promotion programs.

Table 7-2 Test Items for Senior Fitness Test

Test	Physical Fitness Parameter	Test Objective	Equipment
Six-minute walk	Cardiorespiratory endurance	To assess the maximum distance a participant can walk in 6 min along a 50-yd (45.7-m) course	Stopwatch Tally counters Masking tape 4 Cones Adhesive name tags Pen Chairs for rest
Two-minute step	Cardiorespiratory endurance	To assess the maximum number of steps in place a participant can complete in 2 min	2 Stopwatches 2 Tally counters Two 30-in pieces of cord Masking tape
Chair stand	Lower body strength	To complete as many chair stands in 30 s as possible	Stopwatch
Arm curl	Upper body strength	To complete as many correctly executed arm curls as possible in 30 s	Stopwatch 5- and 8-lb Sets of dumbbells
Chair sit-and-reach	Lower body flexibility	To sit in a chair and attempt to touch the toes with the fingers	18-in Ruler (half a yardstick)
Back scratch	Upper body flexibility	To reach behind the back with the hands to touch or overlap the fingers of both hands as much as possible	18-in Ruler (half a yardstick)
Eight-foot up-and-go	Motor agility/balance	To stand, walk 16 ft (4.9 m), and sit back down in the fastest possible time	Stopwatch Cone Measuring tape
Height and weight	Body composition	To measure a person's BMI	Tape measure

Reprinted with permission from Rikli RE, Jones CJ. *Senior Fitness Test Manual.* Champaign (IL): Human Kinetics; 2001.

Interpreting functional fitness test results. In the context of functional fitness, there are several strategies for interpreting test results. One strategy requires little outside knowledge of norm or criterion data, as discussed earlier in this chapter. After accurately following the assessment protocol for the Senior Fitness Test, the health/fitness professional could simply record the baseline (initial) scores for each test item. After setting agreed on dates for subsequent retests, the health/fitness professional would compare the results of the subsequent tests with the initial test to determine progress in each area of functional fitness. A more sophisticated approach requires some knowledge about normative- and criterion-referenced measurements. This strategy groups participants into different levels of functioning by percentile for the purpose of identifying those at risk for losing functional mobility or independence (Tables 7-3 and 7-4). Participants scoring in the middle 50% are considered in the normal range of scores for the functional fitness parameters. Although these scores are used as norm-referenced measurements to compare the participant's score with the scores gathered from the large national survey of older adults, these scores can also be used as a criterion for classifying individuals into either a high functioning or a low functioning group. Placement into the low functioning group (<25th percentile) positions this individual into the "at risk" category for losing functional mobility or independence. A high functioning status (>75th percentile) may indicate that the individual has defied the normal age-related declines in functioning and will face those declines at a later than expected stage of life. Using Tables 7-3 and 7-4 as a reference point for assessing low, normal, or high functioning fitness status, the health/fitness professional should examine the participant's results not only to identify weak

Table 7-3   Senior Fitness Test Normal Range of Scores for Women

	60–64	65–69	70–74	75–79	80–84	85–89	90–94
Chair stand test (number of stands)	12–17	11–16	10–15	10–15	9–14	8–13	4–11
Arm curl test (number of reps)	13–19	12–18	12–17	11–17	10–16	10–15	8–13
Six-minute walk (number of yards)	545–660	500–635	480–615	435–585	385–540	340–510	275–440
Two-minute step (number of steps)	75–107	73–107	68–101	68–100	60–90	55–85	44–72
Chair sit-and-reach (in. [±])	−0.5 to +5.0	−0.5 to +4.5	−1.0 to +4.0	−1.5 to +3.5	−2.0 to +3.0	−2.5 to +2.5	−4.5 to +1.0
Back scratch (in. [±])	−3.0 to +1.5	−3.5 to +1.5	−4.0 to +1.0	−5.0 to +0.5	−5.5 to +0.0	−7.0 to 1.0	−8.0 to 1.0
Eight-foot up-and-go (s)	6.0–4.4	6.4–4.8	7.1–4.9	7.4–5.2	8.7–5.7	9.6–6.2	11.5–7.3

Reprinted with permission from Rikli RE, Jones CJ. *Senior Fitness Test Manual.* Champaign (IL): Human Kinetics; 2001.

Table 7-4	Senior Fitness Test Normal Range of Scores for Men						
	60–64	65–69	70–74	75–79	80–84	85–89	90–94
Chair stand test (number of stands)	14–19	12–18	12–17	11–17	10–15	8–14	7–12
Arm curl test (number of reps)	16–22	15–21	14–21	13–19	13–19	11–17	10–14
Six-minute walk (number of yards)	610–735	560–700	545–680	470–640	445–605	380–570	305–500
Two-minute step (number of steps)	87–115	86–116	80–110	73–109	71–103	59–91	52–86
Chair sit-and-reach (in. [±])	−2.5 to +4.0	−3.0 to +3.0	−3.0 to +3.0	−4.0 to +2.0	−5.5 to +1.5	−5.5 to +0.5	−6.5 to 0.5
Back scratch (in. [±])	−6.5 to +0.0	−7.5 to 1.0	−8.0 to 1.0	−9.0 to 2.0	−9.5 to 2.0	−9.5 to 3.0	−10.5 to 4.0
Eight-foot up-and-go (s)	5.6–3.8	5.9–4.3	6.2–4.4	7.2–4.6	7.6–5.2	8.9–5.5	10.0–6.2

Reprinted with permission from Rikli RE, Jones CJ. *Senior Fitness Test Manual.* Champaign (IL): Human Kinetics; 2001.

functioning areas, but also to maintain high functioning areas. As with all norm-referenced measurements, the data collected for comparison with an individual score are not an all-inclusive and definitive means of declaring a person functionally fit or unfit. It is merely another tool that may assist the health/fitness professional in implementing a physical activity program whose goal is to improve or maintain functional fitness on an individual basis.

Health-related fitness testing for older adults

Health-related fitness assessment consists of tests relevant to disease risk and is generally appropriate for older adults of all ages (except some frail or senior elderly). Health-related fitness is the foundation for improved quality of life and general well-being, and it is an indication of the individual's risk for a variety of morbidities and death. The components of health-related physical fitness are cardiorespiratory endurance, musculoskeletal fitness, and body composition. One of the important uses of health-related fitness assessment is to determine whether the client has sufficient fitness to achieve health benefits or be at a reduced risk for a variety of diseases.

Cardiorespiratory endurance testing. Cardiorespiratory endurance (*i.e.,* aerobic capacity) is commonly quantified as maximal oxygen uptake capacity ($\dot{V}O_{2max}$) measured during maximal (all-out) tests lasting 5 to 15 minutes. However, for older adults who have any cardiovascular disease risk factor other than age (see Table 7-1), which is the majority of this population, a physician should be present during maximal aerobic endurance tests. Since the presence of a physician during testing is generally not feasible in most fitness testing locations, submaximal tests that estimate $\dot{V}O_{2max}$ should be used for measuring aerobic endurance of most older adults. If clients are asymptomatic and have no known cardiac, pulmonary, or metabolic diseases, the presence of a physician is not a requirement during submaximal aerobic tests (see Table 7-5) (20). There is a large assortment of submaximal tests for estimating $\dot{V}O_{2max}$, including cycle ergometer, row ergometer, bench step, and walk/jog tests. In general, these tests use submaximal exercise heart rate, age-predicted maximal heart rate (generally 220-age), and work rate to estimate $\dot{V}O_{2max}$. Submaximal tests are best used as originally designed, but they can be modified to match the capabilities/limitations of older participants. For example, when using tests that require good balance such as treadmill tests, incline rather than speed can be manipulated to increase intensity (see Table 7-5 for additional options for test modifications). It is important to consider that when tests are modified, the ability to accurately predict $\dot{V}O_{2max}$ is greatly

Table 7-5   Exercise Test Modification Options for Older Adults

Characteristics	Suggested test modification
Low $\dot{V}O_{2max}$	Start at low intensity (2–3 METs)
More time required to reach a steady state	Long warm-up (3+ min); small rise in power output (0.5–1 MET) and/or 2–3 min at each stage
Increased fatigability	Reduce total test time to 12–15 min or use an intermittent protocol
Increased need to monitor ECG, BP, and HR	Bike < treadmill < step test
Poor balance	Bike < treadmill < step test; use treadmill built into the floor
Poor strength (especially upper thighs)	Treadmill > bike or step test
Less ambulatory ability	Increase treadmill grade rather than speed (maximum 3–3.5 mph)
Difficulty holding mouthpiece with dentures	Add support or use face mask to measure VO_2
Impaired vision	Bike > treadmill or step test
Impaired hearing	Treadmill > bike or step test, if person needs to follow a cadence; difficulty understanding and responding in a noisy environment (use electronic bike)
Senile gait patterns and foot problems (e.g., bunions and calluses)	Bike < treadmill < step test

From *ACSM's Resource Manual for Guidelines for Exercise Testing and Prescription*. 6th ed. Baltimore (MD): Lippincott Williams & Wilkins; 2010.

diminished; however, this is not necessarily a problem when the tests are used for primarily clinical versus research purposes. For individuals with poor balance, non–weight-bearing test modalities such as cycle ergometers should be used. Continuous monitoring of the heart rate during submaximal aerobic endurance tests is important to ensure that the test does not inadvertently become a maximal test because the work rate was prescribed too high relative to the client's capability. Detailed descriptions of the procedures for submaximal tests of aerobic endurance ($\dot{V}O_{2max}$) can be found elsewhere (1, 14).

Musculoskeletal fitness testing. Musculoskeletal (neuromuscular) strength can be quantified as absolute strength or as strength endurance. Absolute strength and strength endurance are different but related quantities, and the assessment of each offers advantages and disadvantages when used with older adults. Absolute strength is assessed as repetition maximum (RM), the maximum weight that can be lifted a set number of times with proper technique. 1RM (the maximum weight that can be lifted once) is a good and common measurement of strength and can be obtained safely for older adults (9, 16). Direct 1RM testing places high stress (especially compression) on joints and other tissues; therefore, testing with lower loads for a few repetitions such as 3RM (the maximal weight that can be lifted three times) can be used instead of 1RM testing. Proper RM testing involves multiple trials and can thus become very time consuming, especially if the strength in several muscle groups is assessed. Detailed procedures for RM testing have been described by Kraemer and Fry (11).

To assess muscle strength endurance, the number of repetitions to failure at a given weight is measured. For this type of testing, it is very important to monitor technique as it will often deteriorate near fatigue, which can lead to injury. Testing for strength endurance is not, in contrast to what is commonly believed, inherently safer than absolute strength assessment in older adults. Equations have been developed to predict absolute strength (1RM) from strength endurance. These equations are generally not validated for use with older adults, and thus, caution should be used when interpreting the results from such predictions. Knutzen and colleagues (10) found that six different prediction equations for 1RM systematically underestimated (1–10 kg) the actual 1RM of older men and women for 11 different machine resistance exercises. Instead of predicting the 1RM from muscle strength endurance, the change in the number of repetitions that can be completed can be compared to monitor progress in strength capability. When measuring muscle strength, specificity of the testing mode is very important. It is also important to consider the ambulatory abilities of the older adults being tested as many will have compromised balance capabilities; seated exercises are preferred for those who do not have good balance.

In contrast to aerobic assessments, there are no set risk stratifications published by the American College of Sports Medicine or the American Heart Association regarding which neuromuscular assessments should be avoided in older adults or require the presence of a physician when the neuromuscular assessments do not present a cardiorespiratory challenge. The primary medical safety concern during neuromuscular strength testing of older adults is that blood pressure can increase substantially during testing that involves long durations of high force production or contractions such as isometric endurance or multiple repetition testing; this is a particular concern for those who have hypertension. To reduce the risk of large increases in blood pressure during assessment, the technique known as the Valsalva maneuver (forceful attempt to exhale against a closed glottis resulting in increased intrathoracic pressure) and long-duration isometric tests should be avoided. For the same reason when performing repetitions to failure, the load should be selected so that no more than 8 to 10 repetitions are required. As you have learned, familiarization of participants with procedures is needed for a reliable test. For neuromuscular strength assessments, thorough familiarization, especially learning the proper exercise/lifting technique, is also vitally important for safety and thus should always precede initial strength testing visits.

Power testing. Power is the product of force and velocity of movement and can best be described as explosive force production. Among older adults, the power-producing capacity appears to be more strongly associated with functional mobility performance than muscle strength (3, 4, 7). One of the reasons for this is that high power is required to maintain balance in situations such as being tripped or stepping off a curb. Since velocity is a component of power, most power assessment involves fast movements that might not be appropriate for all older adults; therefore, power testing that is more appropriate/relevant for performance testing is included under performance fitness assessment. A stair climb test is a clinically relevant measure of lower body power in older adults and is meaningfully associated with mobility (5). Furthermore, the stair climb test is easy to administer, requires little equipment, and is safe for use in older adults, even those with some mobility limitations as long as they climb a flight of stairs with the use of assistive equipment (*e.g.,* cane and handrail) (5). The use of a stair climb test to measure power was first described by Margaria and colleagues (13), and therefore this type of test is also referred to as the Margaria stair run test. For this test, participants ascend a flight of stairs as quickly as they can two stairs at a time. Maximal power is then calculated on the basis of the mass of the participants, the vertical displacement (height from step 4 to step 6), and the time it took to get from step 4 to step 6. This test can be modified for use in older adults with mobility limitations by having them use every stair; use a handrail, cane, or similar equipment; and/or only ascend partway up a flight of stairs (*e.g.,* 10 stairs).

Body composition testing. Changes in body composition are often a desired outcome from engagement in physical activity. The methods for measuring body composition range from simple measurements using height and weight (body mass index [BMI]), circumferences, waist–hip ratios, and/or skinfold thickness, which require limited equipment, to very demanding measurements using underwater-weighing, X-ray technology, or ingestion of isotopes; the latter methods are often considered the "gold standard" for body composition. For most trainers, it is only feasible to obtain measurements that require limited equipment and that are simple to conduct; therefore, only those measurements will be discussed further here. It is important to remember that all of these measurements are estimates of body composition, since it is not possible to directly measure body composition of living individuals, and thus, there is a substantial potential for prediction error for all of these measurements. Regardless of the measurement technique used, the best use of body composition data for older adults is for tracking progress over time. Although clients might be interested in the absolute measure of body composition (*e.g.*, their current body fat percentage), the focus should be on change in body composition over time (progression) and less on the absolute value, especially when derived using the methods outlined below.

BMI is a commonly used assessment in large-scale epidemiological studies, since it requires only measurement of height and weight (BMI = weight [in kg]/height^2 [in m]). Although BMI is simple to obtain, it is generally not a useful measure of body composition when examining a single or even a small group of individuals. This is because BMI does not consider the muscular build of the individual, but only the total weight. On the basis of BMI, lean muscular individuals can be wrongly classified as overweight or even obese; in contrast, individuals who are not very muscular but have a high body fat percentage can wrongly be classified as neither overweight nor obese. The latter is a particular concern when assessing older adults, since they often have reduced muscle mass and increased fat mass. Furthermore, improvement in body composition from a training program that induces simultaneous increase in muscle mass and reduction in fat mass can be undetectable or underestimated when using BMI.

> **KEY POINT 7-10** BMI Categories from Centers for Disease Control and Prevention
>
> | | |
> |---|---|
> | <18.5 | Underweight |
> | 18.5–24.9 | Normal |
> | 25.0–29.9 | Overweight |
> | ≥30.0 | Obese |

Skinfolds are measured using calipers from various sites on the right side of the body. The sum of the skinfolds is then applied to equations that predict body fat percentage. In general, skinfold measurements do not appear to be a good tool for body composition assessment in older adults (low-to-moderate correlation [$r = 0.39$ and 0.65 for men and women, respectively] with "gold standard" measurement for body composition) (8). This is partly because older adults have more visceral fat than do younger adults, and skinfold thickness is only a measure of subcutaneous fat. In addition, modesty (wearing a limited amount of clothing) and being touched on the bare skin are concerns with skinfold measurements in older adults. Predicting body composition from **circumference** measurements appears to have better validity for use with older adults. The Tran–Weltman (22, 23) equations, which use only circumference measurements, have been validated for older men and women with moderate to high correlations ($r = 0.57$ and 0.87 for men and women, respectively) with the "gold standard" (8).

Performance fitness testing for older adults

The components of performance fitness include those of health-related fitness plus speed, agility, and power and are related to successful performance in games and skill-related activities. Performance-related fitness assessment is useful mainly for older adults who are very active or involved in sport or exercise competitions. When measuring performance-related fitness, specificity of the assessment to the activity or task for which the performance is related is of paramount importance, both for the safety of participants during the testing and for the usefulness of the results obtained. Since there is a large range of sports and activities for which performance fitness is relevant, this section will only provide guidelines for assessments that transcend most sports and activities.

Speed and agility testing. Speed capability and agility (the ability to quickly change direction at high speeds) are meaningful performance fitness assessments in older adults, but these tests should only be used for those who are highly trained and normally engage in activities similar to the tests. Sprinting and most agility tests rely on very fast movements involving high force and power output; those not accustomed to this type of movement are at an increased risk for injury to muscle and connective tissue. Sprint tests such as the 40-, 60-, or 100-yard dash are good measures of straight running speed; however, for performance in most sports, especially for older adults, it is more meaningful to measure agility. There is a large assortment of standard agility tests. These tests are often variations of shuttle-run tests such as the three-cone test and pro-agility test (5 yd-10 yd-5 yd dash) or quick feet movement tests such as "running ladders." For shuttle run tests, the distance run and the number and angles for changes in direction should be chosen to fit the particular activity for which performance is assessed. To validly assess agility, the tests should be short in duration since they will otherwise be heavily influenced by aerobic and/or anaerobic fitness.

Performance power testing. Maximal power capability is correlated with performance on tasks that require quick body accelerations such as change of direction. In fact, maximal lower-body power capability is one of the best predictors of performance capability for tasks/sports that require fast acceleration or change in direction. Power is best measured using advanced and expensive equipment that is often not available outside of research laboratories; however, in recent years, several types of less expensive high-tech equipment (*e.g.*, linear accelerometers) have become available. Although high-tech equipment allows for precise measurement of power in many movements, lower-body power, which is the most important power capability for most performance testing, can be measured using simple and inexpensive tests. One of the simplest tests for lower-body power capability is maximal vertical jump height. Jump height can be used as a measure of relative power capability, or it can be applied to a prediction equation to obtain an estimate of absolute peak power capability for the lower body. Another relatively simple power test for most older adults is the Margaria stair climb test, described under Health-Related Fitness Assessment above. Upper-body power can be assessed using a vertical medicine ball or bench press (in a Smith machine) throws. As with vertical jumps, the vertical displacement of the throw (height) can be used to estimate power, but unlike vertical jump, vertical throws are a measure of absolute power capability.

Assessment considerations for very physically active or fit older adults

When assessing the physical performance capabilities of older adults who are very physically active and therefore substantially more fit than their average peers, different considerations should be used than those suggested above in this chapter for the typical older adult. For example, if participants are avid runners or cyclists, it makes little sense to assess their aerobic fitness using a low-intensity walk test because this test is unlikely to provide a good measurement of their aerobic endurance capacity. Similarly, it is not useful to administer a 30-second chair stand test to measure the neuromuscular strength of an older adult who competes in power lifting competitions. In general, performance assessment for highly trained older adults should be conducted using tests that are specific/similar to the exercise modes they normally engage in and allow for higher absolute intensity. It is important to remember that although these participants are very active and fit, they are still older adults, which by itself is a risk factor for cardiovascular disease. As a result, even fit older adults are at an increased risk for experiencing a cardiovascular event during physical activity/testing, and precautions should still be taken relative to testing of healthy young adults. Although high endurance trained older adults might regularly reach or approach their maximal aerobic capability (*i.e.*, $\dot{V}O_{2max}$) during their normal training routine, maximal aerobic testing should be conducted only without the presence of a physician if no other risk factor for cardiovascular disease than age is present. Even among older adults who are highly active and fit, many, if not most, have additional risk factors and thus a physician should be present (or nearby) during maximal aerobic exercise tests. Finally, keep in mind that someone who engages in a high amount of endurance training might not have high neuromuscular strength; similarly, participants involved in neuromuscular strength training might not have a high aerobic endurance capacity.

Tracking and assessing one's fitness level

We have reviewed the importance of assessing fitness for older adults and have provided various protocols for tester-facilitated functional, health-related, and performance fitness assessments. In this next section, we'll discuss strategies that assist older adults with tracking their own individual progress.

Self-tracking and goal setting

From the onset of this chapter, several methods for assessing progress and performance in older adults have been introduced, described, and justified as a means of evaluating the current functional, health-related, and performance fitness states of the older adult as well as for tracking progress. With each assessment, whether given by a health/fitness professional or self-assessed by the older adult, the need arises for a log of results. Older adults can participate in regularly scheduled assessments and experience the satisfaction of progress, but neglect to record this progress and therefore lose the reference point for future progressions.

Goal setting is an effective way to self-assess one's progress. By recording daily, weekly, monthly, and yearly goals, one can have a reference to compare assessment results with met or unmet goals. If the assessment results yield positive gains in functional, health-related, and performance status, one can look back at the goal sheets to evaluate the influence on physical progress. This situation can work the other way as well. If assessment results yield no gains or a regression in functional, health-related, or performance status, the older adult can review the goal sheets to assess whether the goals need to be modified (*e.g.*, increase days of physical activity or length of walk) to increase the likelihood of positive assessment results in the future.

Self-tracking with pedometers

Pedometers are increasingly used to monitor and track physical activity behaviors. A variety of steps-per-day criteria have been suggested (*e.g.*, 10,000; 8,500; 7,500; and 5,000), but none of these criteria have been well validated in the scientific literature. That is, no controlled studies have been conducted indicating that individuals who achieve a certain number of steps are at reduced risk for different morbidities. Another issue with pedometers is that they do not differentiate between a slow, moderate, brisk, and fast pace. Thus, a step, regardless of the intensity, is recorded as a step. Some newer pedometers can be programmed to provide estimates of moderate and/or vigorous physical activity per day on the basis of the number of steps taken per minute. Moderate and/or vigorous threshold steps per minute are established for each individual and entered into the pedometer. Regardless of the type of pedometer used, they can serve as a good method for determining how much daily physical activity one is conducting. They can also serve as a means of tracking behavior change. For example, some individuals determine a baseline of typical steps per day and then set a goal of increasing the number of steps by 500 per day or by 10% per week until they achieve the desired number of steps. Rowe et al. (21) measured pedometer steps in individuals older than 60 years and found that these men and women averaged about 5,000 steps a day. However, there is considerable variation in the daily number of steps taken (*e.g.*, Sunday was reported as a less active day).

Self-tracking with social networking

Interest in social networking has spread from the youth to both the general and the older adult populations. Just as older adults can update current events happening in their lives, they can also use social networking sites to track physical activity achievements by posting updates on their status. Older adults can organize group physical activity events, update their social contacts on the progress of physical activity endeavors, post pictures of their physical change, and provide a virtual space for shared commentary about events, individual/group challenges, encouragement, and progress.

Self-tracking with journaling

Journaling can provide a means to reflect on not only the physical activity goals themselves, but the actual physical process of setting goals, implementing a strategy to meet those goals, and either celebrating success of a goal achieved or overcoming obstacles that stand in the way of successful assessment and goal results. Depending on individual preferences, journaling can consist of one line describing how one felt before, during, and after exercise or it can serve as a longer collection of written narratives that assist the older adult in reflecting on physical activity behavior at a deeper level. Either way, the older adult can benefit from self-assessing progress through journaling. There are several journaling tips available online and in the health section of your local library or bookstore.

Self-tracking with new technologies: Smart phones and the Internet

Today's smart phones have many technological advances that can assist the older adult with self-assessment. GPS devices imbedded within the phones can track distance traveled or map out areas to walk, jog, hike, or bike. Special smart phone applications

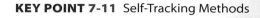

KEY POINT 7-11 Self-Tracking Methods

Diary
Log
Technology
   Cell phone
   Pedometer
   Internet

offer free pedometer, calorie expenditure, and physical activity tracking. This is an assessment technology that offers tremendous and powerful possibilities, and it is expected to grow substantially in the coming years.

The Internet can serve as a useful way of accessing self-assessment tools such as physical activity and goal tracking logs. Among others, the National Institute on Aging offers a comprehensive list of self-assessment worksheets that can be accessed through their Web site: http://www.nia.nih.gov/health/publication/exercise-physical-activity-your-everyday-guide-national-institute-aging/chapter-7

S U M M A R Y

We have provided an overview of the use of physical activity and fitness assessments in older adults. Key concepts are safety in testing, testing concepts, reporting test results, and test selection. The differences in the purpose of testing protocols are important. Functional, health-related, and performance testing result in specific types of assessments that should be considered, depending on your client's needs, abilities, and goals. Specificity of testing is key to test selection. New technology tools are available for recording assessments that help with initial testing, tracking, and goal setting.

QUESTIONS FOR REFLECTION

1. How should an initial assessment differ between an active and a sedentary older adult?

2. What are the primary safety concerns to consider when assessing fitness in older adults?

3. What is the difference between criterion- and norm-referenced evaluations? What information does each of them provide?

4. What should be done before fitness assessment in older adults?

5. When should a physician be present during testing of older adults?

6. Why is it important to test fitness in older adults?

7. What are the differences and similarities between functional, health-related, and performance fitness?

8. What would be an appropriate test of aerobic endurance capacity for a 70-year-old female marathon runner?

9. What would be an appropriate test of neuromuscular strength for a 75-year-old sedentary man?

10. Develop a scenario where you have a new older adult client. Provide an outline of the steps that you would take to assess his or her current fitness level, and provide an overview of the exercise program that you would recommend.

11. Describe the differences between biological and chronological aging, and indicate how this would influence the type of testing you might conduct.

12. Indicate a variety of ways that older adults might track their physical fitness and physical activity levels, keeping in mind their individual preferences and lifestyles.

13. Describe the importance of self-assessment to the older adult.

14. Describe the importance of continual assessments and the role they play in recording progress and influencing exercise program adjustments.

REFERENCES

1. American College of Sports Medicine. *ACSM's Guidelines for Exercise Testing and Prescription.* Baltimore (MD): Lippincott Williams & Wilkins; 2009.
2. Bassett DR Jr, Wyatt HR, Thompson H, Peters JC, Hill JO. Pedometer-measured physical activity and health behaviors in U.S. adults. *Med Sci Sports Exerc.* 2010;42:1819–25.
3. Bean J, Herman S, Kiely DK, Callahan D, Mizer K, Frontera WR, Fielding RA. Weighted stair climbing in mobility-limited older people: A pilot study. *J Am Geriatr. Soc.* 2002;50:663–70.
4. Bean JF, Herman S, Kiely DK, Frey IC, Leveille SG, Fielding RA, Frontera WR. Increased Velocity Exercise Specific to Task (InVEST) training: A pilot study exploring effects on leg power, balance, and mobility in community-dwelling older women. *J Am Geriatr Soc.* 2004;52:799–804.
5. Bean JF, Kiely DK, LaRose S, Alian J, Frontera WR. Is stair climb power a clinically relevant measure of leg power impairments in at-risk older adults? *Arch Phys Med Rehabil.* 2007;88:604–9.
6. Borg GA. *Borg's Perceived Exertion and Pain Scales.* Champaign (IL): Human Kinetics; 1998.
7. American College of Sports Medicine, Chodzko-Zajko WJ, Proctor DN, et al. American College of Sports Medicine position stand. Exercise and physical activity for older adults. *Med Sci Sports Exerc.* 2009;41:1510–30.

8. Clasey JL, Kanaley JA, Wideman L, et al. Validity of methods of body composition assessment in young and older men and women. *J Appl Physiol.* 1999;86:1728–38.

9. Hasten DL, Pak-Loduca J, Obert KA, Yarasheski KE. Resistance exercise acutely increases MHC and mixed muscle protein synthesis rates in 78–84 and 23–32 yr olds. *Am J Physiol Endocrinol Metab.* 2000;278:E620–6.

10. Knutzen KM, Brilla LR, Caine D. Validity of 1RM prediction equations for older adults. *J Strength Cond Res.* 1999;13:242–6.

11. Kraemer WJ, Fry AC. Strength testing: Development and evaluation of methodology. In: Maud PJ, Niemann DC, editors. *Fitness and Sports Medicine: A Health-Related Approach*; 1995.

12. Lemmink KAP, Kemper H. Reliability of the Groningen fitness test for the elderly. *J Aging Phys Act.* 2001;9:194–212.

13. Margaria R, Aghemo P, Rovelli E. Measurement of muscular power (anaerobic) in man. *J Appl Physiol.* 1966;21:1662–4.

14. Maud PJ, Foster C. *Physiological Assessment of Human Fitness.* Champaign (IL): Human Kinetics; 2006.

15. Noble BJ, Borg GA, Jacobs I, Ceci R, Kaiser P. A category-ratio perceived exertion scale: Relationship to blood and muscle lactates and heart rate. *Med Sci Sports Exerc.* 1983;15:523–8.

16. Ploutz-Snyder LL, Giamis EL. Orientation and familiarization to 1RM strength testing in old and young women. *J Strength Cond Res.* 2001;15:519–23.

17. Rikli RE, Jones CJ. Development and validation of a functional fitness test for community-residing older adults. *J Aging Phys Act.* 1999;7:129–61.

18. Rikli RE, Jones CJ. Functional fitness normative scores for community-residing older adults, ages 60–94. *J Aging Phys Act.* 1999;7:162–81.

19. Rikli RE, Jones CJ. *Senior Fitness Test Manual.* Champaign (IL): Human Kinetics; 2001.

20. *ACSM's Resource Manual for Guidelines for Exercise Testing and Prescription.* 6th ed. Baltimore (MD): Lippincott Williams & Wilkins; 2010.

21. Rowe DA, Kemble CD, Robinson TS, et al. Daily walking in older adults: Day-to-day variability and criterion-referenced validity of total daily step counts. *J Phys Act Health.* 2007;4:434–46.

22. Tran ZV, Weltman A. Predicting body composition of men from girth measurements. *Hum Biol.* 1988;60:167–75.

23. Tran ZV, Weltman A. Generalized equation for predicting body density of women from girth measurements. *Med Sci Sports Exerc.* 1989;21:101–4.

CHAPTER 8

Healthy Lifestyles in Old Age: Integrating Physical Activity with Nutrition to Maintain a Healthy Body Composition and Prevent Disability

Ellen M. Evans, Dolores D. Guest, Rudy J. Valentine, and Anne E. O'Brien

● ● ● **CHAPTER OUTLINE**

INTRODUCTION

If an older adult has routine health checkups and good health care, what else can be done to maintain good health? The most important modifiable behaviors that can impact health in older adults are physical activity, nutrition, psychological management (*i.e.*, stress and depression), and alcohol and tobacco use. The benefits and recommendations regarding the first factor, physical activity, have been addressed extensively in the previous chapters and will also be integrated into this chapter. The recommendations for the last two factors are simple: avoid smoking and other tobacco use completely and limit alcohol consumption. Notably, all of the above-listed health behaviors are often related to each other. For example, the diet, especially caloric intake, can greatly influence weight and body composition, which are also impacted by physical activity. In addition, it is well documented that decreased psychological well-being, including anxiety and depression, often triggers poor eating behaviors and greater alcohol intake. On the other hand, increased physical activity is associated with enhanced psychological well-being.

The concept of energy balance with regard to weight management is relatively simple in principle; that is, if a person takes in more calories than they expend, weight gain will occur; alternatively, if expended energy is greater than dietary energy intake, then weight loss will occur. Although understanding the fundamentals of energy balance (*i.e.*, calories in and calories out) is relatively simple, to manage energy intake and expenditure behaviors is very challenging, as evidenced by the growing obesity epidemic. It is appreciated by many that being overweight or obese is not healthy, and being overweight or overfat in older age can have even greater negative consequences on physical and emotional health (27). Indeed, the aging or "graying" of our society along with the obesity epidemic is predicted to overwhelm our health care system with excessive numbers of individuals who have chronic diseases and physical disability (27). In addition to the many known diseases associated with obesity (*e.g.*, cardiovascular disease, diabetes, and cancer), which often occur in older adults, obesity is also strongly associated with physical disability. Unfortunately, there is no well-defined "best practice" regarding weight management in older adults. Aging is also associated with loss of muscle and bone mass, often leading to reductions in strength and physical functional ability and increased risk of bone fractures (1). These collective changes in body composition, increases in fat mass, and reductions in bone and lean mass that typically occur with age are often termed "disordered body composition." Research regarding disordered body composition with age and its link to reduced physical function, risk of physical disability, and ultimately loss of independence is an active area of research, clinical practice, and public health interest.

Lack of physical activity and poor nutrition behaviors can also negatively impact psychological well-being, potentially causing anxiety and depression, poor sleep quality, and ultimately, fatigue. Older individuals have the added challenge of combating fatigue to complete their activities of daily living to remain living independently. This chapter will provide an overview of the importance of both physical activity and nutrition to enhance successful aging using an integrated view of these behaviors to maintain a healthy body composition.

BODY COMPOSITION IN OLDER ADULTS

A healthy body composition is important at all ages; however, the importance of each component on health status changes as an individual becomes older. Oftentimes, the term *body composition* is used interchangeably with *body fat*. However, the definition of body composition is more complex than a way to simply describe fatness. Numerous models of body composition exist (*e.g.*, molecular and chemical); however, conceptually and from a disease perspective, it is useful to think about body composition as the three measurable components of fat, bone, and lean mass of the human body. The technology, dual-energy X-ray absorptiometry (commonly abbreviated as DXA or DEXA), to measure these three components of the body is routinely available in clinics as well as in research laboratories. These measures of body composition also relate to diseases that are most common in older adults. For example, as mentioned previously, it is well established that greater than normal levels of adiposity, being overweight and obese, are related to cardiovascular diseases (*e.g.*, heart disease and hypertension) and metabolic diseases (*e.g.*, Type 2 diabetes mellitus and cancer) (18). Reductions in bone mass are linked to osteoporosis, placing an individual at higher risk for breaking a bone (1). Finally, age-associated loss of muscle mass and strength, termed *sarcopenia,* is also related to morbidity and mortality (6).

In addition to the link between body composition and physical diseases discussed above, physical activity and nutrition behaviors (and their effects on body composition) can also influence psychological well-being. Physical activity is well established as prevention and as a treatment for some types of anxiety and depressive disorders. Nutritional intake can also directly influence the risk of anxiety (*e.g.*, caffeine intake) and depression (*e.g.*, malnutrition). Newer research has focused on the importance of fatigue prevention in older adults, and the link between physical activity, nutrition, and weight status is of high interest (19). Most people think of fatigue as exhaustion or lack of energy. Loss of "vitality" is a common perception of older adults. Fatigue is very prevalent in older adults, with some estimates suggesting as many as 50% of older adults experience fatigue severe enough to negatively impact behaviors, limiting social, physical, and mental activities (29). Physical inactivity and higher levels of body fat are both associated with more fatigue in older adults (19, 29). Maintenance of vigor in late life is another reason to practice good health behaviors, specifically physical activity and nutrition, to maintain a healthy body composition.

Evaluation of weight status and body composition changes with aging

A body mass index (BMI) is a measure that relates a person's weight to his or her height and is commonly expressed in kilograms (weight) to meters squared (height) or $kg \cdot m^{-2}$. Having a BMI between 18.5 and 24.9 $kg \cdot m^{-2}$ is considered normal and healthy, with greater values being defined as overweight or obese (see

Table 8–1 Body Weight–Related Classifications for Older Adults		
	Men	**Women**
BMI (kg·m⁻²)	BMI standards are the same for men and women	
Underweight	<18.5	
Normal	18.5–24.9	
Overweight	25.0–29.9	
Obese	30.0–39.9	
Extreme obesity	40.0 and above	
Relative body fat (%)		
Healthy	10–25	25–38
Obese	>25	>38
Waist circumference (cm or in)		
Unhealthy	>102 or > 40	>88 or >35

Adapted with permission from World Health Organization. *Obesity: Preventing and Managing the Global Epidemic* (Report of a WHO Consultation; World Health Organization Technical Report Series 894). Geneva, Switzerland: World Health Organization; 2000.

Table 8-1), with the latter being related to an increased risk of disease (18). The use of BMI is common in large population studies of health status and is often used by a physician to evaluate the health of his or her patients. However, BMI may not accurately reflect changes in body composition that occur with aging. The amount of body fat that one has is typically expressed in relation to one's body weight or the percentage of one's weight that is fat mass (*i.e.*, %Fat). With the normal aging process, bone and lean mass are lost while fat mass is gained. A person often loses height as well. This means that the relationship between height and weight changes in an older person compared with a younger adult. For example, if a person has a BMI of 25 kg·m⁻² at the age of 30 and this remains constant through the age of 80, he or she will have more body fat late in life for the same BMI. Importantly, this body composition shift is often disguised, and may not be noticed by typical clinical measures. Therefore, assessing body composition is as important as assessing BMI to determine health status, especially for the older adult (1). A summary of BMI, %Fat, and health status classifications for older adults is provided in Table 8-1.

KEY POINT 8-1

Body Mass Index (BMI), a measure that relates a person's weight to their height, is often used to evaluate health; however, with older adults, the accuracy is limited because of changes in height and body composition.

Body composition refers to the various components of the human body and is generally divided into fat, bone, and lean mass. Fat mass can be further divided into essential fat, that which is necessary for normal functioning, and storage fat, that which is issued as an energy source. The role of essential fat is to provide insulation and padding to the internal organs and to maintain body temperature and healthy cell function. As the name implies, it is essential to live. The two primary locations where fat is stored in the body are subcutaneous (or just beneath the skin) and in the visceral or intraabdominal depot (or deep within the abdominal cavity). Nearly all of the minerals of the human body are contained in the bones. In general, higher bone mass and density is associated with higher bone strength. Strong bones protect against fractures. Because bone mass is not fat mass, it is technically considered part of lean mass. Although it is more accurate to label muscle mass as "mineral (or bone) free lean mass," it can be thought of simply as lean mass. Lean mass contains the majority of the protein and water stores of the human body and is greater than 90% skeletal muscle. The DXA allows the body to be quantified into these three components of fat, bone, and lean mass (see Figures 8-1 and 8-3).

The normal aging process is associated with changes in body composition. Bone and lean mass are greatest during young adulthood (~30 yr of age), and thereafter a steady decline occurs in both. Fat mass increases with age, and the location of the fat mass is redistributed such that there is a relative increase in intraabdominal fat along with a decrease in relative subcutaneous fat (1). This redistribution of fat is bad for health because a larger waist girth is associated with increased risk for many diseases, including cardiovascular diseases, diabetes, and some cancers (18). See Table 8-1 for health status classifications related to waist circumference.

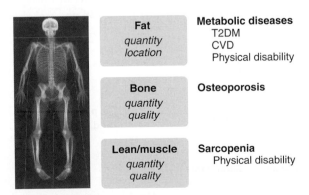

FIGURE 8-1   The link between main components of body composition (fat, bone, and lean mass) and public health challenges. Picture depicts a DXA scan of a young healthy adult

Body composition, physical function, and risk for physical disability

Becoming physically disabled is a major concern for many older adults. Physical disability can be thought of as the inability to fulfill a desired or necessary social or personal role (17). For many older adults, disability means the loss of mobility and independence or the inability to do activities of daily living such as bathing, dressing, cooking, and housework. Changes in all three components of body composition associated with aging can have a significant effect on an individuals' ability to perform activities of daily living. Therefore, a healthy body composition is important for older adults to preserve physical function, as reductions in function are related to falling, injuries, dependency on others, declines in cognition, and ultimately mortality (1, 6).

KEY POINT 8-2

The risk for physical disability is greatly increased when an older adult is overweight or obese, as the available strength cannot move the body weight.

The three-component model of body composition (fat, bone, and lean mass) can also be a useful framework to evaluate the risk for physical disability. The link between bone health and disability is easy to understand. Age-associated loss of bone mass, which reduces bone strength, may result in a bone fracture. Fracture of a bone, especially the hip, immediately reduces physical function and, depending on recovery, can cause a loss of independence (Figure 8-2).

The path from obesity to physical disability can be both indirect and direct. Notably, obesity has been identified as the greatest cause of disability in older adults (5, 27). Excessive body fat can lead to the development of chronic diseases, with the diseases themselves and oftentimes the treatment (*e.g.*, cancer and radiation) negatively impacting body composition and physical function. Higher levels of body fat have also been linked to reductions in lower-extremity physical function, limited mobility, and elevated risk for physical disability in older

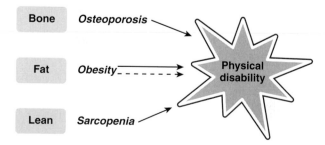

FIGURE 8-2   Pathways from main components of body composition to physical disability in older adults

adults (1, 27). This appears to be particularly true in the initial stages of disability, leading to loss of mobility.

Declines in skeletal muscle mass can also negatively impact physical function in a number of ways. The reduction in muscle mass is associated with declines in strength, muscle power, and endurance in older adults. Furthermore, it is well established that loss of strength often results in functional limitations (1, 28). Lower levels of muscle mass may not be problematic if the load being carried (*i.e.*, total body mass) is relatively low as well. On the other end of the spectrum, an individual with a high level of muscle mass but a disproportionately elevated total body mass will likely be challenged to physically function. In this manner, there is an interaction between amounts of fat mass and muscle mass.

Individuals at greatest risk for disability are those with excess body fat and inadequate muscle mass, termed *sarcopenic obesity,* which unfortunately represents a rapidly growing proportion of the population (1, 5, 28). Simply put, although muscle strength is important, only assessing strength fails to account for the "load" to be moved. In tasks of daily living, this is thought of as total body mass, which is made up largely of fat mass in the older adult. Note that it is very common to have a relative body fat of ~40% to 50% in an older woman, which means that nearly half of the body weight is fat mass.

The sarcopenic obese condition leads to reductions in physical function; moreover, it is a leading cause of frailty in older adults (1, 5, 28). In turn, frailty is a major risk factor for falling and bone fractures. The combined effects of decreasing lean and bone mass with concomitant increases in fat mass represent an ever increasing public health challenge. As the obesity epidemic and graying of America both continue, it is plausible to contend that the physical (physical limitation, physical disabilities, chronic disease states), mental (depression, reductions in quality of life), and financial (indirect and direct costs) burdens of sarcopenic obesity are a foremost health concern for older adults and will likely be the greatest public health challenge (Figure 8-3).

Muscle quality: definitions and importance for successful aging

Both aging and reductions in physical activity (which are related) have been determined to influence muscle mass and strength. These age-related changes are a result of several factors, including muscle fiber atrophy (reduction in fiber size) and hypoplasia (reduction in fiber number). The question remains: Is muscle weakness with aging primarily due to a loss of muscle mass or other factors? Actually, during the aging process, a mismatch between losses in muscle mass and muscle strength begins to occur (6). That is to say, older adults appear to lose more strength than can be accounted for by their loss of muscle mass. Looking at this another way, the remaining muscle is weaker than it should be, or has less ability to produce force. This phenomenon is explained as a loss in muscle quality.

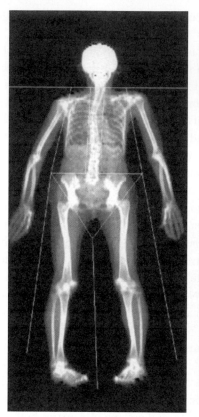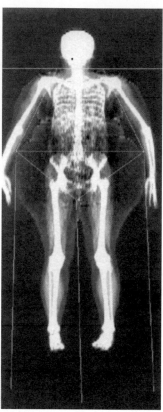

FIGURE 8-3   Examples of DXA scans depicting older women of the same age, but differing in body composition. Figure on the left is a woman who is frail with 18% body fat; figure on the right is a woman who is sarcopenic obese with 52% body fat. Note that both women have similar amounts of lean mass

KEY POINT 8-3

Muscle quality is defined as the amount of force production for a given amount of muscle or muscle strength relative to muscle mass.

Muscle quality is most often defined as muscle strength normalized (or relative) to muscle mass. In clinical research, it is calculated as strength divided by muscle mass (strength/mass). Quantification of muscle quality is dependent on the resources available. The ideal measurement of muscle quality would incorporate the ability to precisely assess muscle cross-sectional area and simultaneously elucidate strength producing capabilities of the measured muscle mass (20). This type of measurement requires imaging techniques such as magnetic resonance imaging (MRI) or computed tomography (CT). Using imaging techniques, muscle quality can also be assessed in terms of the *effective* muscle physiological cross-sectional area, or the composition of the muscle itself. Aging, obesity, and a sedentary lifestyle all contribute to changes in muscle composition, or reductions in muscle quality evidenced by fat infiltration into muscle (giving the muscle a marbling pattern, similar to the appearance of a low-quality steak). Similar to the muscle quality defined above (muscle strength/ muscle mass), this fat infiltration into the muscle and reductions in muscle quality are also related to increased mobility limitations in well-functioning older individuals (Figure 8-4) (28).

A more common approach to obtaining indicators of muscle quality is using DXA to quantify lean tissue (a proxy of muscle mass) and normalizing strength to this measured lean mass. In fact, muscle quality defined using DXA of the legs (the primary muscles used to walk and for most tasks of daily living) has been determined to be the most important factor for physical function in obese frail older individuals (26). The growing availability of DXA instruments, particularly in the clinical set- ting, makes this an available and informative approach to assessing muscle quality. Middle-aged and older adults typically get "bone scans" using DXA to measure bone mass and density to assess the risk of osteoporosis. It is anticipated in the future that whole body scans will also measure fat and lean mass to evaluate the risk of obesity and sarcopenia. Now that it is clear that body composition is important for success- ful aging, guidance regarding how to obtain healthy levels of fat, bone, and lean mass will be explored.

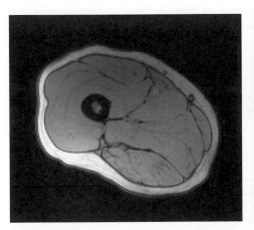 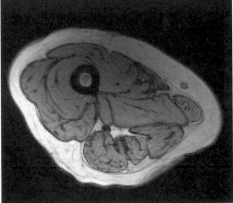

FIGURE 8-4   Examples of MRI images of the thigh for a physically active normal weight young woman (**left**) and an inactive normal weight older woman (**right**). Although the circumferences of the thighs are similar, note the differences in subcutaneous adipose tissue (light-colored band on perimeter of the thigh) and fat within the muscle itself illustrating lower muscle quality in the older woman

STRATEGIES FOR OLDER ADULTS TO OBTAIN A HEALTHY BODY COMPOSITION

Healthy body composition at any age, but especially in late life, is influenced by three main factors: hormones, physical activity, and nutrition. Conceptually, this can be thought of as a "three-legged stool," with the strongest and most stable stool having all three legs in balance and individually strong. The most familiar example relates to bone status and osteoporosis. For example, a typical older woman can have excellent nutritional and physical activity habits; however, owing to reductions in estrogen that occur at menopause she can still become high risk for osteoporosis. The risk of nontraumatic bone fracture can be the result of bone-dependent influences (*e.g.*, bone mass and bone density) or bone-independent influences (*e.g.*, muscle strength, balance, and reaction time), which contribute to fall risk. The International Osteoporosis Foundation has provided recommendations on how to maintain healthy bones (19). However, it should be appreciated that the "three-legged stool" concept applies to all three main body composition components — fat, bone, and lean mass (Table 8-2).

KEY POINT 8-4

All components of body composition (fat, bone, and lean mass) are influenced by three main factors: hormones, physical activity, and nutrition.

Table 8–2   Modifiable Risk Factors for Osteoporosis Prevention

Risk	Facts	How to Modify
Alcohol	● People with excessive alcohol consumption (>2 drinks daily) have a 40% increased risk of sustaining any osteoporotic fracture compared with people with moderate or no alcohol intake.	● Men should consume <3 drinks·day^{-1}; women <2 drinks·day^{-1}.
	● High intakes of alcohol negatively affect bone-forming cells and lead to poor nutritional status.	
Smoking	● People with a past history of cigarette smoking and people who smoke are at increased risk for any fracture compared with nonsmokers	● Do not smoke.
Low BMI	● Leanness (BMI <20 kg·m^{-2}), regardless of age, sex, and weight loss, is associated with greater bone loss and increased risk of fracture.	● Maintain BMI within 20–25 kg·m^{-2}.

Risk	Facts	How to Modify
	• People with a BMI of 20 kg·m⁻² have a two-fold increased risk of fracture compared with people with a BMI of 25 kg·m⁻².	
Poor nutrition	• When insufficient calcium is absorbed from dietary sources, bones break down and sacrifice bone calcium to supply the nerves and muscles with the mineral needed.	• Consume enough calories for optimal nutrition.
	• There are indications that protein is also important in that it may act synergistically with vitamin D and calcium.	• In many cases, supplementation is necessary to take in enough vitamin D and calcium.
Vitamin D deficiency	• Vitamin D helps calcium absorption from the intestines into the blood. Vitamin D is made in our skin with exposure to the sun's ultraviolet rays. In most people, casual exposure to the sun for as little as 10 to 15 minutes a day is usually sufficient. However, for people who do not go outdoors, and during the winter months in northern latitudes, food or supplemental sources of vitamin D are often needed.	• At least 800 international units of vitamin D and 1,000–1,200 mg of calcium daily can protect against osteoporosis.
Eating disorders	• Osteoporosis can also be compounded by eating disorders such as anorexia nervosa and bulimia.	• Seek treatment for any disordered eating behavior.
Estrogen deficiency	• Estrogen acts like a "brake" for bone breakdown and calcium release into the blood. Therefore, if estrogen is not optimal, depending on life stage (puberty, childbearing years, or after menopause), bones will not build as they should prior to ~30 yrs of age, and bone loss will be accelerated after peak bone mass is attained.	• Talk with your doctor about estrogen imbalances to decide the best course of action.
Insufficient exercise	• People with a more sedentary lifestyle are more likely to have a hip fracture than those who are more active. For example, women who sit for more than 9 h a day are 50% more likely to have a hip fracture than those who sit for less than 6 h a day.	• Meet exercise recommendations outlined for your appropriate age group.
Frequent falls	• Visual impairments, loss of balance, neuromuscular dysfunction, dementia, immobilization, and use of sleeping pills are quite common conditions in older persons, significantly increase the risk of falling, and accordingly increase the risk of fracture.	• Treat any underlying issues to minimize the risk and/or frequency of falls.
	• 90% of hip fractures result from falls.	

Adapted with permission from International Osteoporosis Foundation Web site [Internet]. Nyon, Switzerland: International Osteoporosis Foundation; [cited 2010 Dec 27]. Available from: http://www.iofbonehealth.org/patients-public/about-osteoporosis/symptoms-risk-factors/modifiable.html

Hormones

Although hormonal evaluation and treatment is not within the exercise professional's scope of practice, it is beneficial to be aware of the normal changes with aging and the most common clinical abnormality that can influence body composition components. The primary influential hormones on body composition are the growth hormone and the sex steroids (primarily estrogen and testosterone). As part of the normal aging process, reductions in these hormones have profound and well-characterized effects on body composition, including (a) increased whole body fatness, (b) increased fat storage in the central depots (abdomen region), (c) a reduction in bone mass, and (d) a reduction in lean mass.

Although an extensive literature supports the benefits of hormone therapy for body composition in older adults, routine prescriptions are not endorsed by the medical community because of adverse side effects and other health risks. The most common abnormal change that is often seen in older adults, especially women, is alterations in thyroid function. Hypothyroidism can cause weight gain, specifically fat mass, whereas hyperthyroidism can cause weight loss and abnormal reductions in bone mass. Hormone evaluation and potential therapy is a decision between an older adult and his or her physician; however, it is important to recognize that hormones can have major implications for all body composition components.

Physical activity

Physical inactivity is directly linked to reduced muscle mass and quality and reductions in physical functional ability; habitual physical activity has been consistently associated with improvements in physical function (4, 13). The benefits of physical activity have been documented as a prolonged time until mobility disability occurs in the lifespan (and loss of independence) as well as clinically meaningful improvements in physical function testing scores in the research laboratory.

KEY POINT 8-5

Habitual physical activity can reduce feelings of fatigue, thereby giving more vigor for physical activity, resulting in a "positive behavioral cycle."

Many research studies have shown that the muscle of older adults remains highly adaptable to exercise training. Although recommendations regarding other health outcomes (*e.g.*, cardiovascular disease prevention) are well established, the quantity and intensity of physical activity required to obtain benefits in physical function are currently not established. However, several aspects consistently appear across most, if not all, recommendations.

It is unquestionable that muscular strength plays an important role in physical performance, as evidenced by athletic events. However, this relationship extends to less conventional aspects of "performance" for older adults, including daily activities such as getting up and down from a chair or car, walking from the car to the store and back, and carrying and lifting groceries to a countertop or cupboard. It is clear that even light or modest levels of endurance types of physical activity, such as walking, are sufficient to influence physical function performance, with limited added benefit of more intense training (4). This finding has great public health significance, as older adults can positively influence their physical function ability simply by increasing their daily activity levels, without the burden of high-intensity "training."

Some evidence also suggests that muscle power, the ability to produce force quickly, may also be an important predictor of physical functional ability (12). Muscle power appears to decline earlier in life than does muscle strength, likely because of changes in muscle fibers and reduced contractile properties of the muscle. Many of the most challenging tasks for older adults, such as getting off the sofa or out of a chair, require short bursts of strength, or are reliant on muscle power, rather than total muscle strength. Similarly, challenges to balance require a rapid production of strength to quickly regain posture and prevent falling. Incorporating some basic power training into an exercise program is beneficial in this regard.

In addition to resistance training (for muscle strength, endurance, and power) and cardiovascular endurance training, a well-rounded exercise program to prevent physical disability in older adults also includes flexibility, balance, and functional training. The latter includes specificity training such as getting up and out of a chair and other activities that simulate "real life." Activities that challenge balance and coordination using situations potentially encountered in daily life (*e.g.*, recovering from loss of balance) are also important (27).

Real Life Story 8-1   Jean — Resistance Training

Jean, a 74-year-old grandmother of 9, enjoyed an active lifestyle including playing with grandchildren, gardening, and taking care of her husband, David, who had become disabled in a car accident. However, in the past 5 years, Jean noticed increased difficulty when trying to care for her husband, but thought it was inevitable and due to normal aging. With encouragement from friends, Jean decided to join a strength training class for older adults. The class met 3 times a week for an hour each session and included a warm-up, light stretching, and traditional strength training. At first, Jean was discouraged because she was able to lift only a small amount of weight and could not complete three sets of 12 repetitions for each exercise. However, as the class went on, Jean was able to lift more weight and complete more repetitions. By the end of the 6 months, Jean had doubled the amount of weight she was able to lift with her legs! But what really mattered to Jean was that she could see the benefits of the strength training class in her everyday life. She was able to help her husband without becoming out of breath. Jean even noticed that she was able to get down on the floor and play with her grandchildren with less difficulty. As a result of her newfound strength, Jean has once again taken up an old hobby — gardening. As a result of the strength training class, Jean not only developed more confidence and strength, but was also able to continue participating in her favorite activities with people she loved.

In addition to the "physical" importance of physical activity for physical function, it is important to recognize the important psychological aspects as well. Reduced muscle mass and strength decreases the capacity to perform physical work and the relative workload of a given task (*i.e.*, lifting the gallon of milk is "harder") and increases fatigue. As an older adult is more physically active, feelings of fatigue will be reduced and more confidence for future activity will occur, resulting in a "positive behavioral cycle." Alternatively, older adults are much more susceptible to general fatigability, or exercise-induced tiredness. Doing too much too soon could be counterproductive and reduce adherence to any exercise program. Furthermore, older adults must maintain enough energy to be capable of completing their necessary daily tasks. Other chapters in this book outline effective strategies to enhance adherence to physical activity in older adults.

Nutrition

Regarding successful aging, the balance of nutrients is just as important as physical activity to maintain a healthy body composition. The Food and Nutrition Board (FNB) of the Institute of Medicine (IOM), the Department of Health and Human Services (HHS), and the United States Department of Agriculture (USDA), the main governing bodies for nutrition recommendations, have established nutrient intake recommendations across the life-span, including for older adults. For the purposes of these recommendations, all dietary plans are divided by calorie level. These recommendations are further divided into food groups within calorie levels for both men and women to ensure meeting various nutrient needs (24). It is important to note that these recommendations are for relatively healthy older adults. Discussed below are important changes that occur with aging that can alter food intake and cause potential malnourishment, even in the presence of obesity. Finally, a brief discussion of various nutrient recommendations will be presented in Table 8-3.

Physiological changes

There are a number of physiological changes that affect food intake and directly impact nutritional status as one becomes older. First, most people experience a decline in the sense of smell and some also experience a loss of ability to taste, both of which have been shown to affect how much and what foods will be selected by older adults at a given meal (15). Second, changes in oral health can also result in a decreased nutritional status. Tooth loss, ill-fitting dentures, and even swallowing disorders inhibit normal or pleasurable food intake. People frequently eat less or choose different foods (often softer, lower-nutrient foods) to avoid discomfort at meal times (23). Third, there are several appetite-regulating hormones that are altered with age. For example, cholecystokinin (CCK) — a hormone that triggers feelings of fullness — is chronically elevated in older individuals compared with their younger counterparts (11).

Table 8–3 Recommended Daily Food Intake by Food Groups per Calorie Intake Level

Food Group	Calorie Level						
	1,600	1,800	2,000	2,200	2,400	2,600	2,800
Fruits	1.5 c (3 srv)	1.5 c (3 srv)	2 c (4 srv)	2 c (4 srv)	2 c (4 srv)	2 c (4 srv)	2.5 c (5 srv)
Vegetables	2 c (4 srv)	2.5 c (5 srv)	2.5 c (5 srv)	3 c (6 srv)	3 c (6 srv)	3.5 c (7 srv)	3.5 c (7 srv)
Dark green vegetables (c wk^{-1})	2	3	3	3	3	3	3
Orange vegetables (c wk^{-1})	1.5	2	2	2	2	2.5	2.5
Legumes (c wk^{-1})	2.5	3	3	3	3	3.5	3.5
Starchy vegetables (c wk^{-1})	2.5	3	3	6	6	7	7
Other vegetables (c wk^{-1})	5.5	6.5	7.5	7	7	8.5	8.5
Grains (oz-eq)	5	6	6	7	8	9	10
Whole grains	2	3	3	3.5	4	4.5	5
Other grains	2	3	3	3.5	4	4.5	5
Lean meat and beans (oz-eq)	5	5	5.5	6	6.5	6.5	7
Milk (c)	3	3	3	3	3	3	3
Oils (g)	22	24	27	29	31	34	36
Discretionary calories	132	195	267	290	362	410	426

Food group amounts shown in cup (c) or ounce-equivalents (oz-eq), with number of servings (srv) in parentheses when it differs from the other units. See *Dietary Guidelines for Americans, 2005* for more details.

Adapted with permission from U.S. Department of Health and Human Services and U.S. Department of Agriculture. *Dietary Guidelines for Americans, 2005* (HHS Publication number: HHS-ODPHP-2005-01-DGA-A). Washington (DC): U.S. Government Printing Office; 2005.

These circulating indicators of positive energy balance could partially explain decreases in appetite reported by people as they age. Fourth, changes in absorption during digestion may result in changes in proper use of nutrients by the body. For example, older adults have *reduced* intestinal absorption of carbohydrates, proteins and dietary lipids, vitamin D, and calcium (16). The current dietary recommendations for older Americans were developed in part on the basis of these changes in absorption of various nutrients and in part to address the importance of maintaining a healthy body composition.

Key nutrients

To maintain a healthy body composition, the changing role of overall energy (calories), macronutrients (carbohydrates, lipids/fats, protein), and key micronutrients (vitamins: B$_6$, B$_{12}$, folate, and D; minerals: calcium) in the older adult will be the focus.

Energy (calorie) needs. With aging, calorie needs generally decrease; however, this is also related to reductions in energy expenditure because of physical activity (21). Recall from above that to remain in energy balance, dietary caloric intake needs to align with energy expenditure. As expected, the more active a person is, the higher the caloric needs will be at any stage of life. In addition, typically, a larger person will expend more calories for a given activity than a smaller person. Because of these two factors, physical activity levels and body size, it is difficult to estimate total daily energy expenditure precisely. Consultation with a registered dietitian may be appropriate for an older adult if energy balance is an issue. It is also important to balance nutrients (carbohydrate, protein, fat, vitamins, and minerals) within the appropriate calorie level and focus on nutrient dense foods (high nutrients/g) to ensure maximal health and weight management (24). It is critical to note that because the energy intake requirements needed to remain in energy balance are relatively low (see Table 8-3 — discretionary calories), the older adult, especially a smaller-framed female, will have very few discretionary calories (see Tables 8-3 and 8-4), which is one major reason why obesity is a problem in older adults: Calories used in physical activity are not enough to offset the "empty" calories taken in as sweets and snack foods.

Carbohydrate. Carbohydrates are an important part of the diet because they provide the body's cells with energy. Carbohydrates include grains (rice, breads, pasta, etc.), fruits, and some vegetables. In mid- and late life, insulin resistance may start to become an issue, leading to people becoming very "carb-conscious." Although balancing carbohydrate intake with insulin is important, it is not generally recommended that people eliminate carbohydrates from their diet under normal circumstances because of their use by the body (and especially by the brain) as fuel, nor is

Table 8-4 Estimated Calorie Requirements for a "Reference Size" Older Adult Aged 51 and Above

Activity Level	Woman	Man
Sedentary[a]	1,600	2,000
Moderately active[b]	1,800	2,200–2,400
Active[c]	2,000–2,200	2,400–2,800

Note: The calorie ranges shown are to accommodate needs of different aged individuals within the group, with fewer calories being needed at older ages.
[a]Sedentary means a lifestyle that includes only the light physical activity associated with typical day-to-day life.
[b]Moderately active means a lifestyle that includes physical activity equivalent to walking about 1.5 to 3 miles·day^{-1} at 3 to 4 miles·hour^{-1}, in addition to the light physical activity associated with typical day-to-day life.
[c]Active means a lifestyle that includes physical activity equivalent to walking more than 3 miles·day^{-1} at 3 to 4 miles·hour^{-1}, in addition to the light physical activity associated with typical day-to-day life.
Adapted with permission from U.S. Department of Health and Human Services and U.S. Department of Agriculture. *Dietary Guidelines for Americans, 2005* (HHS Publication number: HHS-ODPHP-2005-01-DGA-A). Washington (DC): U.S. Government Printing Office; 2005.

it necessary to increase carbohydrate intake in relation to the rest of the diet (24). A subgroup of carbohydrates is fiber. Fiber is important for maintaining proper gut health (*e.g.*, preventing constipation), and higher intakes have been associated with lower incidence of colon cancer and lower levels of circulating cholesterol, as well as triggering feelings of fullness (9).

Lipids. Lipids (or fats) in the diet are also a key element because they not only provide flavor and texture to foods but are also carriers of fat-soluble vitamins, act as important building blocks for many hormones, and perform other essential functions throughout the body. Even with age, the body may not absorb fats as efficiently as it once could, but by eating a balanced diet, enough is generally absorbed for proper function. Also, owing to lower calorie needs in older age, less fat, which is calorically dense, is needed (22). No matter what age, it is important to focus on higher intake of the healthy fats — monounsaturated fatty acids (MUFAs; olive oil, avocados, etc.), polyunsaturated fatty acids (PUFAs; nuts, seeds, etc.), and specifically omega-3 and -6 oils (found in fatty fish and nuts) — and on lower intake of saturated fats (found in red meat, butter, etc.) and trans-fats (found in processed foods such as shortening and prepackaged crackers, cookies, etc.).

Protein. Protein is a key macronutrient for muscle building and maintenance. Similar to other macronutrients, there is a slightly diminished absorption rate of protein in older adults. However, many studies conclude that there is not necessarily an increased need for protein, above that found in a balanced diet (0.8 g protein per kg body weight), although this level remains an active area of research (21). Considering the importance of muscle maintenance, high-quality lean proteins in the form of fish, poultry, dairy, and soy should be a major focus in the diet of older adults (21).

B Vitamins and folate. Circulating levels of vitamin B_6 appear to diminish with age. This vitamin is important for normal metabolic function and enzymatic activity (14). Because of its importance, people aged 50 and above are encouraged to increase their intake through adequate intake of a varied diet or through supplementation (8). With age, adults also lose the ability to effectively absorb naturally occurring vitamin B_{12}, which can lead to an otherwise rare form of anemia (pernicious anemia), resulting in fatigue. Because of this, it is recommended that adults aged 50 and above focus on eating foods fortified with vitamin B_{12} such as fortified cereals or take crystalline B_{12} supplements ($2.4\ \mu g \cdot d^{-1}$) to ensure adequate intake (24). Folate (or folic acid) is yet another B vitamin, key for optimal cellular function. Folate levels are not affected by aging, but are quickly diminished by consuming a poor diet, often resulting in supplementation. However, elevated folate levels (from fortified food sources or supplementation) can mask B_{12} deficiency, resulting in delayed diagnosis and treatment, which can further compromise health status (25).

Vitamin D and calcium. Adequate vitamin D is important for bone maintenance and hormone function. It is recommended that "older adults, people with dark skin, and people exposed to insufficient ultraviolet band radiation (*i.e.,* sunlight) consume extra vitamin D from vitamin D-fortified foods and/or supplements" (24). Both women and men aged 70 and above should consume 800 IU of vitamin D daily (7). Vitamin D is important not only for bone health, but also for muscle mass and physical function, especially in older adults, as suggested by increasing research (3). Of equal importance to bone health is calcium intake. Calcium is considered a "nutrient of concern" for all adults, but it is highly important that adequate amounts be consumed in either supplement or natural form (*i.e.,* food — dairy, leafy greens, etc.) for bone maintenance. Women aged 50 and above and men aged 70 and above should have 1,200 mg of calcium daily (7). Importantly, upper limits have been set for supplementation for both of these nutrients (vitamin D = 4,000 IU d^{-1} and calcium = 2,000 mg d^{-1}). Excessive intakes of vitamin D can result in kidney and tissue damage, while extreme levels of calcium can lead to kidney stones (7).

Summary of nutrition

The aging process can alter the way a person makes food choices (appetite, pleasure, etc.) and how nutrients are absorbed. The key macronutrients and micronutrients and energy balance needs for a healthy body composition were addressed. For safety reasons, it is critical to seek appropriate expertise and advice from a registered dietitian with regard to the diet before drastically changing behaviors. This is especially important regarding weight management as weight loss is more complicated in older adults.

WEIGHT LOSS IN OLDER ADULTS

Unfortunately, there is no well-defined "best practice" regarding weight management in older adults primarily for two reasons. First, the public health problem of obesity in older adults is a new phenomenon in terms of prevalence, having greatly increased in the past decade or so as the obese "middle-aged" adults became older (2, 5). With the increases in medical technologies, obesity-related diseases can now be cured or managed, enabling the older adult to live a longer life. Consequently, overweight and obese adults are living longer. Second, the typical solution for obesity (*i.e.,* weight loss) is more complicated in older adults compared with their younger counterparts, and best practice is still being established with ongoing research (27).

Body composition changes during weight loss in older adults

The main components of body composition — fat, bone, and lean mass — are all interrelated. For young adults, in general, greater amounts of lean and fat mass are related to greater bone mass and density, with lean mass having a stronger relation to bone status. In older adults, these relations are generally true; however, it also depends on initial bone density and lean mass status, if the person is able to move (*i.e.*, can load the bones with his or her body weight), and the person's hormone status (*e.g.*, estrogen levels).

Similarly, when an individual loses weight, he or she will typically lose bone mass and lean mass. The magnitude of these losses is dependent on how much weight is lost, if a person exercised while losing the weight, the quality of the diet while losing weight (*e.g.*, calcium and protein), and the hormone status of the person (*e.g.*, estrogen levels). Paradoxically, the reduction in fat mass that reduces the risk of cardiovascular and metabolic diseases may increase the risk of osteoporosis and sarcopenia (27).

KEY POINT 8-6

Obese older adults should lose weight but only under medical supervision so as to lose minimal bone and lean muscle mass.

What is not well established is how changes in weight and body composition favorably affect physical function in older adults (1, 28). Theoretically, the small reduction in bone mass, or bone-dependent risk factor for fracture, is more than

Real Life Story 8-2   Linda — Weight Loss and Exercise

Linda is a 68-year-old woman. She is a retired secretary. She has four grown children and nine grandchildren. She is 6'4' tall and weighs 167 lb. She has been treated for hypertension for 6 years now. At her last doctor's appointment, she was told that she is prediabetic. Her doctor wants her to lose about 10 pounds in the next 6 months and then come back to see him. He refers Linda to a dietitian. At her appointment with the dietitian, Linda explains that she does not understand what prediabetes is but that her older sister had high blood pressure and diabetes and died of a heart attack 2 years ago at the age of 71. Linda also states that she never had any issues with her weight until she went through menopause and stopped working — both of which happened when she was 60. She is fearful and willing to do what the doctor wants, so she can avoid more medications and any complications from her diseases.

The dietitian works with Linda to develop a 1,600-calorie diet. She also encourages Linda to find things that she can do to increase her physical activity level. Linda talks to her friends and finds out that there is a program for people 50 years and older that meets every morning during the week where she can use a gym and take different exercise classes. Linda joins this group and begins to attend 3 days a week. She also sticks to her diet — which includes adding more vegetables, fruits, and fish and limiting red meats and fried foods. When Linda goes back to her doctor 6 months later, he is pleased to see that making these simple changes has allowed her to lose 12 pounds. He also sees that her blood pressure is actually low, so he changes her hypertension medication to the lowest possible dose. He tells her to continue on this regimen and come back in 6 more months. They will continue to monitor her hypertension and glucose levels, but for now, she has been able to avoid adding more medications.

offset by the increases in physical function and reductions in the risk of falling, a bone-independent risk factor for fracture. Alternatively, the reductions in lean mass with weight loss could also cause a reduction in strength and subsequently an adverse change in physical function. As the population ages and with the rising rates of obesity, the interactions of the body composition components and their implications for physical function will be an active area of research and of high clinical importance.

Recommended strategies for weight loss

The effect of weight loss on mortality in older adults is not always positive. Most studies indicate that weight loss is associated with an increase in mortality; however, most of these studies do not evaluate whether the older adults were initially lean or obese, nor do they control for *unintentional* weight loss, which is a common complication of serious disease such as cancer. Limited research in older adults, who are at higher risk for metabolic disease or suffering from osteoarthritis, indicates that moderate weight loss is beneficial for both physical and mental health (27).

Research indicates that weight loss treatment programs that focus on lifestyle intervention are as effective with older adults as with younger adults. Limited research also suggests that older adults are more compliant with the weight-reducing lifestyle therapy, losing more weight and maintaining the weight loss to a greater degree than middle-aged adults (27). There are three therapeutic options for weight management: (a) surgery, (b) pharmacotherapy, and (c) lifestyle and behavior modifications involving diet and physical activity. It is critical to note that all weight loss regimens in older adults should be undertaken only after consultation with the individual's personal physician. Obviously, the first two options are in the medical domain, whereas the exercise professional may play a role in the last choice (27).

KEY POINT 8-7

Exercise and optimal nutrition are needed for an older adult to lose weight safely.

The Obesity Society and the American Society for Nutrition have provided a position statement for obesity in older adults (27). Basic energy balance principles apply to the older adult. The most effective strategy to cause weight loss is caloric restriction. Although regular exercise or physical activity is not essential for achieving initial weight loss, abundant research documents that regular exercise is essential for maintaining weight loss and the prevention of weight regain in adults of all ages. Weight loss therapy that minimizes muscle and bone mass losses is recommended for older persons who are obese and who have physical functional impairments or metabolic complications that can benefit from weight loss. It is also recommended that a thorough medical history, physical examination, appropriate laboratory tests, review of medications, and assessment of readiness to lose weight are essential before beginning therapy to reduce weight status. The primary approach is to achieve sustained lifestyle change. Indeed, lifestyle modifications are critical to overcome barriers to comply with dietary and physical activity changes. This will require clinicians and others on the medical team to assist the older adult with the fundamentals of goal setting, self-monitoring strategies, developing social support, and stimulus control.

Older adults have special challenges to adhering to behavior changes required to reduce weight. They often have more chronic diseases to manage, a reduced quality of life, and more depression and cognitive dysfunction compared with younger adults, all of which complicate lifestyle changes. In addition, similar to children, dependency may be common; therefore, the lifestyle change program will need to include participation by family members and care providers. If the person is living in an institution where they do not control their food choices, this will also complicate behavior change strategies. Limited financial resources may also impact the success of the behavioral change program. Older adults may also have challenges to learning incurred with reductions in vision and hearing and comorbidities. Finally, use of medications is common in older adults, and they also have a high risk of medication-related problems. Evaluation of medications is critical as some may cause weight gain (*e.g.*, steroids and antidepressants). Importantly, weight loss–induced improvements in health status may require changes in medications such as insulin for Type 2 diabetes mellitus or hypertension medications.

Specific to caloric restriction, a modest reduction in energy intake (500–750 kcal·d^{-1}) is recommended. Very low calorie diets (<800 kcal·d^{-1}) are not recommended, as they often cause medical complications and also promote greater losses of bone and lean mass. The diet should contain ~1.0 g per kg of body weight of high-quality protein to reduce loss of muscle mass. In addition, multivitamin and mineral supplements will likely be needed to ensure that all daily recommended requirements are met to reduce loss of bone mass. The expertise of a registered dietitian may be needed to provide appropriate nutritional counseling.

The recommendations for an exercise prescription within a weight loss program are similar to general exercise recommendations. For older adults, the goal of the exercise regimen, within the context of a weight loss program, is to reduce loss of bone and muscle mass as well as to maintain or improve physical function. The specific objectives of the exercise program are to increase flexibility, endurance, and strength; therefore, a multicomponent program that includes flexibility and balance challenges, aerobic activity, and resistance exercise is recommended. After medical clearance including undergoing exercise stress testing if needed, the exercise program should be started gradually and progressed individually after considering chronic diseases and level of physical disability.

S U M M A R Y

This chapter highlighted the importance of physical activity and nutrition behaviors to maintain the health of the three main components of body composition (fat, bone, and lean mass) for successful aging. Healthy body composition is of primary importance in preventing reductions in physical function, risk for physical disability, and loss of independence. In addition, a healthy body composition can also enhance psychological well-being, especially reducing fatigue and maintaining vigor. Physical activity provides a proven method to slow the process of physical disability. Good nutrition is also essential. Regarding weight loss, reductions in fat mass, rather than focusing on gains in lean mass, appear to be a worthwhile target to maintain, or possibly regain physical function in older adults; however, care needs to be used to prevent further losses of bone and lean mass. Consulting with medical, exercise, and nutrition experts is essential when attempting changes with regard to physical activity and nutrition behaviors in older adults to prevent any harm to health. However, the human body remains remarkably adaptable to change into old age, and it is never too late to experience the physical and psychological benefits of healthy lifestyle choices.

QUESTIONS FOR REFLECTION

1. How is body composition defined?

2. What are the three main components?

3. How is body composition measured?

4. What are normal changes in body composition with the aging process?

5. How do the main components of body composition influence the risk for physical disability?

6. What is muscle quality and how is it measured?

7. How does muscle quality change with age and influence the risk for physical disability?

8. Discuss the main strategies to maintain a healthy body composition in old age.

9. How do changes with age impact our dietary patterns in terms of food choices, digestion, and nutrient needs?

10. What are the key recommendations for safe and effective weight loss as an older adult?

11. What are the main components of an exercise program to prevent physical disability?

REFERENCES

1. Alley DE, Ferrucci L, Barbagallo M, Studenski SA, Harris, TB. A research agenda: The changing relationship between body weight and health in aging. *J Gerontol A Biol Sci Med Sci.* 2008;63:1257–9.
2. Bouchard DR, Janssen I. Dynapenic-obesity and physical function in older adults. *J Gerontol A Biol Sci Med Sci.* 2010;65(1):71–7.
3. Bouvard B, Annweiler C, Sallé A, Beauchet O, Chappard D, Audran M, Legrand E. Extraskeletal effects of vitamin D: Facts, uncertainties, and controversies. *Joint Bone Spine.* 2011;78(1):10–6.
4. Brach JS, Simonsick EM, Kritchevsky S, Yaffe K, Newman AB. The association between physical function and lifestyle activity and exercise in the health, aging and body composition study. *J Am Geriatr Soc.* 2004;52:502–9.
5. Chen H, Guo X. Obesity and functional disability in elderly Americans. *J Am Geriatr Soc.* 2008;56(4):689–4.
6. Clark BC, Manini TM. Sarcopenia =/= dynapenia. *J Gerontol A Biol Sci Med Sci.* 2008; 63(8):829–34.
7. Food and Nutrition Board, Institute of Medicine. *Dietary Reference Intakes for Calcium and Vitamin D.* Washington (DC): National Academy Press; 2011.
8. Food and Nutrition Board, Institute of Medicine. *Dietary Reference Intakes for Thiamin, Riboflavin, Niacin, Vitamin B6, Folate, Vitamin B12, Pantothenic Acid, Biotin, and Choline.* Washington (DC): National Academy Press; 1998.
9. Gallaher DD, Schneeman BO. Dietary fiber. In: Bowman BA, Russell RM, editors. *Present Knowledge in Nutrition: Eighth Edition* (83-91). Washington (DC): ILSI Press; 2001.
10. International Osteoporosis Foundation Web site [Internet]. Nyon, Switzerland: International Osteoporosis Foundation; [cited 2010 Dec 27]. Available from: http://www.iofbonehealth.org/patients-public/about-osteoporosis/symptoms-risk-factors/modifiable.html
11. MacIntosh CG, Morley JE, Wishart J, Morris H, Jansen JB, Horowitz M, Chapman IM. Effect of exogenous cholecystokinin (CCK)-8 on food intake and plasma CCK, leptin, and insulin concentrations in older and young adults: Evidence for increased CCK activity as a cause of the anorexia of aging. *J Clin Endocrinol Metab.* 2001;86;5830–7.
12. Marsh AP, Miller ME, Saikin AM, et al. Lower extremity strength and power are associated with 400-meter walk time in older adults: The InCHIANTI study. *J Gerontol A Biol Sci Med Sci.* 2006;61:1186–93.
13. Martin HJ, Syddall HE, Dennison EM, Cooper C, Sayer AA. Relationship between customary physical activity, muscle strength and physical performance in older men and women: Findings from the Hertfordshire Cohort Study. *Age Ageing.* 2008;37:589–93.
14. McCormick DB. Vitamin B-6. In: Bowman BA, Russell RM, editors. *Present Knowledge in Nutrition: Eighth Edition* (207–213). Washington (DC): ILSI Press; 2001.
15. Morley JE. Anorexia of aging: Physiologic and pathologic. *Am J Clin Nutr.* 1997;66:760–73.
16. Morley JE. The aging gut: Physiology. *Clin Geriatr Med.* 2007;23:757–67.
17. Nagi S. Some conceptual issues in disability and rehabilitation. In: Sussman M, editor. *Sociology and Rehabilitation.* Washington (DC): American Sociological Association; 1965. p. 100–13.
18. World Health Organization. *Obesity: Preventing and Managing the Global Epidemic* (Report of a WHO Consultation; World Health Organization Technical Report Series 894). Geneva, Switzerland: World Health Organization; 2000.
19. Poluri A, Mores J, Cook DB, Findley TW, Cristian A. Fatigue in the elderly population. *Phys Med Rehabil Clin N Am.* 2005;16:91–108.
20. Reeves ND, Narici MV, Maganaris CN. Myotendinous plasticity to ageing and resistance exercise in humans. *Exp Physiol.* 2006;91:483–98.
21. Russell RM, Rasmussen H. The impact of nutritional needs of older adults on recommended food intakes. *Nutr Clin Care.* 1999;2(3);164–76.
22. Russell RM, Rasmussen H, Lichtenstein AH. Modified food guide pyramid for people over seventy years of age. *J Nutr.* 1999;129(3):751–753.
23. Sullivan DH, Martin W, Flaxman N, Hagen JE. Oral health problems and involuntary weight loss in a population of frail elderly. *J Am Geriatr Soc.*1993;41:725–31.
24. U.S. Department of Health and Human Services and U.S. Department of Agriculture. *Dietary Guidelines for Americans, 2005* (HHS Publication number: HHS-ODPHP-2005-01-DGA-A). Washington (DC): U.S. Government Printing Office; 2005.
25. Vellas BJ, Garry PJ. Aging. In: Bowman BA, Russell RM, editors. *Present Knowledge in Nutrition: Eighth Edition.* Washington (DC): ILSI Press; 2001. p. 439–46.

26. Villareal DT, Banks M, Siner C, Sinacore DR, Klein S. Physical frailty and body composition in obese elderly men and women. *Obes Res.* 2004;12:913–20.

27. Villareal DT, Apovian CM, Kushner RF, Klein S. Obesity in older adults: Technical review and position statement of the American Society for Nutrition and NAASO, The Obesity Society. *Am J Clin Nutr.* 2005;82:923–34.

28. Visser MM, Goodpaster BH, Kritchevsky SB, et al. Muscle mass, muscle strength, and muscle fat infiltration as predictors of incident mobility limitations in well-functioning older persons. *J Gerontol A Biol Sci Med Sci.* 2005;60(3):324–33.

29. Wick JY, LaFleur J. Fatigue: Implications for the elderly. *Consult Pharm.* 2007;22:566–70.

CHAPTER 9

Helping Older Adults Select the Physical Activity Program That's Right for Them

Michael E. Rogers, PhD, CSCS, FACSM, and
Nicole L. Rogers, PhD

CHAPTER OUTLINE

INTRODUCTION

As the previous chapters of this book have discussed, there is a large amount of scientific evidence demonstrating that regular physical activity can provide substantial health benefits to older adults. Physical activity offers one of the greatest opportunities to extend years of active independent life, reduce disability, and improve the quality of life for older adults (1). Despite these clear benefits, the majority of older adults do not participate in regular physical activity, and prescribing physical activity and/or specific exercise programs is not yet common practice (6). To enhance engagement in physical activity among older adults, we recommend a three-step process (11). The first is the screening process before initiating an activity program, the second is the prescription process, and the third is motivating the individual to begin and adhere to the exercise prescription.

PREACTIVITY SCREENING

The purpose of preactivity screening is to: (a) minimize the risk of injury or other serious adverse events such as musculoskeletal injury, falls, or cardiovascular events while achieving maximum benefit from physical activity; (b) identify medical issues so that exercise programs can be appropriately modified for safety and optimal benefit; and (c) identify functional limitations that the activity program will address (2, 3, 10).

Preactivity screening of older adults is a controversial issue, and opinions about the benefits and disadvantages of screening vary widely (4). Serious adverse events associated with physical activity are rare and unpredictable, and neither exercise stress tests nor screening questionnaires such as the Revised Physical Activity Readiness Questionnaire (rPAR-Q) (15) adequately identify the very small number of people at risk for such events (7). However, many guidelines and programs still strongly recommend "see a doctor first" (8), and older adults who want to begin a low- to moderate-level lifestyle activity program such as walking, swimming, or gardening are often reluctant to start if recommended to see a physician (11).

Preactivity screening is sometimes physically or psychologically traumatic and costly for the individual and the health care system, and sometimes prohibits those individuals who are most likely to benefit from low- to moderate-intensity physical activities from participating (12). Although the U.S. Preventative Task Force now advises against the use of exercise stress tests for asymptomatic individuals (16), recent guidelines from the American Heart Association and the American College of Cardiology state that medical screening should not be required for older adults before beginning an activity program (5), and a Best Practices Statement from the American College of Sports Medicine declares that asymptomatic older adults can safely begin a low-intensity activity program even if they have not had a recent medical examination (1), but many older adults still believe that they must "see a doctor a doctor first."

With the lack of evidence to support using cardiac stress testing before starting a light- to moderate-level exercise program, activity participation should not require screening by a physician (1). However, appropriate screening should be conducted before initiating a physical activity program to ensure that older adults engage in appropriate physical activity programs that provide maximum health benefits and prevent injuries. The most commonly used tool in the United States and Canada for this purpose is the rPAR-Q, which focuses on medical history as well as symptoms and risk factors for cardiovascular events associated with exercise but does not address musculoskeletal problems nor does it provide recommendations about appropriate physical activity programs. In addition, this screening tool was designed for individuals up to 69 years of age, and it suggests that anyone beyond this age see a doctor before becoming more active if they are not already used to being "very active." When an individual responds "yes" to any of the tool's questions, the individual is directed to see a health care provider and/or to have the health care provider grant written permission before being allowed into an activity program. Furthermore, for anyone who uses the rPAR-Q, including those who pass the screening, the tool does not give information about the type(s) of programs that would be beneficial. Although practitioners commonly employ this screening tool with older adults, the rPAR-Q has not been rigorously tested in older adult populations, presents several issues that can be a deterrent to physical activity participation, and does not provide guidance regarding appropriate physical activity programs.

EXERCISE AND SCREENING FOR YOU

The Exercise and Screening for You (EASY) tool was developed to screen older adults of any age, including the oldest-old (13), for common health concerns that should be considered before starting an activity program and to guide the individual toward appropriate physical activities (12). The EASY tool is modeled after the commonly used rPAR-Q and was based on prior experience and clinical research. Although the questions within the rPAR-Q (see Key Point 9-1) and the EASY are similar (see Table 9-1), there are significant differences in how the tool guides individuals with respect to their physical activity options.

KEY POINT 9-1 Questions from the Revised Physical Activity Readiness Questionnaire (rPAR-Q)

Has your doctor ever said that you have a heart condition and that you should only do physical activity recommended by a doctor?

Do you feel pain in your chest when you do physical activity?

In the past month, have you had chest pain when you were not doing physical activity?

Do you lose your balance because of dizziness or do you ever lose consciousness?

Do you have a bone or joint problem that could be made worse by a change in your physical activity?

Is your doctor currently prescribing drugs (*e.g.*, water pills) for your blood pressure or heart condition?

Do you know of any other reason why you should not do physical activity?

Table 9-1   Exercise/Physical Activity Assessment and Screening for You (EASY)

For most people, physical activity should not pose any major problems or risks, especially if their physical activity program is started at a low level and increased gradually over time. The EASY has been designed to help you and your health care provider or exercise specialist feel comfortable that you are beginning or increasing an exercise or physical activity program that is safe for you and will help you achieve the best possible health outcomes.

Please read each question carefully and check yes or no opposite the question if it applies to you. Completing this form will give you an idea what you should do before starting a new exercise program.

Yes/No

1. _____ Do you have pains in your heart and chest at least twice a week? (Note: Severe chest pain on the left side is a possible warning sign requiring immediate medical attention)

2. _____ Do you feel faint or have spells of severe dizziness at least twice a week?

3. _____ Have you been told in the past 4 weeks that your blood pressure reading was high, with the top number being greater than 180 or the bottom number being greater than 100?

4. _____ Do you currently have a bone, joint, or muscle problem that causes you pain severe enough that you want to do something to alleviate it (take medication or use heat, ice, or other treatments) at least twice a week?

5. _____ Do you have pain severe enough that you want to do something to alleviate it (take medication or use heat, ice, or other treatments) at least twice a week?

6. _____ Do you feel short of breath doing activities such as walking up a hill, up the stairs, or when making a bed?

7. _____ Do you fall at least twice a week?

8. _____ Is there a physical reason not mentioned why you would be concerned about starting an exercise program?

If you answered NO to all questions...

Congratulations! You can begin the exercise or physical activity program you are planning safely and can expect to achieve positive physical and mental health benefits. To minimize any potential risk, we encourage you to review exercise safety tips and be aware of signs and symptoms indicating need to reduce or terminate activity.

If you answered YES to one or more questions...

If you currently engaged in a physical activity or exercise program several days a week or more and have had no associated health problems in engaging in this activity, feel free to continue with current activities. However, we recommend that you review tips for exercising safely.

Otherwise, if you have not recently done so, consult with your health care provider to determine if the current program you want to begin is going to be good for you, or if you need to be provided with a program that is more suitable to your current health situation. Utilize the following section to guide you in establishing an appropriate exercise program with your health care provider, physical therapist, or exercise trainer.

The rPAR-Q requires just a single yes/no response to each item, and the individual either passes screening or does not. If the individual answers "yes" to any question, then he or she is required to see his or her health care provider before beginning physical activity. With the EASY tool, only in the case of an individual experiencing an acute medical problem that has not been previously evaluated by a health care provider is the individual encouraged to see his or her provider before engaging in physical activity.

The EASY tool follows an algorithm for each question so that the older adult and/or the health care provider is directed to a list of available physical activity programs that are appropriate for a given condition. The EASY tool addresses many of the weaknesses of other screening processes because it incorporates an interactive Web site (www.easyforyou.info) to guide the older adult and/or health care provider toward appropriate physical activities.

The EASY tool contains six questions (Table 9-1) as follows:

1. Do you have pains, tightness, or pressure in your chest during physical activity (walking, climbing stairs, household chores, similar activities)?
2. Do you currently experience dizziness or lightheadedness?
3. Have you ever been told that you have high blood pressure?
4. Do you have pain, stiffness, or swelling that limits or prevents you from doing what you want or need to do?
5. Do you fall, feel unsteady, or use assistive device while standing or walking?
6. Is there a health reason not mentioned why you would be concerned about starting an exercise program?

These questions identify any health problems individuals may have that might affect the type of physical activity they should perform, and guide them to the programs that would be of most benefit given their clinical condition. The recommended activity programs are from respected professional organizations. For example, if an older adult answered "yes" to the question "Do you have pain, stiffness, or swelling that limits or prevents you from doing what you want or need to do?" then he or she is guided to a list of programs developed for those with arthritic conditions. It is also recommended to the older adult that he or she share the results with his or her healthcare provider and ask "Are there any exercises that I should not do?" In addition, the older adult is encouraged to use the comprehensive listing of safety tips provided in the EASY tool before, during, and after physical activity.

It is important to recognize that screening should not be a one-time activity. Rather it is an ongoing process, and individuals need to monitor and attend to changes in their health, be aware of signs and symptoms of potentially harmful events, and be familiar with the safety tips.

FINDING THE RIGHT TYPE OF PROGRAMMING

To prescribe the safest and most appropriate exercise program for older adults, it is important to consider the medical history of the individual with a focus on cardiorespiratory symptoms, such as dizziness or shortness of breath, and musculoskeletal problems, such as degenerative joint disease or musculoskeletal pain. Information from preactivity screening is used for this purpose. If, for example, the older adult has knee pain while performing weight-bearing activity, then weight-bearing exercises may not be appropriate at that time. Table 9-2 provides some guidelines for what types of exercise to recommend in light of various health problems common in older adults. In addition, it is also important to consider the personal physical activity preferences of individuals, as well as their personal health, fitness goals, and aspirations.

Table 9-2 Linking Screening Results to Appropriate Activity Options

EASY Item	Additional Information to Provide	Possible Exercise Options to Discuss
1. Do you have pains in your heart and chest at least two times per week?	• Length of time symptoms have been present. • Are symptoms relieved when medication is used? • Is pain associated with walking, lifting, or any other type of physical activity?	Once any new acute illness is evaluated, plan to start: • Progressive activity as tolerated: • Walking at a comfortable pace for increasing distances • Weight lifting at a comfortable level increasing as tolerated • Balance and flexibility exercises
2. Do you feel faint or have spells of severe dizziness at least two times per week?	• Length of time symptoms have been present? • Are symptoms associated with walking, lifting, or any other type of physical activity?	Once any new or acute illness is evaluated, plan to start: • Progressive activity as tolerated: • Walking at a comfortable pace for increasing distances • Weight lifting at a comfortable level increasing as tolerated • Balance and flexibility exercises
3. Have you been told in the past month that your blood pressure is elevated so that the top number is >180 or the bottom number is >100?	• Do you take medication for high blood pressure? • Have blood pressure checks been in normal range since starting on medication?	Once the top number of your blood pressure is ≤180 and the bottom number is ≤100, you can begin your exercise program
4. Do you currently have a bone, joint, or muscle problem that causes you pain (at least 5 out of 7 d of the week) in your back, legs, arms, shoulder, neck, or other areas?	• Do you have any pain, stiffness, or difficulty walking because of these problems?	• If you have no symptoms associated with the bone or joint problems, you may begin your exercise program • If you have associated pain, proceed to item 5
5. Do you have pain severe enough that you want to do something to alleviate it (take medication or use heat, ice, or other treatments) at least twice a week?	• Does walking increase your pain in any of these areas? • Does lifting any amount of weight increase your pain in any of these areas?	• Avoid exercise programs that are specifically geared toward walking on a hard surface • Avoid resistance exercise activities (lifting weights or using stretchy bands) that increase pain • Discuss options with your health care provider or an exercise trainer. These options might include engaging in pool exercise programs, or utilizing appropriate exercise equipment • Balance and flexibility exercises

EASY Item	Additional Information to Provide	Possible Exercise Options to Discuss
6. Do you feel short of breath doing activities such as walking up a hill, up the stairs, or when making a bed?	• Have you just noticed this within the past few weeks?	Once any new or acute health problems are identified and treated, plan to start: • Progressive activity as tolerated: • Walking at a comfortable pace for increasing distances • Weight lifting at a comfortable level increasing as tolerated • Balance and flexibility exercises
7. Do you fall at least twice a week?	• Provide details about when and under what circumstances falls have occurred. • Review whether falls have resulted in any serious injuries.	• Begin with chair exercises • Try to have person present during exercise activity • Emphasize balance and lower body strength exercises
8. Is there a good physical reason not mentioned here why you would be concerned about starting an exercise program?	• Provide details of what your physical or mental health concerns are related to exercise.	Unless your health care provider feels you should avoid any specific activity: • Progressive activity as tolerated: • Walking at a comfortable pace for increasing distances • Weight lifting at a comfortable level increasing as tolerated • Balance and flexibility exercises

For general health and well-being, a well-rounded physical activity program should consist of endurance, strength, balance, and flexibility (1). Endurance-related physical activity refers to continuous movement that involves large muscle groups and is sustained for a minimum of 10 minutes. Examples of endurance activity include biking, swimming, walking, and lifestyle activities that incorporate large muscle groups. Strength-related activity refers to increasing muscle strength by moving or lifting some type of resistance, such as weights or elastic bands, at a level that requires some physical effort. In general, at least four exercises for both the upper and lower body with one to three sets of 10 to 12 repetitions performed on at least 2 days a week are recommended for increasing muscle strength. Flexibility-related activity facilitates greater range of motion around the joint. These exercises should be performed a minimum of 2 days a week. Balance is the ability to maintain control of the body over the base of support so as to avoid falling. Both static (maintaining balance without moving) and dynamic (moving without losing balance) balance activities should be performed on a regular basis.

One should provide individualized recommendations with specific goals for any physical activity program, based on the abilities and needs of the older adults. Many factors are taken into consideration in prescribing a physical activity program such as safety, physical ability, motivation, support, and goals. For some older adults, simply walking for 10 minutes a day is a start; others who may not be able to walk can implement some upper body strengthening; and others may ready for a well-rounded daily routine (see Key Point 9-2). Emphasize that individuals may start at 5 or 10 minutes of easy and fun activity, and work up to 30 minutes of activity on most days of the week. Individuals may also break up the 30 minutes into smaller, 10-minute segments. They can incorporate other activities they may enjoy such as a sport or strength training program. *The overall goal of the program is to facilitate a behavioral change among older adults to begin some type of physical activity, working toward the recommendations of the ACSM.*

KEY POINT 9-2

Well-Rounded Physical Activity Program Recommendations

   Incorporate moderate activity for a goal of 30 min at least 5 d·wk^{-1}

   Perform strengthening activities at least 2 d·wk^{-1}

   Include warm-up and cool-down with each workout

   Incorporate balance activities into daily activities

Sample prescription

   Monday: Cardiorespiratory activities 10–30 min (walk/jog, bike, swim)

   Tuesday: Strengthening and balance activities

   Wednesday: Cardiorespiratory activities 10–30 min

   Thursday: Strengthening and balance activities

   Friday: Cardiorespiratory activities 10–30 min

   Saturday: Strengthening and balance activities

   Sunday: Gardening, walk in park or mall, or other recreational activity with friends and family 10–30 min

It is critical *not* to overwhelm individuals with physical activity. Remember, this is a behavioral change with many factors to consider. While the ACSM recommendations are ideal, any level of physical activity is beneficial for virtually every older adult.

MOTIVATING OLDER ADULTS TO ADHERE TO A REGULAR EXERCISE PROGRAM

Unfortunately, despite the many known benefits to exercise for all older adults, the majority of these individuals do not regularly exercise. Motivational techniques should be used not only to initiate an exercise program, but also to assure ongoing adherence. The first step to motivating an older adult to exercise is educating the individual about the benefits of exercise (11). It is particularly important to emphasize the immediate benefits that can be expected if physical activity is performed regularly. Many older adults often indicate that they are not interested in exercising to prolong life, but rather for the benefit of improving their health and quality of life (9).

Along with education, an "exercise prescription" should be included that identifies specific activities the individual is to perform. Many older adults focus on immediate and continual benefits in the adoption and maintenance of an exercise program. It is important that exercise prescriptions are related to obtainable goals and desired outcomes. For example, if the individual wants to reduce his or her risk of falls, then balance exercises, along with muscle strengthening of the lower body, should be included. For an individual suffering from osteoarthritis-related knee pain, water exercises are one way to help reduce symptoms. In addition, land-based exercises such as aerobic walking, resistance exercise, and tai chi reduce pain and disability from knee osteoarthritis (14). Knowledge of these options might serve to assist an older adult with the adoption of an exercise program.

Older adults tend to be more compliant with a physical activity program if they have individualized programs based on their needs and specific goals. It is important to use the results of a physical ability assessment as well as their subjective functional limitations in determining individual goals and exercise needs. Activities should be recommended to individuals who are safe and efficient to address their limitations. By including specific activities to address specific conditions, individuals should be able to see improvement in their functional levels, thus promoting compliance.

Individual goal-setting should precede physical activity prescription to facilitate compliance, and goals should be SMART — *specific, measurable, attainable, relevant, and time-dependent.*

Specific: specific reference to functional activities should be listed
Measurable: goals that can be measured should be included
(not "I will feel better")
Attainable: goals should be realistic and attainable by the individual
Relevant: goals should be relevant to the individuals' daily
activities
Time-dependent: time frames should be provided

For example, "After 8 weeks of strength training, I will be able to walk up and down a flight of stairs 3 times." A chart is useful in motivating individuals to continue participation to reach their goals.

My goals:

Area to Improve	Specific Goal	Target Date
Lower body strength	Walk up and down my stairs 3 times	8 wk

Daily goals can be written out for the individual to clarify exactly what activities should be done on a daily basis. Long-term goals, such as decreasing pain or falls, can be placed on the daily goal sheet as a reminder of what he or she ultimately hopes to achieve through exercise.

The 5 *As* of behavioral counseling are also a useful framework for helping to design goals:

- *Assess* current activities
- *Advise* on specific goals
- *Agree* on collaborative goals
- *Assist* with understanding how to meet challenges and address barriers
- *Arrange* the most appropriate follow-up care

An individualized physical activity program should include specific activities for specific impairments or limitations. A goal-based physical activity program designed to improve function and decrease disability is important for compliance. Use of an "activity log" to track progress by noting the specific activity performed, as well as the intensity and duration of each activity, can also be helpful. This chart is used to document progress toward goals and to show a health care provider. Either a weekly or monthly chart (below) can be used to track progress.

WEEKLY (indicate the type of activity you performed each day)

Activity	Sunday	Monday	Tuesday	Wednesday	Thursday	Friday	Saturday
Cardio	10,000 steps	20 min swim		10,000 steps		30 min bike	
Stretch	✓	✓	✓	✓	✓	✓	
Strength			✓		✓		
Balance	✓			✓			✓

MONTHLY (indicate days that you did some type of physical activity with a check, and note the activity)

Week	Sunday	Monday	Tuesday	Wednesday	Thursday	Friday	Saturday
1							
2							
3							
4							

Once the physical activity program has been established (including exercise prescription and goals) and the program has begun, individuals must learn how to progress the activities. Progression is the key to improving fitness over time and can be achieved by gradually increasing any of the following:

- *Frequency:* The number of times per week
- *Duration:* The length or number of the activity per exercise (time, sets, repetitions)
- *Intensity:* The level of the activity (noted by resistance or RPE)

Although there is little research to support that there is a significant risk associated with physical activity, many older adults may be fearful that exercise may worsen conditions such as arthritis or cardiovascular disease, and therefore, they are unwilling to exercise. As with the prescription for any medication, a prescription for exercise should also include potential exercise side effects. These might be sensations associated with actually doing the exercise (*e.g.*, shortness of breath when walking), or they may be things that occur the day after exercise (*e.g.*, muscle soreness). The older adult should be informed of these potential sensations and be informed of how to prevent and/or treat them if they occur. They should also be assured that these are common issues and do not typically indicate an acute medical problem. They should also be informed that the occurrence of these side effects tends to decrease with regular activity. To further ensure safe exercise activities, older adults should be given a list of safety tips (Table 9-3) to follow. These safety tips that are part of the EASY tool kit help individuals know when it may not be safe to initiate their activity program, when they should stop exercising, and what to expect as normal at the end of an activity session.

For some older adults, seeing others their age exercise or hearing testimonials and anecdotal stories from others their age who are exercising and improving their health can be very motivating. Share stories with participants and give examples of your own exercise activities and how you benefit from them. Finally, make sure you ask each individual about his or her exercise program on a regular basis. Showing them that you care about their exercise program and that you believe it is important for their health can be a very important factor in the ongoing maintenance of older adults' activity program (Key Point 9-3).

Table 9-3   EASY Safety Tips for Exercise Initiation

Exercise safety tips to always consider before starting exercise
 Always wear comfortable, loose-fitting clothing and appropriate shoes for your activity.
 Warm-up: Perform a low- to moderate-intensity warm-up for 5–10 min.
 Drink water before, during, and after your exercise session.
 When exercising outdoors, evaluate your surroundings for safety: traffic, pavement, weather, and strangers.
 Wear clothes made of fabrics that absorb sweat and remove it from your skin.
 Never wear rubber or plastic suits. These could hold the sweat on your skin and make your body overheat.
 Wear sunscreen when you exercise outdoors.
Exercise safety tips for when to STOP exercising
 Stop exercising right away if you:
 Have pain or pressure in your chest, neck, shoulder, or arm.
 Feel dizzy or sick.
 Break out in a cold sweat.
 Have muscle cramps.
 Feel acute (not just achy) pain in your joints, feet, ankles, or legs.
 Slow down if you are out of breath. You should be able to talk while exercising without gasping for breath.
Exercise safety tips to recognize days/times when exercise should NOT be initiated:
 Do not do hard exercise for 2 h after a big meal.
 Do not exercise when you have a fever and/or viral infection accompanied by muscle aches.
 Do not exercise if your systolic blood pressure is >200 and your diastolic is >100.
 Do not exercise if your resting heart rate is >120.
 Do not exercise if you have a joint that you are using to exercise (such as a knee or an ankle) is red, warm, and painful.
 Stop exercising if you experience severe pain or swelling in a joint. Discomfort that persists should always be evaluated.
 Do not exercise if you have a new symptom that has not been evaluated by your health care provider such as pain in your chest, abdomen, or a joint; swelling in an arm, leg, or joint; difficulty catching your breath at rest; or a fluttering feeling in your chest.

S U M M A R Y

The chapter covered three important areas that can help older adults engage in appropriate physical activity: conducting preactivity screening, developing an exercise prescription, and motivating the individual to begin and adhere to an exercise prescription. Preactivity screening helps minimize the risk of injury or other adverse health events when engaging in physical activity, identifies medical issues so that exercise programs can be modified for safety and optimal benefit, and identifies functional limitations that the activity program can address. The EASY tool was developed specifically for older adults and is an excellent preactivity screening method that identifies health concerns that should be considered and guides the individual toward appropriate activities. Developing a specific, goal-oriented exercise prescription that provides a well-rounded program consisting of endurance, strength, flexibility, and balance is important, but should be done so with the individual's activity preferences, personal health, fitness goals, and aspirations in mind. Such an individualized program will not only be safer, but also be much more appealing, thus increasing the likelihood of sustained participation.

KEY POINT 9-3 Putting It All Together

Determine safety of physical activity (risk factors) and diseases

Assess individual ability and reported limitations

Discuss personal goals, preferences, and resources for physical activity

Determine activities that are appropriate for the individual on the basis of abilities, needs, and goals

Determine appropriate frequency, intensity, and duration for each activity

Establish weekly program and discuss progression

Instruct in use of tracking logs

Follow up and assess activity levels, and progress or modify activities

 # QUESTIONS FOR REFLECTION

1. What are the three purposes of preactivity screening?

2. Do all older adults need to see a physician before starting any type of activity program? Why or why not?

3. What are the advantages of the EASY screening tool compared with the r-PARQ?

4. Is screening a one-time only event? Why or why not?

5. What should a well-rounded activity program consist of?

6. What factors should be considered when prescribing physical activity to an older adult?

7. What should initially be done to motivate an older adult to engage in physical activity?

8. What components are included when developing SMART goals?

9. Describe the 5 As behavioral counseling.

10. How can progression of physical activity be achieved?

11. Describe the physical activity safety tips that should be considered for older adults.

REFERENCES

1. American College of Sports Medicine. Physical activity programs and behavior counseling in older adult populations. *Med Sci Sports Exerc.* 2004;36:1997–2003.
2. Balady GJ, Driscoll D, Foster C, et al. Recommendations for cardiovascular screening, staffing, and emergency policies at health/fitness facilities. *Med Sci Sports Exerc.* 1998;30:1009–18.

3. Bean J, Vora A, Frontera WR. Benefits of exercise for community-dwelling older adults. *Arch Phys Med Rehabil.* 2004;85:S31–42.

4. Chodzko-Zajko W, Ory MG, Resnick B. Beyond screening: The need for new pre-activity counseling protocols to assist older adults transition from sedentary living to physically active lifestyles. *J Active Aging.* 2004;3(4):26.

5. Gibbons RJ, Balady GJ, Beasley JW, et al. ACC/AHA guidelines for exercise testing: Executive summary. A report of the American College of Cardiology/American Heart Association Task Force on Practice Guidelines (Committee on Exercise Testing). *Circulation.* 1997;96:345–54.

6. Glasgow R, Eakin EG, Fisher EB, Bacak SJ, Brownson RC. Physician advice and support for physical activity: Results from a national survey. *Am J Prev Med.* 2001;21:189–96.

7. Morey MC, Sullivan RJ Jr. Medical assessment for health advocacy and practical strategies for exercise initiation. *Am J Prev Med.* 2003;25:204–8.

8. Ory M, Resnick B, Jordan PJ, et al. Screening, safety, and adverse events in physical activity interventions: Collaborative experiences from the behavior change consortium. *Ann Behav Med.* 2005;29(suppl):20–8.

9. Resnick B, Spellbring AM. Understanding what motivates older adults to exercise. *J Gerontol Nurs.* 2000;26:34–42.

10. Resnick B, Ory M, Coday M, Riebe D. Older adults' perspectives on screening prior to initiating an exercise program. *Prev Sci.* 2005;6:203–11.

11. Resnick B, Ory MG, Rogers ME, Page P, Lyle RM, Chodzko-Zajko W, Bazzarre TL. Screening for and prescribing exercise for older adults. *Geriatrics Aging.* 2006;9:174–82.

12. Resnick B, Ory MG, Hora K, et al. A proposal for a new screening paradigm and tool called Exercise Assessment and Screening for You (EASY). *J Phys Act Aging.* 2008;16:231–49.

13. Resnick B, Ory MG, Hora K, Rogers ME, Page P, Chodzko-Zajko W, Bazzarre TL. The Exercise Assessment and Screening for You (EASY) Tool: Application in the oldest old population. *Am J Lifestyle Med.* 2008;2:432–40.

14. Ringdahl E, Pandit S. Treatment of knee osteoarthritis. *Am Fam Physician.* 2011;83:1287–92.

15. Thomas S, Reading J, Shepard RJ. Revision of the Physical Activity Readiness Questionnaire (PAR-Q). *Can J Sports Sci.* 1992;17:338–45.

16. US Preventive Services Task Force. Screening for coronary heart disease: Recommendation statement. *Ann Intern Med.* 2004;140:569–72.

CHAPTER 10

Frequently Asked Questions about Physical Activity

Wojtek Chodzko-Zajko

CHAPTER OUTLINE

- **Introduction**
- **Ten frequently asked questions**
  - FAQ 1: Why should I be physically active?
  - FAQ 2: How much physical activity do I need?
  - FAQ 3: What is the best exercise for older adults?
  - FAQ 4: How many times a week should I exercise?
  - FAQ 5: I have not exercised for many years, where should I start?
  - FAQ 6: Will physical activity help reduce my risk for specific diseases and conditions?
  - FAQ 7: Do I need to see a doctor before beginning a program of physical activity?
  - FAQ 8: Is exercise safe?
  - FAQ 9: Am I too old to exercise?
  - FAQ 10: Do I need special clothing and equipment?
- **Online resources for older adults interested in increasing physical activity**
  - Department of Health and Human Services Physical Activity Guidelines Web Site Materials
  - National Institutes of Health Resources
  - Administration on Aging
  - President's Council on Fitness, Sports, and Nutrition
  - National Physical Activity Plan
  - AARP Health and Fitness
  - ACSM/AMA
  - Online Exercise Screening Tool
  - National Council on Aging

INTRODUCTION

In the chapters of this book, you have read about the many reasons why older adults should be regularly physically active. The expert chapter authors have presented a compelling case for physical activity, summarizing the physiological, psychological, social, and other benefits that accrue to people of all ages who are able to maintain a physically active lifestyle. There can be little doubt that there is a substantial body of scientific evidence that indicates that regular physical activity can bring dramatic health benefits to people of all ages and abilities and that these benefits extend over the entire life-course. Physical activity offers one of the greatest opportunities to extend years of active independent life, reduce disability, and improve the quality of life for midlife and older persons.

Unfortunately, despite a wealth of evidence about the benefits of physical activity for midlife and older persons, there has been little success in convincing Americans aged 50 and older to adopt physically active lifestyles. For example, the Centers for Disease Control and Prevention estimates that between one-third to one-half of Americans older than 50 years get no leisure time physical activity at all (see Chapters 1 and 2). One of the goals of the *ACSM Guide to Exercise and Physical Activity for Older Adults* has been to assist exercise professionals to identify and understand some of the barriers faced by older adults when they attempt to increase their physical activity, and to outline specific strategies for helping them to overcome these barriers. In this book, you will find a number of strategies designed to help you become a physical activity professional who is comfortable and effective working with seniors of all ages and ability levels.

For those of us who make our living advocating for healthy and physically active lifestyles, it may come as a surprise to realize how little many older adults know about physical activity. However, most older adults were educated at a time and in a culture in which little was known about the health benefits of physical activity, and professionals and members of the public were skeptical about the need to remain physically active after retirement. In this final chapter we review some frequently asked questions that older adults ask about exercise and physical activity, with the goal of assisting you to provide succinct but accurate responses that will serve to motivate and inform your older clients.

TEN FREQUENTLY ASKED QUESTIONS

FAQ 1: Why should I be physically active?

Response. There are many reasons you should build physical activity into your everyday life. Regular physical activity can help improve quality of life in old age. Physical activity can help you stay active and engaged with your family and community. It can help you manage or postpone some of the chronic diseases and conditions many of us have come to expect from old age. Aging does not have to be something that "happens to us" — on the contrary, being physically active can help us play a more active role in our own aging. Physical activity can help us live happier, healthier, and more productive lives.

Advice to exercise professionals. For many years, exercise professionals have tended to focus on the health or medical benefits of exercise and physical activity when trying to motivate sedentary individuals to become more active. For some individuals, motives such as decreasing cholesterol levels, improving cardiac output, and increasing bone mineral density are effective motivators, but for many seniors, they are not. As an exercise professional, you should also stress that regular physical activity can be fun, can increase quality of life, and can help seniors continue to do the things that they like to do. In Chapter 4, Diane Whaley and Agnes Schrider describe a number of evidence-based strategies that can be used to help motivate people to be physically active. It is doubtful that a single motivational strategy will work for all older adults. Exercise professionals should ensure that they are familiar with a variety of motivational strategies so as to find the technique that works best for each of their clients.

FAQ 2: How much physical activity do I need?

Response. Ideally, you should aim to do at least 150 minutes of moderate-intensity aerobic activity per week as well as 2 days per week of resistance exercises. However, start by doing what you can, and gradually look for ways to do more. If you have not been active for a while, start out slowly. After several weeks or months, build up your activities — do them longer and more often.

Advice to exercise professionals. In Chapters 2, 3, 5, and 9 specific guidelines and recommendations regarding the quantity and quality of physical activity needed to ensure significant outcomes are discussed in detail. It is important for all exercise professionals to know and understand these guidelines. The current Physical Activity Guidelines for Americans summarize the best available scientific recommendations, and we should certainly be prepared to summarize this information for our clients. However, it is important to understand that for many older adults, 150 minutes of moderate-intensity aerobic activity per week can be an extremely intimidating target that may leave them discouraged or unwilling to even try to increase their physical activity. As an exercise professional, it is important that you help older clients understand that it is perfectly acceptable to gradually increase physical activity levels, starting at easily achievable, nonthreatening levels and slowly increasing as the older adult becomes more comfortable with exercise and physical activity.

FAQ 3: What is the best exercise for older adults?

Response. There is no single best exercise that works for all older persons. Depending on how you define it, "old age" can cover as much as a 50-year age span, ranging from 50 to 100 years of age and older. For this reason, it is impossible to recommend a single set of activities that is best for all older persons. Some seniors can run marathons or compete in triathlons, whereas others may be more comfortable walking, gardening, or doing tai chi. Still others will get their exercise in a chair or in bed! The most important thing to do, regardless of your age, is to avoid inactivity. The specific type of physical activity will always vary from person to person. A good idea is to select activities you enjoy. If possible, mixing up activities that promote stamina, strength, flexibility, and balance is a good idea.

Advice to exercise professionals. The best exercise or physical activity program is the one that your clients are willing and able to do regularly, that they enjoy, and that adds to their quality of life. For some individuals, this will be a structured group exercise program at the local senior center or YMCA, but for others, it will be something much less structured, possibly involving activities such as healthy commuting, gardening, or walking the dog. Many exercise professionals grew up enjoying games and sports and are extremely comfortable "working out" in traditional exercise environments. It is important to remember that not all older adults have enjoyed similar positive experiences with traditional exercise programs. Work with your clients to understand their goals, aspirations, and personal preferences. For some individuals, identifying options for active living (see Chapter 3) may be a much more successful strategy than simply referring an individual to an exercise program at a local fitness center or community agency. An extremely important aspect of your role as an exercise professional is to help your clients to identify the physical activity program that's right for them (see Chapter 9).

FAQ 4: How many times a week should I exercise?

Response. Generally, it is better to spread physical activity out throughout the week, with a goal of being active on at least 3 to 5 days·week^{-1}. By choosing activities that you enjoy and that are convenient and affordable, you may be able to find a way to be active on almost all days of the week. Try to mix up your physical activity program, so you are not doing the same thing every day. On some days you might go for a walk in your neighborhood with a friend or family member; on other days you might take advantage of a more structured exercise program at the senior center or church. Many people find that wearing a step counter can help them keep track of their activity levels. On days when you have not accumulated many steps, an afterdinner walk can help you maintain your commitment to an active lifestyle.

Advice to exercise professionals. As an exercise professional, one of the most important things you can do for your clients is to empower them to be independently physically active and not to depend solely on you for their physical activity. Relatively few people have the time or desire to participate in a structured exercise program 7 days a week. You should work with your clients to help them develop activities that they can do on their own time and in their own space. By helping seniors understand that there are many different ways to be active, you can help them develop a well-rounded, personalized activity program that selects from a menu of physical activity choices and helps them to be active on most, if not all, days of the week.

FAQ 5: I have not exercised for many years, where should I start?

Response. Forget the old saying "no pain, no gain"—it is simply not true! Too many of us learned in childhood that physical activity has to be painful or exhausting if it is going to do us any good. There are many excellent options for those of us who cannot or do not want to exercise vigorously. Walking is a wonderful way to increase your activity level. Stretching, tai chi, and water exercise are also good options. For example, the Arthritis Foundation offers excellent aqua exercise programs specially designed for those with arthritis and joint disorders. Gardening and working outdoors can also be a good form of physical activity. Remember, the most important thing is not what you do; rather it is most important to avoid complete inactivity.

Advice to exercise professionals. Prescribing exercise and physical activity is as much an art as it is a science. The most successful exercise professionals are those who have mastered both of these elements. Simply informing clients about the current scientific guidelines may not be sufficient to motivate them to change their behavior. Understanding some of the principles of behavioral change discussed in Chapter 4 can help you develop greater insight into how to identify the right place for an individual to start on their journey toward an active lifestyle. Many years ago, when I was a young assistant professor, my mother called me from her home in England and asked me to help her with her wish to be more physically active. At that time, she was in her early 60s, a widow living alone, working full-time as a teacher. Mom told me that she knew that she was supposed to do 30 minutes of aerobic exercise at least three times a week, but by the time she got home from a long day at school, she was too tired to imagine doing 30 minutes of physical activity. For her, the current physical activity guidelines seemed like an impossible mountain to climb. In my advice to mom, I suggested that when she got home from work, before she took off her coat, she ask herself a simple question "Do I have the energy to walk to the shops at the end of the road?" The shops were about 100 yards from her home, and she often walked there to buy milk and other groceries. If the answer to the question was "yes," she simply had to walk to the shops and come back. If the answer was "no," it was perfectly fine to take off her coat and relax. I asked her to mark her wall calendar each day that she decided to walk to the corner store. We agreed that I would call back in a couple of weeks (this was before the era of Skype and cheap international phone calls). Two weeks later when I called back, the first words out of her mouth were "I had three check marks on the calendar last week and four this week." She was ecstatic; she had broken through a barrier. A few weeks later, I suggested that when she got to the corner store, she ask herself another question "Am I ready to go back home, or do I want to walk around the block?" Twenty years later, my mom is an active and energetic 80-year-old woman who still lives alone in the same house. She maintains a routine of regular physical activity that she credits for her independence and high quality of life. Her physically active lifestyle consists mostly of walking in her neighborhood and doing calisthenics and exercises at home. I am not suggesting that the strategy I used with my mom will work for all seniors. However, it is clear that if we are to be successful in motivating sedentary individuals to change their behavior, we will need to pay close attention to their goals and preferences as we work with them to develop a program that is meaningful and that helps them to overcome their personal obstacles and barriers.

FAQ 6: Will physical activity help reduce my risk for specific diseases and conditions?

Response. Physical inactivity is a major risk factor for many physical and psychological conditions. Sedentary living is associated with heart disease, obesity, diabetes, and many other conditions. Inactivity is also linked to low self-esteem and psychological depression. Regular physical activity can positively influence all the above conditions. Many studies have shown that activity can also help slow the loss of muscle and bone mass that often occurs with advancing age. In addition to these physical and psychological benefits, physical activity can often have significant social benefits. Many seniors enjoy group exercise programs where they have a chance to interact with fellow exercisers of all ages. Even for those individuals who prefer to be active alone or with a partner, physical activity can help them retain the strength and stamina necessary for playing an active role in everyday life.

Advice to exercise professionals. One of the areas in which more scientific research is needed pertains to the specific mode, intensity, and duration of exercise and physical activity needed to bring about a particular clinical outcome. When approached by an older person with a specific disease or condition, it is especially important for an exercise professional to recommend an exercise or activity program that has been shown to be effective in the treatment and management of that particular condition. In Chapter 6, Bo Fernhall, Abbi Lane, and Huimin Yan provide an overview of physical activity options for older adults with special issues and concerns. Similarly, in Chapter 9, Michael and Nicole Rogers propose some strategies to help older adults identify the program that is best for them. It is important for exercise professionals to have a good sense of who the target audience is for a particular exercise or physical activity program and feel comfortable discussing the advantages and disadvantages of a specific program with their individual clients. For example, when approached by an older woman with osteoporosis who was looking for an exercise program to increase her bone mineral density, it would probably not be optimal to recommend a low-intensity walking and calisthenics program conducted at the local senior center. Exercise professionals should familiarize themselves with the variety of exercise and physical activity options available in their community and be prepared to work together with their clients to help identify the most appropriate choice for each individual. The online EASY Screening Tool (http://www.easyforyou.info/) is an excellent resource for exercise professionals wishing to tailor physical activity to the needs of a particular client.

FAQ 7: Do I need to see a doctor before beginning a program of physical activity?

Response. Regular visits to your doctor are always a good idea. In an ideal world, everyone would discuss any proposed change in activity level with his or her doctor. Unfortunately, for many Americans, regular visits to physicians are not always possible. Not having a doctor should not be an excuse for inactivity and sedentary living. The vast majority of older Americans can find a safe and effective activity program that works for them. If you do not have a doctor, you should consider consulting an exercise specialist or other health professionals. In most communities, you can visit a gym, YMCA, or health club to get advice about what kind of activity program is best for you.

Advice to exercise professionals. Although there are some risks associated with participation in regular physical activity, the risks associated with a sedentary lifestyle far exceed them. Physical activity risks are related to level of intensity, with lower-intensity physical activity being associated with the lowest risk. Low-intensity physical activity reduces the risks of injury and muscle soreness and may be perceived as less threatening than moderate-to-high intensity routines. Although lower risk is associated with lower-intensity exercise, the consensus is that moderate physical activity has a better risk/benefit ratio, and moderate-intensity physical activity should be the goal for older adults. Although having an ongoing dialogue with a health care provider is recommended, the involvement of a primary care provider before beginning a program of physical activity depends on a person's health condition and the level of intensity and mode of physical activity. The ACSM Best Practice Statement recommends that before starting or increasing their level of physical activity, older adults should have a strategy for risk management and prevention of activity-related injuries. The most important strategy is to start with low-intensity physical activity and increase intensity gradually. Whenever possible, physical activity bouts should include a warm-up and cool-down component. Increasing muscular strength around weight-bearing joints, particularly the knee, also reduces the risk of musculoskeletal injury.

FAQ 8: Is exercise safe?

Response. Yes! Almost everyone can find a safe and effective exercise program tailored toward his or her health status, physical activity goals, and personal preferences. It is far more risky to your health to be sedentary than it is to begin a program of light-to-moderate intensity physical activity. The greatest risk is that your muscles will be sore in the first few weeks of an exercise program. There are some things that you can do to reduce these risks. Learn to read your body's signals. On days that your body feels tired or weary, take it easy. On good days, take advantage of your body and enjoy yourself! Once we learn how to read our body's signals and respect its needs, we get a better sense of how to adjust our activity programs as we grow older. Very few individuals will be able to (or would want to) run or dance as energetically in their 70s as they could in their 20s. Many believe that the secret of successful aging is learning how to adjust to changing needs and circumstances while remaining an active and vibrant member of society.

Advice to exercise professionals. Although some experts and organizations recommend having a physical examination and exercise test before beginning or increasing physical activity, exercise tests have a substantial level of false positives for heart disease that may lead to unnecessary further testing and in turn increase the risk to older adults. Requiring a physician approval may impose a barrier that reduces the number of people who will begin a program. Because all physical activity is associated with a slight increase in acute injury risk, this small increase must be weighed against the more substantial benefits associated with long-term physical activity. For healthy, asymptomatic adults of any age, the U.S. Preventive Services Task Force does not recommend any type of cardiac screening (ECG, exercise test) before the initiation of physical activity. Although ongoing dialogue between patients and their health professionals is always desirable, the ACSM Best Practice statement recommends that preexercise screening by a physician should not be a prerequisite for participation in low-intensity physical activity. For sedentary older people who are asymptomatic, low-intensity physical activity can be safely initiated regardless of whether an older person has had a recent medical evaluation. As an exercise professional, you will need to work within the rules and regulations set by your employers and the facilities in which you work; however, you should not assume that mandatory preexercise screening is always necessary, especially for relatively healthy, community dwelling seniors.

FAQ 9: Am I too old to exercise?

Response. No! You are never too old to exercise! Physical activity has been shown to be of benefit for individuals of all ages, including persons as old as 90 and 100 years of age. Many people just like you are active on a daily basis. You can find a physical activity program that you will enjoy, will make you feel better, and will increase your quality of life. Think about what you most like to do in life and what you hope to gain from being active. An exercise professional can help you develop a physical activity program that will help you achieve these goals.

Advice to exercise professionals. It is increasingly clear that beneficial effects of regular physical activity can be observed at all stages of the life-course, ranging from the very young to the oldest old. In recent years, many excellent and well-publicized studies have focused our attention on the benefits of regular physical activity in those cohorts of seniors who were previously thought to be "too old" or "too frail" to partake in physical activity. There are a number of reasons why the frail and the oldest old tend to be the most sedentary members of society. First, many of the oldest old do not think of themselves as candidates for physical activity. They are unaware of the many benefits that can accrue to them if they increase their physical activity levels, and they do not realize that many people just like them enjoy activity on a regular basis. Second, for many years, exercise and physical activity professionals were reluctant to expose the oldest old to the rigors of even the most modest physical activity regimens. It is only recently that professional organizations and Institutional Review Boards have begun to recognize that the benefits of physical activity are much greater than the very small risks they pose. Third, many of the exercise and physical activity programs traditionally employed with the middle-aged and young-old are poorly suited for use with the frail and the oldest old. However, there are now an ample number of effective evidence-based programs that have been proven to work in frail and older adult populations. In the chapters of this book, you will have read about many different strategies that are available to you to help engage the oldest members of society in safe, effective, and enjoyable physical activity.

FAQ 10: Do I need special clothing and equipment?

Response. No! Special clothing and equipment are seldom needed. Safe and effective physical activity can be performed wearing comfortable street shoes and loose-fitting everyday clothes. Effective strength training can be achieved with inexpensive equipment such as elastic bands and water-filled jugs.

Advice to exercise professionals. Many older adults have significant discretionary income and are ready and willing to spend it on club memberships, exercise equipment, and clothing; however, many others are in less fortunate financial circumstances and do not have a lot of money to invest in physical activity. I encourage exercise professionals to be sensitive to the resources available to their older clients and to tailor their advice and recommendations accordingly. In my own clinical experience, probably the most important equipment needed to maintain an active lifestyle is a well-fitting pair of shoes that are comfortable and provide adequate cushioning to minimize the risk of muscle and joint injuries.

ONLINE RESOURCES FOR OLDER ADULTS INTERESTED IN INCREASING PHYSICAL ACTIVITY

Department of Health and Human Services Physical Activity Guidelines Web Site Materials

PAG Homepage: **http://www.health.gov/paguidelines/**
Be Active Your Way: **http://www.health.gov/paguidelines/adultguide/default. aspx**
PAG Blog: **http://www.health.gov/paguidelines/blog/default.aspx**
PAG Toolkit: **http://www.health.gov/paguidelines/toolkit.aspx**

National Institutes of Health Resources

Exercise & Physical Activity: Your Everyday Guide from the National Institute on Aging: **http://www.nia.nih.gov/HealthInformation/Publications/ExerciseGuide/**
NIH Senior Health: **http://nihseniorhealth.gov/**

Administration on Aging

Evidence-Based Prevention Program: **http://www.aoa.gov/AoA_Programs/ HPW/Evidence_Based/index.aspx**

President's Council on Fitness, Sports, and Nutrition

Fitness.Gov: **http://www.fitness.gov/**

National Physical Activity Plan

National Plan Homepage: **http://physicalactivityplan.org/**
National Plan Mission and Vision: **http://www.physicalactivityplan.org/vision.htm**

AARP Health and Fitness

AARP Fitness Resources: **http://products.aarp.org/discounts/fitness/**

ACSM/AMA

Exercise is Medicine Homepage: **http://www.exerciseismedicine.org/**

Online Exercise Screening Tool

EASY Screening Tool: **http://www.easyforyou.info/**

National Council on Aging

Center for Healthy Aging Homepage: **http://www.healthyagingprograms.org/**
Evidence-Based Programs: **http://www.healthyagingprograms.org/content. asp?sectionid=32**

Exercise and Physical Activity for Older Adults

Wojtek J. Chodzko-Zajko, Ph.D., FACSM, (Co-Chair)

David N. Proctor, Ph.D., FACSM, (Co-Chair)

Maria A. Fiatarone Singh, M.D.

Christopher T. Minson, Ph.D., FACSM

Claudio R. Nigg, Ph.D.

George J. Salem, Ph.D., FACSM

James S. Skinner, Ph.D., FACSM.

SUMMARY

The purpose of this Position Stand is to provide an overview of issues critical to understanding the importance of exercise and physical activity in older adult populations. The Position Stand is divided into three sections: Section 1 briefly reviews the structural and functional changes that characterize normal human aging, Section 2 considers the extent to which exercise and physical activity can influence the aging process, and Section 3 summarizes the benefits of both long-term exercise and physical activity and shorter-duration exercise programs on health and functional capacity. Although no amount of physical activity can stop the biological aging process, there is evidence that regular exercise can minimize the physiological effects of an otherwise sedentary lifestyle and increase active life expectancy by limiting the development and progression of chronic disease and disabling conditions. There is also emerging evidence for significant psychological and cognitive benefits accruing from regular exercise participation by older adults. Ideally, exercise prescription for older adults should include aerobic exercise, muscle strengthening exercises, and flexibility exercises. The evidence reviewed in this Position Stand is generally consistent with prior American College of Sports Medicine statements on the types and amounts of physical activity recommended for older adults as well as the recently published *2008 Physical Activity Guidelines for Americans*. All older adults should engage in regular physical activity and avoid an inactive lifestyle.

In the decade since the publication of the first edition of the American College of Sports Medicine (ACSM) Position Stand "Exercise and Physical Activity for Older Adults," a significant amount of new evidence has accumulated regarding the benefits of regular exercise and physical activity for older adults. In addition to new evidence regarding the importance of exercise and physical activity for healthy older adults, there is now a growing body of knowledge supporting the prescription of exercise and physical activity for older adults with chronic diseases and disabilities. In 2007, ACSM, in conjunction with the American Heart Association (AHA), published physical activity and public health recommendations for older adults (see Table 1 for a summary of these recommendations) (167). Furthermore, the College has now developed best practice guidelines with respect to exercise program structure, behavioral recommendations, and risk management strategies for exercise in older adult populations (46). Recently, the Department of Health and Human Services published for the first time national physical activity guidelines. The *2008 Physical Activity Guidelines for Americans* (50) affirms that regular physical activity reduces the risk of many adverse health outcomes. The guidelines state that all adults should avoid inactivity, that some physical activity is better than none, and that adults who participate in any amount of physical activity gain some health benefits. However, the guidelines emphasize that for most health outcomes, additional benefits occur as the amount of physical activity increases through higher intensity, greater frequency, and/or longer duration. The guidelines stress that if older adults cannot do 150 min of moderate-intensity aerobic activity per week because of chronic conditions, they should be as physically active as their abilities and conditions allow.

This revision of the ACSM Position Stand "Exercise and Physical Activity for Older Adults" updates and expands the earlier Position Stand and provides an overview of issues critical to exercise and physical activity in older adults. The Position Stand is divided into three sections: Section 1 briefly reviews some of the structural and functional changes that characterize normal human aging. Section 2 considers the extent to which exercise and/or physical activity can influence the aging process through its impact on physiological function and through its impact on the development and progression of chronic disease and disabling conditions. Section 3 summarizes the benefits of both long-term exercise and physical activity and shorter-duration exercise programs on health and functional capacity. The benefits are summarized primarily for the two exercise modalities for which the most data are available: 1) aerobic exercise and 2) resistance exercise. However, information about the known benefits of balance and flexibility exercise is included whenever sufficient data exist. This section concludes with a discussion of the benefits of exercise and physical activity for psychological health and well-being.

Definition of terms. Throughout the review, the Institute of Medicine's definitions of physical activity and exercise and related concepts are adopted, where *physical activity* refers to body movement that is produced by the contraction of skeletal

Table A-1 Summary of ACSM/AHA Physical Activity Recommendations for Older Adults

The current consensus recommendations of the ACSM and AHA with respect to the frequency, intensity, and duration of exercise and physical activity for older adults are summarized below. The ACSM/AHA Physical Activity Recommendations are generally consistent with the 2008 *DHHS Physical Activity Guidelines for Americans*, which also recommend 150 *min.wk*$^{-1}$ of physical activity for health benefits. However, the DHHS Guidelines note that additional benefits occur as the amount of physical activity increases through higher intensity, greater frequency, and/or longer duration. The DHHS Physical Activity Guidelines stress that if older adults cannot do 150 min of moderate-intensity aerobic activity wk^{-1} because of chronic conditions, they should be as physically active as their abilities and conditions allow.

Endurance exercise for older adults:
Frequency: For moderate-intensity activities, accumulate at least 30 or up to 60 (for greater benefit) min·d^{-1} in bouts of at least 10 min each to total 150–300 min·wk^{-1}, at least 20–30 min·d^{-1} or more of vigorous-intensity activities to total 75–150 min·wk^{-1}, an equivalent combination of moderate and vigorous activity.
Intensity: On a scale of 0 to 10 for level of physical exertion, 5 to 6 for moderate-intensity and 7 to 8 for vigorous intensity.
Duration: For moderate-intensity activities, accumulate at least 30 min·d^{-1} in bouts of at least 10 min each or at least 20 min·d^{-1} of continuous activity for vigorous-intensity activities.
Type: Any modality that does not impose excessive orthopedic stress; walking is the most common type of activity. Aquatic exercise and stationary cycle exercise may be advantageous for those with limited tolerance for weight bearing activity.

Resistance exercise for older adults:
Frequency: At least 2 d·wk^{-1}.
Intensity: Between moderate- (5–6) and vigorous-(7–8) intensity on a scale of 0 to 10.
Type: Progressive weight training program or weight bearing calisthenics (8–10 exercises involving the major muscle groups of 8–12 repetitions each), stair climbing, and other strengthening activities that use the major muscle groups.

Flexibility exercise for older adults:
Frequency: At least 2 d·wk^{-1}.
Intensity: Moderate (5–6) intensity on a scale of 0 to 10.
Type: Any activities that maintain or increase flexibility using sustained stretches for each major muscle group and static rather than ballistic movements.

Balance exercise for frequent fallers or individuals with mobility problems:
ACSM/AHA Guidelines currently recommend balance exercise for individuals who are frequent fallers or for individuals with mobility problems. Because of a lack of adequate research evidence, there are currently no specific recommendations regarding specific frequency, intensity, or type of balance exercises for older adults. However, the ACSM Exercise Prescription Guidelines recommend using activities that include the following: 1) progressively difficult postures that gradually reduce the base of support (*e.g.*, two-legged stand, semitandem stand, tandem stand, one-legged stand), 2) dynamic movements that perturb the center of gravity (*e.g.*, tandem walk, circle turns), 3) stressing postural muscle groups (*e.g.*, heel stands, toe stands), or 4) reducing sensory input (*e.g.*, standing with eyes closed).
The ACSM/AHA Guidelines recommend the following special considerations when prescribing exercise and physical activity for older adults. The intensity and duration of physical activity should be low at the outset for older adults who are highly deconditioned, functionally limited, or have chronic conditions that affect their ability to perform physical tasks. The progression of activities should be individual and tailored to tolerance and preference; a conservative approach may be necessary for the most deconditioned and physically limited older adults. Muscle strengthening activities and/or balance training may need to precede aerobic training activities among very frail individuals. Older adults should exceed the recommended minimum amounts of physical activity if they desire to improve their fitness. If chronic conditions preclude activity at the recommended minimum amount, older adults should perform physical activities as tolerated so as to avoid being sedentary.

muscles and that increases energy expenditure. *Exercise* refers to planned, structured, and repetitive movement to improve or maintain one or more components of physical fitness. Throughout the Position Stand, evidence about the impact of exercise training is considered for several dimensions of exercise: *aerobic exercise training* (AET) refers to exercises in which the body's large muscles move in a rhythmic manner for sustained periods; *resistance exercise training* (RET) is exercise that causes muscles to work or hold against an applied force or weight; *flexibility* exercise refers to activities designed to preserve or extend range of motion (ROM) around a joint; and *balance* training refers to a combination of activities designed to increase lower body strength and reduce the likelihood of falling. Participation in exercise and the accumulation of physical activity have been shown to result in improvements in *Physical fitness*, which is operationally defined as a state of well-being with a low risk of premature health problems and energy to participate in a variety of physical activities. *Sedentary living* is defined as a way of living or lifestyle that requires minimal physical activity and that encourages inactivity through limited choices, disincentives, and/or structural or financial barriers. There is no consensus in the aging literature regarding when *old age* begins and no specific guidelines about the *minimum age* of participants in studies that examine the various aspects of the aging process. The recently published ACSM/ AHA physical activity and public health recommendations (167) for older adults suggest that, in most cases, "old age" guidelines apply to individuals aged 65 yr or older, but they can also be relevant for adults aged 50–64 yr with clinically significant chronic conditions or functional limitations that affect movement ability, fitness, or physical activity. Consistent with this logic, in the present review, most literatures cited are from studies of individuals aged 65 yr and older; however, occasionally, studies of younger persons are included when appropriate.

Process. In 2005, the writing group was convened by the American College of Sports Medicine and charged with updating the existing ACSM Position Stand on exercise for older adults. The panel members had expertise in public health, behavioral science, epidemiology, exercise science, medicine, and gerontology. The panel initially reviewed the existing ACSM Position Stand and developed an outline for the revised statement. Panel members next wrote background papers addressing components of the proposed Position Stand, using their judgment to develop a strategy for locating and analyzing relevant evidence. The panelists relied as appropriate on both original publications and earlier reviews of evidence, without repeating them. Because of the breadth and diversity of topics covered in the Position Stand and the ACSM requirement that Position Stands be no longer than 30 pages and include no more than 300 citations, the panel was not able to undertake a systematic review of all of the published evidence of the benefits of physical activity in the older population. Rather, thePosition Stand presents a critical and informed synthesis of the major published work relevant to exercise and physical activity for older adults.

Strength of evidence. In accordance with ACSM Position Stand guidelines, throughout this Position Stand, we have attempted to summarize the strength of the available scientific evidence underlying the relationships observed in the various subsections of the review. An Agency for Health Care Research and Quality (AHRQ) report notes that no single approach is ideally suited for assessing the strength of scientific evidence particularly in cases where evidence is drawn from a variety of methodologies (260). The AHRQ report notes that significant challenges arise when evaluating the strength of evidence in a body of knowledge comprising of combinations of observational and randomized clinical trial (RCT) data as frequently occurs in aging research. The AHRQ consensus report notes that although many experts would agree that RCTs help to ameliorate problems related to selection bias, others note that epidemiological studies with larger aggregate samples or with samples that examine diverse participants in a variety of settings can also enhance the strength of scientific evidence. Consistent with this approach, in this Position Stand, the writing group adopted a taxonomy in which both RCT and observational data were considered important when rating the strength of available evidence into one of four levels. In each case, the writing group collectively evaluated the strength of the published evidence in accordance with the following criteria:

1. *Evidence Level A.* Overwhelming evidence from RCTs and/or observational studies, which provides a consistent pattern of findings on the basis of substantial data.
2. *Evidence Level B.* Strong evidence from a combination of RCT and/or observational studies but with some studies showing results that are inconsistent with the overall conclusion.
3. *Evidence Level C.* Generally positive or suggestive evidence from a smaller number of observational studies and/or uncontrolled or nonrandomized trials.
4. *Evidence Level D.* Panel consensus judgment that the strength of the evidence is insufficient to place it in categories A through C.

SECTION 1: NORMAL HUMAN AGING

Structural and functional decline. With advancing age, structural and functional deterioration occurs in most physiological systems, even in the absence of discernable disease (152). These age-related physiological changes affect a broad range of tissues, organ systems, and functions, which, cumulatively, can impact activities of daily living (ADL) and the preservation of physical independence in older adults. Declines in maximal aerobic capacity ($\dot{V}O_{2max}$) and skeletal muscle performance with advancing age are two examples of physiological aging (98). Variation in each of these measures are important determinants of exercise tolerance (245) and functional abilities (16, 41) among older adults. Baseline values in middle-aged women and men predict future risks of disability (19, 192), chronic disease (18) and death (18, 160). Age-related reductions in $\dot{V}O_{2max}$ and strength also suggest that at any submaximal exercise load, older adults are often required to exert a higher percentage of their maximal capacity (and effort) when compared with younger persons.

Changing body composition is another hallmark of the physiological aging process, which has profound effects on health and physical function among older adults. Specific examples include the gradual accumulation of body fat and its redistribution to central and visceral depots during middle age and the loss of muscle (sarcopenia) during middle and old age, with the attendant metabolic (113, 190) and cardiovascular (123, 222) disease risks. A summary of these and other examples of physiological aging, the usual time course of these changes, and the potential functional and clinical significance of these changes are provided in Table 2.

Evidence statement and recommendation. *Evidence category A.* Advancing age is associated with physiologic changes that result in reductions in functional capacity and altered body composition.

Declining physical activity. Older populations are generally less physically active than young adults, as indicated by self-report and interview, body motion sensors, and more direct approaches for determining daily caloric expenditure (53, 216, 261) Although the total time spent per day in exercise and lifestyle physical activities by some active older adults may approach that of younger normally active adults (11, 217), the types of physical activities most popular among older adults are consistently of lower intensity (walking, gardening, golf, low-impact aerobic activities) (191, 209) compared with those of younger adults (running, higher- impact aerobic activities) (209). A detailed breakdown of physical activity participation data by age groups and physical activity types is beyond the scope of this review; however, the National Center for Health Statistics maintains a database of the most recent monitoring data for tracking Healthy People 2010 objectives including physical activity. Data are included for all the objectives and subgroups identified in the Healthy People 2010, including older adults (166).

Evidence statement and recommendation. *Evidence category A/B.* Advancing age is associated with declines in physical activity volume and intensity.

Increased chronic disease risk. The relative risk of developing and ultimately dying from many chronic diseases including cardiovascular disease, type 2 diabetes, obesity, and certain cancers increases with advancing age (137, 217, 222). Older populations also exhibit the highest prevalence of degenerative musculoskeletal conditions such as osteoporosis, arthritis, and sarcopenia (176, 179, 217). Thus, age is considered a primary risk factor for the development and progression of most chronic degenerative disease states. However, regular physical activity substantially modifies these risks. This is suggested by studies demonstrating a statistically significant decrease in the relative risk of cardiovascular and all-cause mortality among persons who are classified as highly fit (and/or highly active) compared with those in a similar age range who are classified as moderately fit (and/or normally active) or low fit (and/or sedentary). The largest increment in mortality benefit is seen when comparing sedentary adults with those in the next highest physical activity level (19). Additional evidence suggests that muscular strength and power also predict allcause and cardiovascular mortality, independent of cardiovascular fitness (69, 122). Thus, avoidance of a sedentary lifestyle by engaging in at least some daily physical activity is a prudent recommendation for reducing the risk of developing chronic diseases and postponing premature mortality at any age. Although a detailed breakdown of the impact of physical activity

Table A-2 Summary of Typical Changes in Physiological Function and Body Composition with Advancing Age in Healthy Humans

Variables	Typical Changes	Functional Significance[a]
Muscular function		
Muscle strength and power	Isometric, concentric, and eccentric strength decline from age ~40 yr, accelerate after age 65–70 yr. Lower body strength declines at a faster rate than upper body strength. Power declines at faster rate than strength.	Deficits in strength and power predict disability in old age and mortality risk.
Muscle endurance and fatigability	Endurance declines. Maintenance of force at a given relative intensity may increase with age. Age effects on mechanisms of fatigue are unclear and task-dependent.	Unclear but may impact recovery from repetitive daily tasks.
Balance and mobility	Sensory, motor, and cognitive changes alter biomechanics (sit, stand, locomotion). These changes + environmental constraints can adversely affect balance and mobility.	Impaired balance increases fear of falling and can reduce daily activity
Motor performance and control	Reaction time increases. Speed of simple and repetitive movements slows. Altered control of precision movements. Complex tasks affected more than simple tasks.	Impacts many IADL and increases risk. of injury and task learning time.
Flexibility and joint ROM	Declines are significant for hip (20%–30%), spine (20%–30%), and ankle(30%–40%) flexion by age 70 yr, especially in women. Muscle and tendon elasticity decreases.	Poor flexibility may increase risks of injury, falling, and back pain.
Cardiovascular function Cardiac function	Max HR ($208 - 0.7 \times$ age), stroke volume, and cardiac output decline. Slowed HR response at exercise onset. Altered diastolic filling pattern (rest, ex). Reduced left ventricular ejection fraction %. Decreased HR variability.	Major determinant of reduced exercise capacity with aging.
Vascular function	Aorta and its major branches stiffen. Vasodilator capacity and endothelium-dependent dilation of most peripheral arteries (brachial, cutaneous) decrease.	Arterial stiffening and endothelial dysfunction increase CVD risk.
Blood pressure	BP at rest (especially systolic) increases. BP during submaximal and maximal exercise are higher in old vs young, especially in older women.	Increased systolic BP reflects increased work of the heart
Regional blood flow	Leg blood flowisgenerally reducedatrest, submaximal, and maximal exercise. Renal and splanchnic vasoconstriction during submaximal exercise may be reduced with age.	May influence exercise, ADL, and BP regulation in old age
O_2 extraction	Systemic: same at rest and during submaximal exercise, same or slightly lower at maximal exercise. Legs: no change at rest or during submaximal exercise exercise; decreased slightly at maximal exercise.	Capacity for peripheral O_2 extraction is relatively maintained.
Blood volume and composition	Reduced total and plasma volumes; small reduction in hemoglobin concentration.	May contribute to reduced max stroke volume via reduced cardiac preload.

(Cont.,)

Table A-2 Summary of Typical Changes in Physiological Function and Body Composition with Advancing Age in Healthy Humans (Continued)

Variables	Typical Changes	Functional Significance[a]
Body fluid regulation	Thirst sensation decreases. Renal sodium- and water-conserving capacities are impaired. Total body water declines with age.	May predispose to dehydration and impaired exercise tolerance in the heat.
Pulmonary function Ventilation	Chest wall stiffens. Expiratory muscle strength decreases. Older adults adopt different breathing strategy during exercise. Work of breathing increases.	Pulmonary aging not limiting to exercise capacity, except in athlete.
Gas exchange	Loss of alveoli and increased size of remaining alveoli; reduces surface area for O_2 and CO_2 exchange in the lungs.	Arterial blood gases usually well-maintained up to maximal exercise.
Physical functional capacities Maximal O_2 uptake	Overall decline averages 0.4–0.5 mL kg^{-1} min^{-1} yr^{-1} (9% per decade) in healthy sedentary adults. Longitudinal data suggest rate of decline accelerates with advancing age.	Indicates functional reserve; disease and mortality risk factor.
O_2 uptake kinetics	Systemic O_2 uptake kinetics at exercise onset is slowed in old vs young, but this may be task specific. Prior warm-up exercise may normalize age difference.	Slow VO_2 kinetics may increase O2 deficit and promote early fatigue.
Lactate and ventilatory thresholds	Ventilatory thresholds (expressed as a percentage of $VO2_{max}$) increase with age. Maximal lactate production, tolerance, and clearance rate postexercise decline.	Indicative of reduced capacity for high intensity exercise.
Submaximal work efficiency	Metabolic cost of walking at a given speed is increased. Work efficiency (cycling) is preserved, but O_2 debt may increase in sedentary adults.	Implications for caloric cost and VO2 prediction in older adults.
Walking kinematics	Preferred walking speed is slower. Stride length is shorter; double-limb support duration is longer. Increased gait variability. These age differences are exaggerated when balance is perturbed.	Implications for physical function and risk of falling.
Stair climbing ability	Maximal step height is reduced, reflects integrated measure of leg strength, coordinated muscle activation, and dynamic balance.	Implications for mobility and physically demanding ADL.
Body composition/ metabolism Height	Height declines approximately 1 cm per decade during the 40s and 50s, accelerated after age 60 yr (women > men). Vertebral disks compress; thoracic curve becomes more pronounced.	Vertebral changes can impair mobility and other daily tasks.
Weight	Weight steadily increases during the 30s, 40s, and 50s, stabilizes until ~ age 70 yr, then declines. Age-related changes in weight and BMI can mask fat gain/muscle loss.	Large, rapid loss of weight in old age can indicate disease process.
FFM	FFM declines 2%–3% per decade from 30 to 70 yr of age. Losses of total body protein and potassium likely reflect the loss of metabolically active tissue (i.e., muscle).	FFM seems to be an important physiological regulator.

Table A-2 Summary of Typical Changes in Physiological Function and Body Composition with Advancing Age in Healthy Humans

Variables	Typical Changes	Functional Significance[a]
Muscle mass and size	Total muscle mass declines from age ~40 yr, accelerated after age 65–70 yr (legs lose muscle faster). Limb muscles exhibit reductions in fiber number and size (Type II > I).	Loss of muscle mass, Type II fiber size = reduced muscle speed/power.
MQ	Lipid and collagen content increase. Type I MHC content increases, type II MHC decreases. Peak-specific force declines. Oxidative capacity per kg muscle declines.	Changes may be related to insulin resistance and muscle weakness.
Regional adiposity	Body fat increases during the 30s, 40s, and 50s, with a preferential accumulation in the visceral (intra-abdominal) region, especially in men. After age 70 yr, fat (all sites) decreases.	Accumulation of visceral fat is linked to CV and metabolic disease.
Bone density	Bone mass peaks in the mid to late 20s. BMD declines 0.5% yr^{-1} or more after age 40 yr. Women have disproportionate loss of bone (2%–3% yr^{-1}) after menopause.	Osteopenia (1–2.5 SD below young controls) elevates fracture risk.
Metabolic changes	RMR (absolute and per kg FFM), muscle protein synthesis rates (mitochondria and MHC), and fat oxidation (during submaximal exercise) all decline with advancing age.	These may influence substrate utilization during exercise.

Typical changes generally reflect age-associated differences on the basis of cross-sectional data, which can underestimate changes followed longitudinally.

[a] The strength of existing evidence for the functional associations identified in the far right column ranges between A and D.
BMI, body mass index; BP, blood pressure; CVD, cardiovascular disease; IADL, instrumental ADL; MHC, myosin heavy chain; Peak, peak or maximal exercise responses; RMR, resting metabolic rate.

on the reduction in risk of developing and dying from chronic diseases is beyond the scope of this review, the recently published *Physical Activity Guidelines Advisory Committee Report* (51) by the Department of Health and Human Services (DHHS) provides a comprehensive summary of the evidence linking physical activity with the risk of developing and dying from a variety of different conditions. The report contains information for the general population as well as for older adults in particular.

Evidence statement and recommendation. *Evidence category B.* Advancing age is associated with increased risk for chronic diseases, but physical activity significantly reduces this risk.

SECTION 2: PHYSICAL ACTIVITY AND THE AGING PROCESS

Physical activity and the aging process. Aging is a complex process involving many factors that interact with one another, including primary aging processes, "secondary aging" effects (resulting from chronic disease and lifestyle behaviors), and genetic factors

(152, 258). The impact of physical activity on primary aging processes is difficult to study in humans because cellular aging processes and disease mechanisms are highly intertwined (137). There are currently no lifestyle interventions, including exercise, which have been shown to reliably extend maximal lifespan in humans (98, 175). Rather, regular physical activity increases average life expectancy through its influence on chronic disease development (via reduction of secondary aging effects). Physical activity also limits the impact of secondary aging through restoration of functional capacity in previously sedentary older adults. AET and RET programs can increase aerobic capacity and muscle strength, respectively, by 20%–30% or more in older adults (101, 139).

Evidence statement and recommendation. *Evidence category A.* Regular physical activity increases average life expectancy through its influence on chronic disease development, through the mitigation of age-related biological changes and their associated effects on health and well-being, and through the preservation of functional capacity.

Factors influencing functional decline in aging. Although the pattern of age-related change for most physiological variables is one of decline, some individuals show little or no change for a given variable, whereas others show some improvement with age (119). There are also individuals for whom physical functioning oscillates, exhibiting variable rates of change over time (120, 187, 192), possibly reflecting variable levels of physical activity and other cyclical (seasonal) or less predictable (sickness, injuries) influences. However, even after accounting for the effect of different levels of physical activity, there is still substantial between- subject variability (at a given point in time and in rates of change over time) for most physiological measures, and this variability seems to increase with age (231). Individual variation is also apparent in the adaptive responses to a standardized exercise training program; some individuals show dramatic changes for a given variable (responders), whereas others show minimal effects (nonresponders) (24).

Determining the extent to which genetic and lifestyle factors influence age-associated functional declines and the magnitude of the adaptive responses to exercise (i.e., trainability) of both younger and older individuals is an area of active investigation. Exercise training studies involving families and twin pairs report a significant genetic influence on baseline physiological function (explaining ~30% to 70% of between-subjects variance) and trainability of aerobic fitness (24), skeletal muscle properties (199), and cardiovascular risk factors (24). Although the role of genetic factors in determining changes in function over time and in response to exercise training in older humans is not well understood, it is likely that a combination of lifestyle and genetic factors contribute to the wide interindividual variability seen in older adults.

Evidence statement and recommendation. *Evidence category B.* Individuals differ widely in how they age and in how they adapt to an exercise program. It is likely that a combination of genetic and lifestyle factors contribute to the wide interindividual variability seen in older adults.

Exercise and the aging process. The acute physiological adjustments of healthy sedentary older men and women to submaximal aerobic exercise are qualitatively similar to those of young adults and are adequate in meeting the major regulatory demands of exercise, which include the control of arterial blood pressure and vital organ perfusion, augmentation of oxygen and substrate delivery and utilization within active muscle, maintenance of arterial blood homeostasis, and dissipation of heat (213). The acute cardiovascular and neuromuscular adjustments to resistance exercise (both isometric and dynamic) also seem to be well preserved in healthy older adults (213). Accordingly, the normal age-associated reductions in functional capacity discussed in Section 1 should not limit the ability of healthy older adults to engage in aerobic or resistance exercise. In addition, long-term adaptive or training responses of middle-aged and nonfrail older adults to conventional AET or RET programs (i.e., relative intensity-based, progressive overload) are qualitatively similar to those seen in young adults. Although absolute improvements tend to be less in older versus young people, the relative increases in many variables, including $\dot{V}O_{2max}$ (100), submaximal metabolic responses (211), and exercise tolerance with AET and limb muscle strength (139), endurance (255), and size (203) in response to RET, are generally similar. Physiological aging alters some of the mechanisms and time course (174, 253) by which older men and women adapt to a given training stimulus (i.e., older adults may take longer to reach the same level of improvement), and sex differences are emerging with respect to these mechanisms (16), but the body's adaptive capacity is reasonably well-preserved, at least through the seventh decade (98, 217). During the combined demands of large muscle exercise and heat and/or cold stress, however, older individuals do exhibit a greater reduction in exercise tolerance and an increased risk of heat and cold illness/injury, respectively, compared with young adults (126). Age differences in exercise tolerance at higher ambient temperatures may be at least partially due to the lower aerobic fitness levels in older adults (126). Cessation of aerobic training by older adults leads to a rapid loss of cardiovascular (184, 210) and metabolic (201) fitness, whereas strength training-induced (neural) adaptations seem more persistent (139), similar to what has been observed in younger populations (44, 139).

Evidence statement and recommendation. *Evidence category A.* Healthy older adults are able to engage in acute aerobic or resistance exercise and experience positive adaptations to exercise training.

Physical activity and successful aging. When centenarians and other long-lived individuals are studied, their longevity is often attributed to a healthy lifestyle. Three characteristic behaviors are routinely reported; these include exercising regularly, maintaining a social network, and maintaining a positive mental attitude (214, 231). Physiological factors that are most frequently associated with longevity and successful aging include low blood pressure, low body mass index and central adiposity, preserved glucose tolerance (low plasma glucose and insulin concentrations), and an atheroprotective blood lipid profile consisting of low triglyceride and LDL-cholesterol and high HDL-cholesterol concentrations (97, 231). Regular physical activity seems to be the only lifestyle behavior identified to date, other than perhaps caloric restriction, which can favorably influence a broad range of physiological systems and chronic disease risk factors (97, 98), and may also be associated with better mental health (154) and social integration (155). Thus, despite large differences in genetic background among those of a given age cohort, it seems that physical activity may be a lifestyle factor that discriminates between individuals who have and have not experienced successful aging (207, 214, 258).

Evidence statement and recommendation. *Evidence category B/C.* Regular physical activity can favorably influence a broad range of physiological systems and may be a lifestyle factor that discriminates between those individuals who have and have not experienced successful aging.

Physical activity and the prevention, management, and treatment of diseases and chronic conditions. There is growing evidence that regular physical activity reduces risk of developing numerous chronic conditions and diseases including cardiovascular disease, stroke, hypertension, type 2 diabetes mellitus, osteoporosis, obesity, colon cancer, breast cancer, cognitive impairment, anxiety, and depression. In addition, physical activity is recommended as a therapeutic intervention for the treatment and management of many chronic diseases including coronary heart disease (70, 185, 242), hypertension (37, 183, 241), peripheral vascular disease (157), type 2 diabetes (220), obesity (252), elevated cholesterol (165, 241), osteoporosis (75, 251), osteoarthritis (1, 3), claudication (232), and chronic obstructive pulmonary disease (170). Furthermore, clinical practice guidelines also identify a role for physical activity in the treatment and management of conditions such as depression and anxiety disorders (26), dementia (54), pain (4), congestive heart failure (197), syncope (25), stroke (79), back pain (85), and constipation (142). Although a detailed review of the impact of regular physical activity on the development, treatment, and management of chronic diseases is beyond the scope of this Position Stand, Table 3 summarizes a growing body of evidence that regular physical activity reduces the risk of developing a large number of chronic diseases and is valuable in the treatment of numerous diseases.

Evidence statement and recommendation. *Evidence category A/B.* Regular physical activity reduces the risk of developing a large number of chronic diseases and conditions and is valuable in the treatment of numerous diseases.

SECTION 3: BENEFITS OF PHYSICAL ACTIVITY AND EXERCISE

This section summarizes published research with respect to the known benefits of exercise on functional capacity, chronic disease risk, and quality of life (QOL) in adults of various ages. The review considers first the effects of long-term participation in exercise by aerobic- and resistance-trained athletes, followed by a summary of the benefits of various modes of exercise training in previously sedentary individuals. The section concludes with a discussion of the benefits of physical activity and exercise training for psychological health, cognitive functioning, and overall QOL.

Table A-3 Summary of the Role of Physical Activity in the Prevention, Management, and Treatment of Chronic Disease and Disability

Disease State	Preventive Role	Therapeutic Role	Effective Exercise Modality	Other Considerations
Arthritis	Possible, via prevention of obesity	Yes	AET RET Aquatic exercise	Low impact
Cancer	Yes, AET in epidemiological studies	Yes, for QOL, wasting, lymphedema, psychological functioning, breast cancer survival	AET RET	Sufficient volume to achieve healthy weight if obese
Chronic obstructive pulmonary disease	No	Yes, for extrapulmonary manifestations	AET RET	RET may be more tolerable in severe disease; combined effects complementary if feasible Time exercise sessions to coincide with bronchodilator medication peak Use oxygen during exercise as needed
Chronic renal failure	Possible, via prevention of diabetes and hypertension	Yes, for exercise capacity, body composition, sarcopenia, cardiovascular status, QOL, psychological function, inflammation, etc.	AET RET	Exercise reduces cardiovascular and metabolic risk factors; improves depression RET offsets myopathy of chronic renal failure
Cognitive impairment	Yes, AET in epidemiological studies	Yes	AET RET	Mechanism unknown Supervision needed for dementia
Congestive heart failure	Possible, via prevention of coronary artery disease and hypertension	Yes, for exercise capacity, survival, cardiovascular risk profile, symptoms, QOL	AET RET	RET may be more tolerable if dyspnea severely limits AET activity Cardiac cachexia targeted by RET
Coronary artery disease	Yes AET and RET now shown to be protective	Yes	AET RET	Complementary effects on exercise capacity and metabolic profile from combined exercise modalities Resistance may be more tolerable if ischemic threshold is very low because of lower HR response to training
Depression	Yes, AET in epidemiological studies	Yes	AET RET	Moderate- to high-intensity exercise more efficacious than low-intensity exercise in major depression Minor depression may respond to wider variety of exercise modalities and intensities
Disability	Yes, AET in epidemiological studies, muscle strength protective	Yes	AET RET	Choice of exercise should be targeted to etiology of disability

(Cont.,)

Table A-3 Summary of the Role of Physical Activity in the Prevention, Management, and Treatment of Chronic Disease and Disability (Continued)

Disease State	Preventive Role	Therapeutic Role	Effective Exercise Modality	Other Considerations
Hypertension	Yes, AET in epidemiological studies	Yes	AET RET	Small reductions in systolic and diastolic pressures seen Larger changes if weight loss occurs
Obesity	Yes, AET in epidemiological studies	Yes	AET RET	Sufficient energy expenditure to induce deficit
Osteoporosis	Yes, AET in epidemiological studies	Yes	AET RET Balance training High-impact exercise	RET maintains lean tissue (muscle and bone) better than AET during weight loss AET should be weight-bearing High-impact, high-velocity activity (*e.g.*, jumping) if tolerable RET effects are local to muscles contracted Balance training should be added to prevent falls
Peripheral vascular disease	Yes, AET via treatment of risk factors for PVD related to exercise	Yes	AET Resistance	Vascular effect is systemic; upper limb ergometrymay be substituted for leg exercise if necessary RET has positive but less robust effect on claudication May need to exercise to the limits of pain tolerance each session to extend time to claudication
Stroke	Yes, AET in epidemiological studies	Yes	AET, treadmill training RET (treatment)	Most effective treatment modality not clear
Type 2 diabetes	Yes, AET in epidemiological studies RET protective for impaired glucose tolerance	Yes	AET RET (treatment)	Exercise every 72 h Moderate- to high-intensity exercise most effective

AET, aerobic exercise training; RET, resistance exercise training; QOL, quality of life.

Studies of Long-Term Physical Activity in Athletes

Aerobic athletes. Compared to their sedentary, age- matched peers, older athletes exhibit a broad range of physiological and health advantages. These benefits include, but are not limited to the following: 1) a more favorable body composition profile, including less total and abdominal body fat (76, 98), a greater relative muscle mass (% of body mass) in the limbs (235), and higher bone mineral density (BMD) at weight bearing sites (78, 164); 2) more oxidative and fatigue-resistant limb muscles (98, 188, 247); 3) a higher capacity to transport and use oxygen (173, 189, 206); 4) a higher cardiac stroke volume at peak exertion (77, 173) and a "younger" pattern of left ventricular filling (increased early-to-late inflow velocity, E/A ratio) (55, 98); 5) less cardiovascular (83) and metabolic (38, 206, 211, 212) stress during exercise at any given submaximal work intensity; 6) a significantly reduced coronary risk profile (lower blood pressure, increased HR variability, better endothelial reactivity, lower systemic inflammatory markers, better insulin sensitivity and glucose homeostasis, lower triglycerides, LDL, and total cholesterol, higher HDL, and smaller waist circumference) (264); 7) faster nerve conduction velocity (253); and 8) slower development of disability in old age (257).

Evidence statement and recommendation. *Evidence category B.* Vigorous, long-term participation in AET is associated with elevated cardiovascular reserve and skeletal muscle adaptations that enable the aerobically trained older individual to sustain a submaximal exercise load with less cardiovascular stress and muscular fatigue than their untrained peers. Prolonged aerobic exercise also seems to slow the age-related accumulation of central body fat and is cardioprotective.

Resistance-trained athletes. The number of laboratory- based physiological comparisons of resistance-trainedathletes at various ages is small by comparison to the literature on aging aerobic athletes. Nevertheless, older RET athletes tend to have a higher muscle mass (131), are generally leaner (217), and are ~30%–50% stronger (131) than their sedentary peers. Compared to age-matched AET athletes, RET athletes have more total muscle mass (131), higher bone mineral densities (236), and maintain higher muscle strength and power (131).

Evidence statement and recommendation. *Evidence category B.* Prolonged participation in RET has clear benefits for slowing the loss of muscle and bone mass and strength, which are not seen as consistently with aerobic exercise alone.

BENEFITS OF EXERCISE TRAINING IN PREVIOUSLY SEDENTARY INDIVIDUALS

AET

Aerobic exercise capacity. Supervised AET programs of sufficient intensity ($\geq$60% of pretraining $\dot{V}O_{2max}$), frequency ($\geq$3 d.wk^{-1}), and length ($\geq$16 wk) can significantly increase $\dot{V}O_{2max}$ in healthy middle-aged and older adults. The average increase in $\dot{V}O_{2max}$ reported in well- controlled studies lasting 16 to 20 wk is +3.8 m.L kg^{-1} min^{-1} or 16.3% when compared with nonexercise control subjects during the same period. Larger improvements in $\dot{V}O_{2max}$ are typically observed with longer training periods (20 to 30 wk) but not necessarily higher training intensities (i.e., >70% of & $\dot{V}O_{2max}$)

(100), unless an interval-type training regimen is used (5, 145). Significant AET-induced increases in $\dot{V}O_{2max}$ have also been reported in healthy subjects older than 75 yr, but the magnitude of improvement is significantly less (60, 146). Although men and women in their 60s and early 70s show similarly relative (% above pretraining) increases in $\dot{V}O_{2max}$ after AET compared with younger adults, there seems to be a sex difference in the underlying mechanisms of adaptation; older men exhibit increases in maximal cardiac output and systemic arteriovenous O_2 difference, whereas older women rely almost exclusively on widening the systemic arteriovenous O_2 difference (228).

Evidence statement and recommendation. *Evidence category A.* AET programs of sufficient intensity ($\geq 60\%$ of pretraining $\dot{V}O_{2max}$), frequency, and length (≥ 3 d.wk^{-1} for ≥ 16 wk) can significantly increase $\dot{V}O_{2max}$ in healthy middle- aged and older adults.

Cardiovascular effects. Three or more months of moderate-intensity AET (*e.g.,* $\geq 60\%$ of $\dot{V}O_{2max}$) elicits several cardiovascular adaptations in healthy (normoten- sive) middle-aged and older adults, which are evident at rest and in response to acute dynamic exercise. The most consistently reported adaptations include the following: 1) a lower HR at rest (101) and at any submaximal exercise workload (84); 2) smaller rises in systolic, diastolic, and mean blood pressures during submaximal exercise (212); 3) improvements in the vasodilator and O_2 uptake capacities of the trained muscle groups (116, 149, 267); and 4) numerous cardioprotective effects, including reductions in atherogenic risk factors (reduced triglyceride and increased HDL concentrations), reductions in large elastic artery stiffness (239), improved endothelial (49) and baroreflex (174) function, and increased vagal tone (174). Evidence for improved myocardial contractile performance (i.e., left ventricular systolic and diastolic function), increased maximal exercise stroke volume, and cardiac hypertrophy after AET has generally been limited to studies involving men (59, 210, 229, 234) and at higher intensities of training (145).

Evidence statement and recommendation. *Evidence category A.* Three or more months of moderate-intensity AET elicits cardiovascular adaptations in healthy middle- aged and older adults, which are evident at rest and in response to acute dynamic exercise.

Body composition. Sedentary Americans typically gain 8 to 9 kg of body weight (mostly fat gain) between the ages of 18 and 55 yr (98); this is followed by additional gains of 1 to 2 kg over the next decade and declining body weight thereafter (76). In studies involving overweight middle-aged and older adults, moderate-intensity AET ($\geq 60\%$ of $\dot{V}O_{2max}$) without dietary modification has generally been shown to be effective in reducing total body fat. Average losses during 2to 9 months ranged from 0.4 to 3.2 kg (1%–4% of total body weight) (123, 244) with the magnitude of total fat loss related to the total number of exercise sessions (80), just as in younger overweight populations. Although these reductions in total fat may seem modest in relation to age-related weight gain, AET can have significant effects on fat loss from the intra-abdominal (visceral) region (*e.g.,* $>20\%$) (107).

In contrast to its effects on body fat, most studies report no significant effect of AET on fat-free mass (FFM). A meta-analysis identified significant increases in total FFM in only 8 of 36 studies that involved AET, and these increases were generally less than 1 kg (244). The lack of impact on FFM accretion by AET reflects the fact that this form of training, which involves repetitive, but low-force muscular contractions, does not generally stimulate significant skeletal muscle growth or improve strength.

Evidence statement and recommendation. *Evidence category A/B.* In studies involving overweight middle- aged and older adults, moderate-intensity AET has been shown to be effective in reducing total body fat. In contrast, most studies report no significant effect of AET on FFM.

Metabolic effects. AET, independent of dietary changes, can induce multiple changes that enhance the body's ability to maintain glycemic control at rest (98, 129), to clear atherogenic lipids (triglycerides) from the circulation after a meal (121), and to preferentially use fat as a muscular fuel during submaximal exercise (219). Healthy men and women in their 60s and 70s seem to retain the capacity to upregulate the cellular processes that facilitate these respective training effects. However, the impact of AET on metabolic control measured at the whole body level and the residual metabolic effects after exercise (throughout the day) may depend on the *intensity* of the training stimulus. For example, although both moderate- (218) and high-intensity (43) AET are shown to increase glucose transporter content in the muscles of older humans, it is the higher-intensity AET programs that may result in greater improvement in whole-body insulin action (52).

Evidence statement and recommendation. *Evidence category B.* AET can induce a variety of favorable metabolic adaptations including enhanced glycemic control, augmented clearance of postprandial lipids, and preferential utilization of fat during submaximal exercise.

Bone health. Low-intensity weight bearing activities such as walking (3–5 d.wk^{-1}) for periods of up to 1 yr have modest, if any, effect on BMD in postmenopausal women (0%–2% increase in hip, spine BMD) (132). However, such activities seem beneficial from the standpoint of counteracting age-related losses (0.5 to 1%yr^{-1} in sedentary controls) and lowering hip fracture risk (7, 132). Studies involving higher-intensity bone loading activities such as stair climbing/descending, brisk walking, walking with weighted vests, or jogging, generally report more significant effects on BMD in postmenopausal women (132), at least during the short term (1 to 2 yr). Research on the effectiveness of exercise for bone health in older men is still emerging (125), but one prospective study found that middle aged and older men who ran nine or more times per month exhibited lower rates of lumbar bone loss than men who jogged less frequently (161).

Evidence statement and recommendation. *Evidence category B.* AET may be effective in counteracting age-related declines in BMD in postmenopausal women.

RET

Muscular strength. Changes in strength after RET are assessed using a variety of methods, including isometric, isokinetic, one-repetition maximum (1-RM), and multiple- repetition (*e.g.,* 3-RM) maximum-effort protocols. In general, strength increases after RET in older adults seem to be greater with measures of 1-RM or 3-RM performance compared with isometric or isokinetic measures (64, 73, 102, 172). Older adults can substantially increase their strength after RET—with reported increases ranging from less than 25% (34, 64, 82, 89, 91) to greater than 100% (63, 66, 73, 140). The influence of age on the capacity to increase strength after RET is complex. Several studies have demonstrated similar percent strength gains between older and younger participants (89, 91, 99, 114, 169), whereas others have reported that percent strength increases are less for older compared with younger adults (139, 144). Additional reports suggest that the effects of age on strength adaptations may be influenced by gender (109), duration of the training intervention (112), and/or the specific muscle groups examined (259).

Evidence statement and recommendation. *Evidence category A.* Older adults can substantially increase their strength after RET.

Muscle power. Power production is equivalent to the force or torque of a muscular contraction multiplied by its velocity. Studies suggest that *power* -producing capabilities are more strongly associated with functional performance than *muscle strength* in older adults (11, 57, 60, 71, 227). Moreover, the age-related loss of muscle power occurs at a greater rate than the loss of strength (23, 88, 93, 111, 159) most likely owing to a disproportionate reduction in the size of Type II fibers (130, 140). However, substantial increases in power (measured using isokinetic, isotonic, stair climbing, and vertical jumping protocols) are demonstrated after RET in older adults (58, 64, 67, 68, 112, 169). Several earlier studies reported greater increases in maximum strength compared with power (67, 115, 227); however, the training protocols in these studies used traditional, slower- movement speeds. More recent studies, incorporating higher-velocity training protocols, suggest that the gains in power may be either comparable (58, 112, 169) or greater (68) to gains in maximum strength/force production.

Evidence statement and recommendation. *Evidence category A.* Substantial increases in muscular power have been demonstrated after RET in older adults.

Muscle quality. Muscle quality (MQ) is defined in muscular performance (strength or power) per unit muscle volume or mass. Understanding the effects of RET on MQ in older adults is important because most studies suggest that increases in strength and power after RET are greater than would be expected based upon changes in muscle mass alone (8, 73, 110, 246). These findings are magnified during the earlier phases of training (91, 163). Although increased motor unit recruitment and/or discharge rates are thought to be the primary contributors to increased MQ after RET (42, 82, 89, 91, 144), other factors including decreased activation of antagonistic muscle groups (89, 91), alterations in muscle architecture and tendon stiffness (193–195), and selective hypertrophy of Type II muscle fiber areas (36, 92, 148) may also influence MQ. Although the hypertrophic response is diminished in older adults, increases in MQ are similar between older and younger men (110, 259) but may be greater in younger women compared with older women (90). Improvements in MQ do not seem to be sex- specific, and adaptations after RET seem to be similar between older men and women (91, 246).

Evidence statement and recommendation. *Evidence category B.* Increases in MQ are similar between older and younger adults, and these improvements do not seem to be sex-specific.

Muscle endurance. Although the ability to repeatedly produce muscular force and power over an extended period may determine an older adult's travel range and functional independence, the effects of RET on muscular endurance are relatively understudied. Increases in muscular strength, secondary to neurological, metabolic, and/or hypertrophic adaptations, are likely to translate into increased muscular endurance by 1) reducing the motor-unit activation required to complete submaximal tasks (104, 136), 2) reducing the coactivation of antagonistic muscles (75, 91), 3) increasing high-energy phosphate (adenosine triphosphate and creatine phosphate) availability (103), 4) shifting the expression of myosin heavy chain isoforms from IIb (IIx) to IIa (215), 5) increasing mitochondrial density and oxidative capacity (116), and 6) reducing the percent of available myofiber volume required to complete submaximal tasks. Marked improvements (34%–200%) in muscular endurance have been reported after RET using moderate- to higher-intensity protocols (2, 82, 255).

Evidence statement and recommendation. *Evidence category C.* Improvements in muscular endurance have been reported after RET using moderate- to higher- intensity protocols, whereas lower-intensity RET does not improve muscular endurance.

Body composition. Most studies report an increase in FFM with high-intensity RET. Men tend to have greater increase in FFM after RET than women, but these sex differences are no longer seen when FFM is expressed relative to initial FFM (102). Although some have suggested that this increase in FFM is primarily due to an increase in total body water (33), both muscle tissue and bone are also affected by RET. Increases in FFM can be attributed to increases in muscle cross-sectional areas (203, 248) and volumes (203). These changes seem to be a result of an increase in Type IIa fiber areas, with a decrease in Type IIx fiber area (8) and no change in Type I fiber area (36). A recent review (103) of 20 studies found that older adults demonstrate hypertrophy of muscle tissue of between 10% and 62% after RET.

Several studies have found that moderate- or high-intensity RET decreases total body fat mass (FM), with losses ranging from 1.6% to 3.4% (8, 33, 102, 105, 106, 108, 114, 249). Recently, investigators have attempted to determine the effect of RET on *regional* FM—specifically subcutaneous adipose tissue (SAT) and intra-abdominal adipose tissue (IAAT). Binder et al. (17) reported no change in IAAT or SAT in frail older adults after 12 wk of RET; however, Hunter et al. (102) reported sex-specific effects—demonstrating that elder women, but not men, lost IAAT (12%) and SAT (6%) after 25 wk of moderate-intensity (65%–80% 1-RM) RET. Others reported that both older men and women decreased IAAT by 10% (108, 248) after 16 wk of RET.

Evidence statement and recommendation. *Evidence category B/C.* Favorable changes in body composition, including increased FFM and decreased FM have been reported in older adults who participate in moderate or high intensity RET.

Bone health. Several meta-analyses have concluded that RET as well as AET have significant positive effects on BMD in most sites in both pre- and postmenopausal women (124, 125, 256, 266). In general, 1%–2% differences between RET and sedentary controls are seen in RCTs in which RET conforms to the principles known to be associated with skeletal adaptation, namely, higher intensity, progressive, and novel loading, as well as high strain rates. For example, Vincent and Braith (254) reported a 1.96% increase in BMD at the femoral neck, with no significant changes in total body, spine, or Ward's Triangle BMD—after high-intensity, low-volume RET of 24 wk in duration. However, other studies have demonstrated more modest effects. For example, Stewart et al. (233) reported that group data inferred a *decrease* in average BMD with combined low-intensity RET and aerobic training; however, regression modeling revealed a positive relation between increases in strength and increases in femoral BMD. Rhodes et al. (198) also reported significant correlations (0.27–0.40) between changes in leg strength and femoral and lumbar BMD changes; however, they too found no between-group differences in controls and exercisers who performed 12 months of RET (75% 1-RM;3 d.wk^{-1}).

Evidence statement and recommendation. *Evidence category B.* High-intensity RET preserves or improves BMD relative to sedentary controls, with a direct relationship between muscle and bone adaptations.

Metabolic and endocrine effects. The effects of short- and long-term RET programs on basal metabolic rate (BMR) in older adults are not clear. Some investigations have reported increases of 7%–9% in BMR after 12–26 wk of exercise (33, 105, 139, 249), whereas other studies of similar duration have not demonstrated changes (158, 237). RET programs can enhance older adults' use of fat as a fuel, as indicated by increased lipid oxidation and decreased carbohydrate and amino acid oxidation at rest (105, 249). Serum cholesterol and triglycerides are also influenced by RET, and reports suggest that training can increase HDL cholesterol by 8%–21%, decrease LDL cholesterol by 13%–23%, and reduce triglyceride levels by 11%–18% (62, 86, 114).

Resting testosterone is lower in older adults, and acute responses of total and free testosterone to weight lifting are blunted in seniors after RET. Neither short- (10–12 wk) (45, 112, 135) nor longer-term (21–24 wk) (22, 87) RET increases resting concentrations of total or free testosterone. A decrease in resting cortisol (15%–25%) (112, 133), however, has previously been observed, which may create a favorable environment for muscle hypertrophy. Peptide hormones, including growth hormone and insulin-like growth factor 1 (IGF-1) also have important anabolic action. Circulating growth hormone stimulates synthesis of IGF-1 in the liver, and circulating IGF-1 promotes differentiation of satellite cells into myotubes (95). Another IGF, mechanogrowth factor, is synthesized locally in muscle and signals the proliferation of satellite cells (94). Although one report suggests that RET may increase circulating IGF-1 in participants with low baseline serum IGF-1 levels (178), most investigations suggest that RET does not alter circulating IGF-1 (8, 15, 22, 89). RET also seems to have no effect on free IGF-1 (15) and does not decrease IGF-1 binding proteins (22, 178)

Evidence statement and recommendation. *Evidence category B/C.* Evidence of the effect of RET on metabolic variables is mixed. There is some evidence that RET can alter the preferred fuel source used under resting conditions, but there is inconsistent evidence regarding the effects of RET on BMR. The effect of RET on a variety of different hormones has been studied increasingly in recent years; however, the exact nature of the relationship is not yet well understood.

Balance Training

Several studies have examined relationships among age, exercise, and balance with the most research having been conducted in populations at risk for falling (i.e., osteoporotic women, frail older adults, subjects with a previous fall history) (231). Several large prospective cohort studies link higher levels of physical activity, particularly walking, with 30%–50% reduction in the risk of osteoporotic fractures (74). However, these studies do not provide data on the utility of balance training alone for achieving this outcome. Nonetheless, balance training activities such as lower body strengthening and walking over difficult terrain have been shown to significantly improve balance in many studies, and are thus recommended as part of an exercise intervention to prevent falls (74, 21, 181, 204). Older adults identified at the highest risk for falls seem to benefit from an individually tailored exercise program that is embedded within a larger, multifactorial falls-prevention intervention (243, 48, 202). Multimodal programs of balance, strength, flexibility, and walking (3032, 171) are shown to reduce the risk of both noninjurious and injurious falls. In addition, there is some evidence that tai chi programs can be effective in reducing the risk of both noninjurious and injurious falls (141, 265).

Evidence statement and recommendation. *Evidence category C.* Multimodal exercise, usually including strength and balance exercises, and tai chi have been shown to be effective in reducing the risk of noninjurious and sometimes injurious falls in populations who are at an elevated risk of falling.

Stretching and flexibility training. Despite decrements in joint ROM with age and established links among poor flexibility, mobility, and physical independence (16, 222, 262), there remains a surprisingly small number of studies that have documented or compared the effects of specific ROM exercises on flexibility outcomes in older populations. One well-controlled study of 70-yr-old women reported significant improvements in low back/hamstring flexibility (+25%) and spinal extension (+40%) after 10 wk of a supervised static stretching program (3 d.wk^{1}) that involved a series of low back and hip exercises (200). Improvements of a similar magnitude have been documented for upper body (i.e., shoulder) and lower body (ankle, knee) flexibility in older men and women using a combination of stretching and rhythmic movements through full ROM (*e.g.,* stretching + yoga or tai chi) (231). Collectively, these results suggest that flexibility can be increased in the major joints by ROM exercises *per se* in healthy older adults. However, there is little consensus regarding how much (frequency, duration) and what types of ROM exercises (static vs dynamic) are the safest and most effective for older adults.

Evidence statement and recommendation. *Evidence category D.* Few controlled studies have examined the effect of flexibility exercise on ROM in older adults. There is some evidence that flexibility can be increased in the major joints by ROM exercises; however, how much and what types of ROM exercises are most effective have not been established.

Effect of exercise and physical activity on physical functioning and daily life activities. The degree to which participation in exercise and physical activity translates into improved physical functioning and enhanced performance of everyday life activities is not yet clear. Contrasting findings of *improved* versus *unchanged* physical performance after a variety of exercise activities (*e.g.,* walking, stair climbing, balance, chair standing) have been reported, and there is not a simple linear relationship between participation in physical activity and changes in disability (i.e., dependence in ADL). For example, improvements of between 7% and 17% have been demonstrated for self-selected and/or maximum-effort walking velocity after a variety of RET programs (13, 90, 96, 99, 118, 208, 226); however, nonsignificant changes have also been reported after lower- and higher-intensity interventions (27, 28, 58, 80, 117). Although some studies demonstrated improvements across a variety of functional tasks (12, 13, 96, 99, 162, 255), other studies suggest functional performance adaptations are more specific, resulting in changes in one functional measure (*e.g.,* walking) but not others (*e.g.,* chair-rise or stair climb performance) (208). Nonetheless, there does seem to be a relationship between maintaining cardiovascular fitness levels and the likelihood of becoming functionally dependent in an 8-yr follow-up study of older adults (180). The nature and strength of the relationship between physical activity and functional performance are likely to vary as a function of the specific physical activity functional measures selected (205, 227). Furthermore, because *specificity of training* principles suggest that performance adaptations will be greatest for those activities that mimic the kinematics, resistances, and movement speeds used in the training program, many authors have emphasized the importance of prescribing higher-velocity movements using activities that mimic ADL (10, 13, 47, 60, 162).

Evidence statement and recommendation. *Evidence category C/D.* The effect of exercise on physical performance is poorly understood and does not seem to be linear. RET has been shown to favorably impact walking, chair stand, and balance activities, but more information is needed to understand the precise nature of the relationship between exercise and functional performance.

BENEFITS OF EXERCISE AND PHYSICAL ACTIVITY FOR PSYCHOLOGICAL HEALTH AND WELL-BEING

In addition to its effects on physiological variables and a variety of chronic diseases and conditions, there is now strong evidence that exercise and physical activity have a significant impact on several psychological parameters. In this revision of the ACSM Position Stand "Exercise and Physical Activity for Older Adults," we update the previous edition of the Position Stand with respect to new evidence regarding the effect of participation in regular physical activity on overall psychological health and well-being, the effect of exercise and physical activity on cognitive functioning, and the impact of exercise and physical activity on overall QOL. In addition, for the first time, we include a separate section that focuses on a relatively new literature that examines the effect of RET on psychological health and well-being.

Physical activity and psychological well-being in aging. There is now considerable evidence that regular physical activity is associated with significant improvements in overall psychological health and well-being (155, 231). Both higher physical fitness (20, 29, 221) and participation in AET are associated with a decreased risk for clinical depression or anxiety (20, 56, 153). Exercise and physical activity have been proposed to impact psychological well-being through their moderating and mediating effects on constructs such as self-concept and self-esteem (72). However, other pathways may also be operative, such as reduction in visceral adiposity along with associated elevation in cortisol (186) and inflammatory adipokines (263, 269) that have been implicated in hippocampal atrophy, cognitive, and affective impairments (143). In addition, for many seniors, aging is associated with a loss of perceived control (9). Because perceptions of control over one's own life are known to be related to psychological health and well-being, exercise scientists have begun to focus on the relationship between activity and various indices of psychosocial control, self-efficacy, and perceived competency (156). McAuley and Katula (155) reviewed the literature examining the relationship between physical activity and self-efficacy in older adults. They conclude that most well-controlled exercise training studies result in significant improvements in both physical fitness and selfefficacy for physical activity in older adults. Several studies suggest that moderate-intensity physical activity may be more effective than either low- or high-intensity training regimens (128, 154). There is growing recognition that physical activity self-efficacy is not only an important outcome measure as a result of participation in activity, it may also be an important predictor of sustained behavioral change in sedentary populations (56).

Evidence statement and recommendation. *Evidence category A/B.* Regular physical activity is associated with significant improvements in overall psychological wellbeing. Both physical fitness and AET are associated with a decreased risk for clinical depression or anxiety. Exercise and physical activity have been proposed to impact psychological well-being through their moderating and mediating effects on constructs such as self-concept and self-esteem.

Physical activity, cognitive functioning, and aging. Both cross-sectional and prospective cohort studies have linked participation in regular physical activity with a reduced risk for dementia or cognitive decline in older adults. Examples include the Study of Osteoporotic Fractures (268), which reported that activity level was linked to changes in Mini-Mental Status Examination scores, and the Canadian Study of Health and Aging, which demonstrated that physical activity was associated with lower risk of cognitive impairment and dementia (138). It also seems that decreases in physical mobility are linked to cognitive decline (127). The InCHIANTI study reported an association between physical mobility, specifically walking speed and ability to walk 1 km, with signs of neurological disease (65). Similarly, the Oregon Brain Aging Study reported an association between walking speed and onset of cognitive impairment (147) Finally, the MacArthur Research Network on Successful Aging Community Study reported associations between declines in cognitive performance and routine physical tasks including measures of grip strength and mobility (i.e., walking speed, chair stands) (238).

Experimental trials of exercise interventions in older adults demonstrate that acute exposure to a single bout of aerobic exercise can result in short-term improvements in memory, attention, and reaction time (39), but more importantly, participation in both AET and RET alone, and in combination, leads to sustained improvements in cognitive performance, particularly for executive control tasks (39). Several studies have compared the individual and combined effects of physical and mental exercise interventions (61, 177). These studies found cognitive benefits to be larger with the combined cognitive and aerobic training paradigms. The mechanism for the relationship between physical activity and exercise and cognitive functioning is not well understood; however, several researchers have suggested that enhanced blood flow, increased brain volume, elevations in brain-derived neurotrophic factor, and improvements in neurotransmitter systems and IGF-1 function may occur in response to behavioral and aerobic training (40, 134).

Evidence statement and recommendation. *Evidence category A/B.* Epidemiological studies suggest that cardiovascular fitness and higher levels of physical activity reduce the risk of cognitive decline and dementia. Experimental studies demonstrate that AET, RET, and especially combined AET and RET can improve cognitive performance in previously sedentary older adults for some measures of cognitive functioning but not others. Exercise and fitness effects are largest for tasks that require complex processing requiring executive control.

Physical activity and QOL in old age. QOL is a psychological construct, which has commonly been defined as a conscious judgment of the satisfaction an individual has with respect to his/her own life (182). In a review of the literature that has examined the relationship between physical activity and QOL in old age, Rejeski and Mihalko (196) conclude that the bulk of the evidence supports the conclusion that physical activity seems to be positively associated with many but not all domains of QOL. Researchers have consistently shown that when physical activity is associated with significant increases in self-efficacy, improvements in health-related QOL are most likely to occur (155).

Evidence statement and recommendation. *Evidence category D.* Although physical activity seems to be positively associated with some aspects of QOL, the precise nature of the relationship is poorly understood.

Effects of RET on psychological health and wellbeing .Recent reviews suggest that RET can improve several indices of psychological health and well-being including anxiety, depression, overall well-being, and QOL (6, 168, 230, 240). The randomized controlled trial evidence for RET as an isolated intervention for the treatment of clinical depression in both younger and older cohorts is robust and consistent. Both AET (81, 151, 153) and RET (150, 224, 225) produce clinically meaningful improvements in depression in clinical patients, with response rates ranging from 25% to 88%. Studies are less consistent among seniors without clinical depression. For example, symptoms of depression did not improve after light-resistance elastic band training in frail community- dwelling seniors without clinical symptoms (35). Mean depression scores also did not improve in healthy, independent but sedentary older women after either moderate- or higher-intensity RET using weight machines; however, anxiety levels did decreased after moderate-intensity RET (250). Improvements in overall well-being and QOL measures (*e.g.,* body pain, vitality, social functioning, morale, and/or sleep quality) have also been reported after RET using moderate- and higher-intensity protocols in community-dwelling seniors with minor or major depression (223) and in independent sedentary older women (250). In contrast, low-intensity task-unspecific protocols may not be effective in improving QOL measures in healthy independent seniors (80, 154).

Evidence statement and recommendation. *Evidence category A/B.* There is a strong evidence that high-intensity RET is effective in the treatment of clinical depression. More evidence is needed regarding the intensity and frequency of RET needed to elicit specific improvements in other measures of psychological health and well-being.

CONCLUSIONS

Although no amount of physical activity can stop the biological aging process, there is evidence that regular exercise can minimize the physiological effects of an otherwise sedentary lifestyle and increase active life expectancy by limiting the development and progression of chronic disease and disabling conditions. There is also emerging evidence for psychological and cognitive benefits accruing from regular exercise participation by older adults (Table 4). It is not yet possible to describe in detail exercise

Table A-4 Summary of the SORT Evidence Strength Taxonomy

Evidence Statements	Evidence Strength A = Highest, D = Lowest
Section 1 — Normal human aging	
Advancing age is associated with physiologic changes that result in reductions in functional capacity and altered body composition.	A
Advancing age is associated with declines in physical activity volume and intensity.	A/B[a]
Advancing age is associated with increased risk for chronic diseases but physical activity significantly reduces this risk.	B
Section 2 — Physical activity and the aging process	
Regular physical activity increases average life expectancy through its influence on chronic disease development, through the mitigation of age-related biological changes and their associated effects on health and well-being, and through the preservation of functional capacity.	A
Individuals differ widely in how they age and in how they adapt to an exercise program. It is likely that lifestyle and genetic factors contribute to the wide interindividual variability seen in older adults.	B
Healthy older adults are able to engage in acute aerobic or resistance exercise and experience positive adaptations to exercise training.	A
Regular physical activity can favorably influence a broad range of physiological systems and may be a major lifestyle factor that discriminates between those individuals who have and have not experienced successful aging.	B/C[a]
Regular physical activity reduces the risk of developing a large number of chronic diseases and conditions and is valuable in the treatment of numerous diseases.	A/B[a]
Section 3 — Benefits of physical activity and exercise	
Vigorous, long-term participation in AET is associated with elevated cardiovascular reserve and skeletal muscle adaptations, which enable the aerobically trained older individual to sustain a submaximal exercise load with less cardiovascular stress and muscular fatigue than their untrained peers. Prolonged aerobic exercise also seems to slow the age-related accumulation of central body fat and is cardioprotective.	B
Prolonged participation in RET is consistently associated with higher muscle and bone mass and strength, which are not seen as consistently seen with prolonged AET alone.	B
AET programs of sufficient intensity ($\geq 60\%$ of pretraining $\dot{V}O_{2max}$), frequency, and length (≥ 3 d.wk^{-1} for ≥ 16 wk) can significantly increase $\dot{V}O_{2max}$ in healthy middle-aged and older adults.	A
Three or more months of moderate-intensity AET elicits cardiovascular adaptations in healthy middle-aged and older adults, which are evident at rest and in response to acute dynamic exercise.	A/B[a]
In studies involving overweight middle-aged and older adults, moderate-intensity AET has been shown to be effective in reducing total body fat. In contrast, most studies report no significant effect of AET on FFM.	A/B[a]
AET can induce a variety of favorable metabolic adaptations including enhanced glycemic control, augmented clearance of postprandial lipids, and preferential utilization of fat during submaximal exercise.	B
AET may be effective in counteracting age-related declines in BMD in postmenopausal women	B
Older adults can substantially increase their strength after RET.	A

Table A-4 Summary of the SORT Evidence Strength Taxonomy

Evidence Statements	Evidence Strength A = Highest, D = Lowest
Substantial increases in muscular power have been demonstrated after RET in older adults.	A
Increases in MQ are similar between older and younger adults, and these improvements do not seem to be sex-specific.	B
Improvements in muscular endurance have been reported after RET using moderate- to higher-intensity protocols, whereas lower-intensity RET does not improve muscular endurance.	C
The effect of exercise on physical performance is poorly understood and does not seem to be linear. RET has been shown to favorably impact walking, chair stand, and balance activities, but more information is needed to understand the precise nature of the relationship between exercise and functional performance	C/D[a]
Favorable changes in body composition, including increased FFM and decreased FM have been reported in older adults who participate in moderate or high intensity RET.	B/C
High-intensity RET preserves or improves BMD relative to sedentary controls, with a direct relationship between muscle and bone adaptations.	B
Evidence of the effect of RET on metabolic variables is mixed. There is some evidence that RET can alter the preferred fuel source used under resting conditions, but there is inconsistent evidence regarding the effects of RET on BMR. The effect of RET on a variety of different hormones has been studied increasingly in recent years; however, the exact nature of the relationship is not yet well understood.	B/C
Multimodal exercise, usually including strength and balance exercises, and tai chi have been shown to be effective in reducing the risk of noninjurious and sometimes injurious falls in populations who are at an elevated risk of falling.	C
Few controlled studies have examined the effect of flexibility exercise on ROM in older adults. There is some evidence that flexibility can be increased in the major joints by ROM exercises; however, how much and what types of ROM exercises are most effective have not been established.	D
Regular physical activity is associated with significant improvements in overall psychological well-being. Both physical fitness and AET are associated with a decreased risk for clinical depression or anxiety. Exercise and physical activity have been proposed to impact psychological well-being through their moderating and mediating effects on constructs such as self-concept and self-esteem.	A/B
Epidemiological studies suggest that cardiovascular fitness and higher levels of physical activity reduce the risk of cognitive decline and dementia. Experimental studies demonstrate that AET, RET, and especially combined AET and RET can improve cognitive performance in previously sedentary older adults for some measures of cognitive functioning but not others. Exercise and fitness effects are largest for tasks that require complex processing requiring executive control.	A/B
Although physical activity seems to be positively associated with some aspects of QOL, the precise nature of the relationship is poorly understood.	D
There is a strong evidence that high-intensity RET is effective in the treatment of clinical depression. More evidence is needed regarding the intensity and frequency of RET needed to elicit specific improvements in other measures of psychological health and well-being.	A/B

[a] Any review of evidence pertaining to exercise and physical activity in older adult populations will necessarily be interdisciplinary and subject to differences in research design across various subdisciplines within exercise science. Whenever possible, a single SORT rating is provided; however, occasionally, when the strength of evidence varies across studies, a composite rating is provided.

programs that will optimize physical functioning and health in all groups of older adults. New evidence also suggests that some of the adaptive responses to exercise training are genotype-sensitive, at least in animal studies (14). Nevertheless, several evidence-based conclusions can be drawn relative to exercise and physical activity in the older adult population: 1) A combination of AET and RET activities seems to be more effective than either form of training alone in counteracting the detrimental effects of a sedentary lifestyle on the health and functioning of the cardiovascular system and skeletal muscles. 2) Although there are clear fitness, metabolic, and performance benefits associated with higher-intensity exercise training programs in healthy older adults, it is now evident that such programs do not need to be of high intensity to reduce the risks of developing chronic cardiovascular and metabolic disease. However, the outcome of treatment of some established diseases and geriatric syndromes is more effective with higher-intensity exercise (*e.g.,* type 2 diabetes, clinical depression, osteopenia, sarcopenia, muscle weakness). 3) The acute effects of a single session of aerobic exercise are relatively short-lived, and the chronic adaptations to repeated sessions of exercise are quickly lost upon cessation of training, even in regularly active older adults. 4) The onset and patterns of physiological decline with aging vary across physiological systems and between sexes, and some adaptive responses to training are age- and sex-dependent. Thus, the extent to which exercise can reverse age- associated physiological deterioration may depend, in part, on the hormonal status and age at which a specific intervention is initiated. 5) Ideally, exercise prescription for older adults should include aerobic exercise, muscle strengthening exercises, and flexibility exercises. In addition, individuals who are at risk for falling or mobility impairment should also perform specific exercises to improve balance in addition to the other components of health-related physical fitness. The conclusions of this Position Stand are highly consistent with the recently published *2008 Physical Activity Guidelines for Americans,* which state that regular physical activity is essential for healthy aging. Adults aged 65 yr and older gain substantial health benefits from regular physical activity, and these benefits continue to occur throughout their lives. Promoting physical activity for older adults is especially important because this population is the least physically active of any age group (50).

The writing group would like to acknowledge the contributions of Drs. Loren Chiu (Metabolic Effects), Sean Flanagan (Body Composition), Beth Parker (Stretching and Flexibility training), and Kevin Short (Metabolic effects) who provided assistance in the preparation of sections of the Position Stand.

This pronouncement was reviewed by the American College of Sports Medicine Pronouncements Committee and by Gareth R. Jones, Ph.D.; Priscilla G. MacRae, Ph.D., FACSM; Miriam C. Morey, Ph.D.; Anthony A. Vandervoort, Ph.D., FACSM; and Kevin R. Vincent, M.D., Ph.D.

This Position Stand replaces the 1998 ACSM Position Stand, "Exercise and Physical Activity for Older Adults." *Med Sci. Sports Exerc.* 1998;30(6):992-1008.

REFERENCES

1. ACRSO. Recommendations for the medical management of osteoarthritis of the hip and knee: 2000 update. American College of Rheumatology Subcommittee on Osteoarthritis Guidelines. *Arthritis Rheum.* 2000;43(9):1905–15.
2. Adams KJ, Swank AM, Berning JM, Sevene-Adams PG, Barnard KL, Shimp-Bowerman J. Progressive strength training in sedentary, older African American women. *Med Sci Sports Exerc.* 2001;33(9):1567–76.
3. AGS. American Geriatrics Society Panel on Exercise and Osteoarthritis. Exercise prescription for older adults with osteoarthritis pain: consensus practice recommendations. A supplement to the AGS Clinical Practice Guidelines on the management of chronic pain in older adults. *J Am Geriatr Soc.* 2001;49(6):808–23.
4. AGS. American Geriatrics Society Panel on Persistent Pain in Older Persons. The management of persistent pain in older persons. *J Am Geriatr Soc.* 2002;50(Suppl 6):S205–24.
5. Ahmaidi S, Masse-Biron J, Adam B, et al. Effects of interval training at the ventilatory threshold on clinical and cardiorespiratory responses in elderly humans. *Eur J Appl Physiol Occup Physiol.* 1998;78:170–6.
6. Arent SM, Landers DM, Etnier JL. The effects of exercise on mood in older adults: a meta-analytic review. *J Aging Phys Act.* 2000;8:407–30.
7. Asikainen TM, Kukkonen-Harjula K, Miilunpalo S. Exercise for health for early postmenopausal women: a systematic review of randomised controlled trials. *Sports Med.* 2004;34:753–78.
8. Bamman MM, Hill VJ, Adams GR, et al. Gender differences in resistance-training-induced myofiber hypertrophy among older adults. *J Gerontol A Biol Sci Med Sci.* 2003;58(2):108–16.
9. Bandura A. *Self-efficacy: The Exercise of Control.* New York (NY): W.H. Freeman and Company; 1997.
10. Barry BK, Carson RG. Transfer of resistance training to enhance rapid coordinated force production by older adults. *Exp Brain Res.* 2004;159(2):225–38.
11. Bassett DR, Schneider PL, Huntington GE. Physical activity in an Old Order Amish community. *Med Sci Sports Exerc.* 2004;36(1):79–85.
12. Bean J, Herman S, Kiely DK, et al. Weighted stair climbing in mobility-limited older people: a pilot study. *J Am Geriatr Soc.* 2002;50(4):663–70.
13. Bean JF, Herman S, Kiely DK, et al. Increased Velocity Exercise Specific to Task (InVEST) training: a pilot study exploring effects on leg power, balance, and mobility in community-dwelling older women. *J Am Geriatr Soc.* 2004;52(5):799–804.
14. Belter JG, Carey HV, Garland T Jr. Effects of voluntary exercise and genetic selection for high activity levels on HSP72 expression in house mice. *J Appl Physiol.* 2004;96(4):1270–6.
15. Bermon S, Ferrari P, Bernard P, Altare S, Dolisi C. Responses of total and free insulin-like growth factor-I and insulin-like growth factor binding protein-3 after resistance exercise and training in elderly subjects. *Acta Physiol Scand.* 1999;165(1):51–6.
16. Binder EF, Birge SJ, Spina R, et al. Peak aerobic power is an important component of physical performance in older women. *J Gerontol A Biol Sci Med Sci.* 1999;54:M353–6.
17. Binder EF, Yarasheski KE, Steger-May K, et al. Effects of progressive resistance training on body composition in frail older adults: results of a randomized, controlled trial. *J Gerontol A Biol Sci Med Sci.* 2005;60(11):1425–31.
18. Blair SN, Kampert JB, Kohl HW 3rd, et al. Influences of cardiorespiratory fitness and other precursors on cardiovascular disease and all-cause mortality in men and women. *JAMA.* 1996;276:205–10.
19. Blair SN, Wei M. Sedentary habits, health, and function in older women and men. *Am J Health Promot.* 2000;15(1):1–8.
20. Blumenthal JA, Babyak MA, Moore KA, et al. Effects of exercise training on older patients with major depression. *Arch Intern Med.* 1999;159(19):2349–56.
21. Booth FW, Weeden SH, Tseng BS. Effect of aging on human skeletal muscle and motor function. *Med Sci Sports Exerc.* 1994;26(5):556–60.
22. Borst SE, Vincent KR, Lowenthal DT, Braith RW. Effects of resistance training on insulin-like growth factor and its binding proteins in men and women aged 60 to 85. *J Am Geriatr Soc.* 2002;50(5):884–8.
23. Bosco C, Komi PV. Influence of aging on the mechanical behavior of leg extensor muscles. *Eur J Appl Physiol Occup Physiol.* 1980;45:209–19.
24. Bouchard C, Rankinen T. Individual differences in response to regular physical activity. *Med Sci Sports Exerc.* 2001;33(6 suppl):S446–51; discussion S452–3.
25. Brignole M, Alboni P, Benditt D, et al. Guidelines on management (diagnosis and treatment) of syncope. *Eur Heart J.* 2001;22(15):1256–306.
26. Brosse A, Sheets E, Lett H, Blumenthal J. Exercise and the treatment of clinical depression in adults: recent findings and future directions. *Sports Med.* 2002;32(12):741–60.
27. Brown M, Holloszy JO. Effects of a low intensity exercise program on selected physical performance characteristics of 60- to 71-year olds. *Aging.* 1991;3(2):129–39.
28. Buchner DM, Cress ME, de Lateur BJ, et al. The effect of strength and endurance training on gait, balance, fall risk, and health services use in community-living older adults. *J Gerontol A Biol Sci Med Sci.* 1997;52(4):M218–24.

29. Camacho TC, Roberts RE, Lazarus NB, Kaplan GA, Cohen RD. Physical activity and depression: evidence from the Alameda County Study. *Am J Epidemiol.* 1991;134(2):220–31.

30. Campbell AJ, Robertson MC, Gardner MM, Norton RN, Buchner DM. Falls prevention over 2 years: a randomized controlled trial in women 80 years and older. *Age Ageing.* 1999;28(6):513–8.

31. Campbell AJ, Robertson MC, Gardner MM, Norton RN, Buchner DM. Psychotropic medication withdrawal and a home-based exercise program to prevent falls: a randomized, controlled trial. *J Am Geriatr Soc.* 1999;47(7):850–3.

32. Campbell AJ, Robertson MC, Gardner MM, Norton RN, Tilyard MW, Buchner DM. Randomised controlled trial of a general practice programme of home based exercise to prevent falls in elderly women. *BMJ.* 1997;315(7115):1065–9.

33. Campbell WW, Crim MC, Young VR, Evans WJ. Increased energy requirements and changes in body composition with resistance training in older adults. *Am J Clin Nutr.* 1994; 60(2):167–75.

34. Carmeli E, Reznick AZ, Coleman R, Carmeli V. Muscle strength and mass of lower extremities in relation to functional abilities in elderly adults. *Gerontology.* 2000;46(5):249–57.

35. Chandler JM, Duncan PW, Kochersberger G, Studenski S. Is lower extremity strength gain associated with improvement in physical performance and disability in frail, community-dwelling elders? *Arch Phys Med Rehabil.* 1998;79:24–30.

36. Charette SL, McEvoy L, Pyka G, et al. Muscle hypertrophy response to resistance training in older women. *J Appl Physiol.* 1991;70:1912–6.

37. Chobanian A, Bakris G, Black H, et al. The Seventh Report of the Joint National Committee on Prevention, Detection, Evaluation, and Treatment of High Blood Pressure: the JNC 7 report. *JAMA.* 2003;289(19):2560–72.

38. Coggan AR, Abduljalil AM, Swanson SC, et al. Muscle metabolism during exercise in young and older untrained and endurance-trained men. *J Appl Physiol.* 1993;75:2125–33.

39. Colcombe S, Kramer AF. Fitness effects on the cognitive function of older adults: a meta-analytic study. *Psychol Sci.* 2003;14(2):125–30.

40. Colcombe SJ, Erickson KI, Scalf PE, et al. Aerobic exercise training increases brain volume in aging humans. *J Gerontol A Biol Sci Med Sci.* 2006;61(11):1166–70.

41. Conley KE, Cress ME, Jubrias SA, Esselman PC, Odderson IR. From muscle properties to human performance, using magnetic resonance. *J Gerontol A Biol Sci Med Sci.* 1995;50 Spec No:35–40.

42. Connelly DM, Vandervoort AA. Effects of isokinetic strength training on concentric and eccentric torque development in the ankle dorsiflexors of older adults. *J Gerontol A Biol Sci Med Sci.* 2000;55A(10):B465–B72.

43. Cox JH, Cortright RN, Dohm GL, Houmard JA. Effect of aging on response to exercise training in humans: skeletal muscle GLUT-4 and insulin sensitivity. *J Appl Physiol.* 1999;86:2019–25.

44. Coyle EF, Martin WHr, Sinacore DR, Joyner MJ, Hagberg JM, Holloszy JO. Time course of loss of adaptations after stopping prolonged intense endurance training. *J Appl Physiol.* 1984; 57:1857–64.

45. Craig BW, Brown R, Everhart J. Effects of progressive resistance training on growth hormone and testosterone levels in young and elderly subjects. *Mech Ageing Dev.* 1989;49:159–69.

46. Cress ME, Buchner DM, Prohaska T, et al. Best practices for physical activity programs and behavior counseling in older adult populations. *J Aging Phys Act.* 2005;13(1):61–74.

47. Cress ME, Conley KE, Balding SL, Hansen-Smith F, Konczak J. Functional training: muscle structure, function, and performance in older women. *J Orthop Sports Phys Ther.* 1996;24(1):4–10.

48. Day L, Fildes B, Gordon I, Fitzharris M, Flamer H, Lord S. Randomised factorial trial of falls prevention among older people living in their own homes. *BMJ.* 2002;325(7356):128.

49. DeSouza CA, Shapiro LF, Clevenger CM, et al. Regular aerobic exercise prevents and restores age-related declines in endothelium-dependent vasodilation in healthy men. *Circulation.* 2000; 102:1351–7.

50. DHHS. *2008 Physical Activity Guidelines for Americans.* Rockville (MD): U.S. Department of Health and Human Services; 2008.

51. DHHS. *Physical Activity Guidelines Advisory Committee Report.* Rockville (MD): U.S. Department of Health and Human Services; 2008.

52. DiPietro L, Dziura J, Yeckel CW, Neufer PD. Exercise and improved insulin sensitivity in older women: evidence of the enduring benefits of higher intensity training. *J Appl Physiol.* 2006;100:142–9.

53. DiPietro L, Williamson DF, Caspersen CJ, Eaker E. The descriptive epidemiology of selected physical activities and body weight among adults trying to lose weight: the Behavioral Risk Factor Surveillance System survey, 1989. *Int J Obes Relat Metab Disord.* 1993;17:69–76.

54. Doody R, Stevens J, Beck C, et al. Practice parameter: management of dementia (an evidence-based review). Report of the Quality Standards Subcommittee of the American Academy of Neurology. *Neurology.* 2001;56(9):1154–66.

55. Douglas PS, O'Toole M. Aging and physical activity determine cardiac structure and function in the older athlete. *J Appl Physiol.* 1992;72:1969–73.

56. Dunn AL, Blair SN, Marcus BH, Carpenter RA, Jaret P. *Active Living Everyday.* Champaign (IL): Human Kinetics; 2001.

57. Earles DR, Judge JO, Gunnarsson OT. Power as a predictor of functional ability in community dwelling older persons. *Med Sci Sports Exerc.* 1997;29(5 suppl):S11.

58. Earles DR, Judge JO, Gunnarsson OT. Velocity training induces power-specific adaptations in highly functioning older adults. *Arch Phys Med Rehabil.* 2001;82:872–8.

59. Ehsani AA, Spina RJ, Peterson LR, et al. Attenuation of cardiovascular adaptations to exercise in frail octogenarians. *J Appl Physiol.* 2003;95:1781–8.

60. Evans WJ. Exercise strategies should be designed to increase muscle power. *J Gerontol A Biol Sci Med Sci.* 2000;55A: M309–M10.

61. Fabre C, Chamari K, Mucci P, Masse-Biron J, Prefaut C. Improvement of cognitive function by mental and/or individualized aerobic training in healthy elderly subjects. *Int J Sports Med.* 2002;23(6):415–21.

62. Fahlman MM, Boardley D, Lambert CP, Flynn MG. Effects of endurance training and resistance training on plasma lipoprotein profiles in elderly women. *J Gerontol A Biol Sci Med Sci.* 2002;57A(2):B54–60.

63. Ferketich AK, Kirby TE, Alway SE. Cardiovascular and muscular adaptations to combined endurance and strength training in elderly women. *Acta Physiol Scand.* 1998;164(3):259–67.

64. Ferri A, Scaglioni G, Pousson M, Capodaglio P, Van Hoecke J, Narici MV. Strength and power changes of the human plantar flexors and knee extensors in response to resistance training in old age. *Acta Physiol Scand.* 2003;177(1):69–78.

65. Ferrucci L, Bandinelli S, Cavazzini C, et al. Neurological examination findings to predict limitations in mobility and falls in older persons without a history of neurological disease. *Am J Med.* 2004;116(12):807–15.

66. Fiatarone MA, Marks EC, Ryan ND, Meredith CN, Lipsitz LA, Evans WJ. High-intensity strength training in nonagenarians. Effects on skeletal muscle. *JAMA.* 1990;263:3029–34.

67. Fiatarone MA, O'Neill EF, Ryan ND, et al. Exercise training and nutritional supplementation for physical frailty in very elderly people. *N Engl J Med.* 1994;330:1769–75.

68. Fielding RA, LeBrasseur NK, Cuoco A, Bean J, Mizer K, Fiatarone Singh MA. High-velocity resistance training increases skeletal muscle peak power in older women. *J Am Geriatr Soc.* 2002;50:655–62.

69. FitzGerald SJ, Barlow CE, Kampert JB, Morrow JR, Jackson AW, Blair SN. Muscular fitness and all-cause mortality: prospective observations. *J Phys Act Health.* 2004;1(1):7–18.

70. Fletcher G, Balady G, Amsterdam E, et al. Exercise standards for testing and training: a statement for healthcare professionals from the American Heart Association. *Circulation.* 2001;104 (14):1694–740.

71. Foldvari M, Clark M, Laviolette LC, et al. Association of muscle power with functional status in community-dwelling elderly women. *J Gerontol A Biol Sci Med Sci.* 2000;55A: M192–9.

72. Folkins CH, Sime WE. Physical fitness training and mental health. *Am Psychol.* 1981;36(4):373–89.

73. Frontera WR, Meredith CN, O'Reilly KP, Knuttgen HG, Evans WJ. Strength conditioning in older men: skeletal muscle hypertrophy and improved function. *J Appl Physiol.* 1988;64: 1038–44.

74. Gillespie LD, Gillespie WJ, Robertson MC, Lamb SE, Cumming RG, Rowe BH. Interventions for preventing falls in elderly people. *Cochrane Database Syst Rev.* 2003;(4): CD000340.

75. Going S, Lohman T, Houtkooper L, et al. Effects of exercise on bone mineral density in calcium-replete postmenopausal women with and without hormone replacement therapy. *Osteoporos Int.* 2003;14(8):637–43.

76. Going S, Williams D, Lohman T. Aging and body composition: biological changes and methodological issues. *Exerc Sport Sci Rev.* 1995;23:411–58.

77. Goldspink D. Ageing and activity: their effects on the functional reserve capacities of the heart and vascular smooth and skeletal muscles. *Ergonomics.* 2005;48:1334–51.

78. Goodpaster BH, Costill DL, Trappe SW, et al. The relationship of sustained exercise training and bone mineral density in aging male runners. *Scand J Med Sci Sports.* 1996;6:216–21.

79. Gordon N, Gulanick M, Costa F, et al. Physical activity and exercise recommendations for stroke survivors: an American Heart Association scientific statement from the Council on Clinical Cardiology, Subcommittee on Exercise, Cardiac Rehabilitation, and Prevention; the Council on Cardiovascular Nursing; the Council on Nutrition, Physical Activity, and Metabolism; and the Stroke Council. *Circulation.* 2004;109 (16):2031–41.

80. Greendale GA, Salem GJ, Young JT, et al. A randomized trial of weighted vest use in ambulatory older adults: strength, performance, and quality of life outcomes. *J Am Geriatr Soc.* 2000; 48(3):305–11.

81. Greist JH, Klein MH, Eischens RR, Faris J, Gurman AS, Morgan WP. Running as treatment for depression. *Compr Psychiatry.* 1979;20(1):41–54.

82. Grimby G, Aniansson A, Hedberg M, Henning GB, Grangard U, Kvist H. Training can improve muscle strength and endurance in 78- to 84-yr-old men. *J Appl Physiol.* 1992;73(6):2517–23.

83. Hagberg JM, Allen WK, Seals DR, Hurley BF, Ehsani AA, Holloszy JO. A hemodynamic comparison of young and older endurance athletes during exercise. *J Appl Physiol.* 1985;58: 2041–6.

84. Hagberg JM, Graves JE, Limacher M, et al. Cardiovascular responses of 70- to 79-yr-old men and women to exercise training. *J Appl Physiol.* 1989;66:2589–94.

85. Hagen K, Hilde G, Jamtvedt G, Winnem M. The Cochrane review of advice to stay active as a single treatment for low back pain and sciatica. *Spine.* 2002;27(16):1736–41.

86. Hagerman FC, Walsh SJ, Staron RS, et al. Effects of high- intensity resistance training on untrained older men: I. Strength, cardiovascular, and metabolic responses. *J Gerontol A Biol Sci Med Sci.* 2000;55A(7):B336–46.

87. Hakkinen K, Pakarinen A, Kraemer WJ, Newton RU, Alen M. Basal concentrations and acute responses of serum hormones and strength development during heavy resistance training in middle-aged and elderly men and women. *J Gerontol A Biol Sci Med Sci.* 2000;55A(2):B95–105.

88. Hakkinen K, Hakkinen A. Muscle cross-sectional area, force production and relaxation characteristics in women at different ages. *Eur J Appl Physiol Occup Physiol.* 1991;62:410–4.

89. Hakkinen K, Kraemer WJ, Newton RU, Alen M. Changes in electromyographic activity, muscle fibre and force production characteristics during heavy resistance/power strength training in middle-aged and older men and women. *Acta Physiol Scand.* 2001;171:51–62.

90. Hakkinen K, Alen M, Kallinen M, Newton RU, Kraemer WJ. Neuromuscular adaptation during prolonged strength training, detraining and re-strength-training in middle-aged and elderly people. *Eur J Appl Physiol.* 2000;83(1):51–62.

91. Hakkinen K, Newton RU, Gordon SE, et al. Changes in muscle morphology, electromyographic activity, and force production characteristics during progressive strength training in young and older men. *J Gerontol A Biol Sci Med Sci.* 1998;53(6): B415–23.

92. Hakkinen K, Pakarinen A, Newton RU, Kraemer WJ. Acute hormone responses to heavy resistance lower and upper extremity exercise in young versus old men. *Eur J Appl Physiol Occup Physiol.* 1998;77(4):312–9.

93. Hakkinen K, Kraemer WJ, Kallinen M, et al. Bilateral and unilateral neuromuscular function and muscle cross-sectional area in middle-aged and elderly men and women. *J Gerontol A Biol Sci Med Sci.* 1996;51A:B21–9.

94. Hameed M, Lange KH, Andersen JL, et al. The effect of recombinant human growth hormone and resistance training on IGF-I mRNA expression in the muscles of elderly men. *J Physiol.* 2004;555(Pt 1):231–40.

95. Hameed M, Orrell RW, Cobbold M, Goldspink G, Harridge SD. Expression of IGF-I splice variants in young and old human skeletal muscle after high resistance exercise. *J Physiol.* 2003; 547(Pt 1):247–54.

96. Henwood TR, Taaffe DR. Improved physical performance in older adults undertaking a short-term programme of high- velocity resistance training. *Gerontology.* 2005;51(2):108–15.

97. Holloszy J. The biology of aging. *Mayo Clin Proc.* 2000; 75(Suppl):S3-8; discussion S8–9.

98. Holloszy JO, Kohrt WM. Sect. 11. Chapt. 24: Exercise. In: *Handbook of Physiology. Aging.* Bethesda (MD): American Physiological Society; 1995. p. 633-66.

99. Holviala JH, Sallinen JM, Kraemer WJ, Alen MJ, Hakkinen KK. Effects of strength training on muscle strength characteristics, functional capabilities, and balance in middle-aged and older women. *J Strength Cond Res.* 2006;20(2):336-44.

100. Huang G, Gibson CA, Tran ZV, Osness WH. Controlled endurance exercise training and VO_{2max} changes in older adults: a meta-analysis. *Prev Cardiol.* 2005;8:217–25.

101. Huang G, Shi X, Davis-Brezette JA, Osness WH. Resting heart rate changes after endurance training in older adults: a metaanalysis. *Med Sci Sports Exerc.* 2005;37(8):1381–6.

102. Hunter GR, Bryan DR, Wetzstein CJ, Zuckerman PA, Bamman MM. Resistance training and intra-abdominal adipose tissue in older men and women. *Med Sci Sports Exerc.* 2002; 34(6):1023–8.

103. Hunter GR, McCarthy JP, Bamman MM. Effects of resistance training on older adults. *Sports Med.* 2004;34(5):329–48.

104. Hunter GR, Treuth MS, Weinsier RL, et al. The effects of strength conditioning on older women's ability to perform daily tasks. *J Am Geriatr Soc.* 1995;43(7):756–60.

105. Hunter GR, Wetzstein CJ, Fields DA, Brown A, Bamman MM. Resistance training increases total energy expenditure and free-living physical activity in older adults. *J Appl Physiol.* 2000; 89:977–84.

106. Hunter GR, Wetzstein CJ, McLafferty CL, Zuckerman PA, Landers KA, Bamman MM. High-resistance versus variable-resistance training in older adults. *Med Sci Sports Exerc.* 2001;33(10):1759–64.

107. Hurley BF, Hagberg JM. Optimizing health in older persons: aerobic or strength training? *Exerc Sport Sci Rev.* 1998; 26:61–89.

108. Ibanez J, Izquierdo M, Arguelles I, et al. Twice-weekly progressive resistance training decreases abdominal fat and improves insulin sensitivity in older men with type 2 diabetes. *Diabetes Care.* 2005;28(3):662–7.

109. Ivey FM, Roth SM, Ferrell RE, et al. Effects of age, gender, and myostatin genotype on the hypertrophic response to heavy resistance strength training. *J Gerontol A Biol Sci Med Sci.* 2000;55:M641–8.

110. Ivey FM, Tracy BL, Lemmer JT, et al. Effects of strength training and detraining on muscle quality: age and gender comparisons. *J Gerontol A Biol Sci Med Sci.* 2000;55(3):B152–7.

111. Izquierdo M, Ibanez J, Gorostiaga E, et al. Maximal strength and power characteristics in isometric and dynamic actions of the upper and lower extremities in middle-aged and older men. *Acta Physiol Scand.* 1999;167:57–68.

112. Izquierdo M, Hakkinen K, Ibanez J, et al. Effects of strength training on muscle power and serum hormones in middle-aged and older men. *J Appl Physiol.* 2001;90(4):1497–507.

113. Janssen I, Ross R. Linking age-related changes in skeletal muscle mass and composition with metabolism and disease. *J Nutr Health Aging.* 2005;9:408–19.

114. Joseph LJO, Davey SL, Evans WJ, Campbell WW. Differential effect of resistance training on the body composition and lipoprotein—lipid profile in older men and women. *Metabolism.* 1999;48(11):1474–80.

115. Jozsi AC, Campbell WW, Joseph L, Davey SL, Evans WJ. Changes in power with resistance training in older and younger men and women. *J Gerontol A Biol Sci Med Sci.* 1999;54A: M591–6.

116. Jubrias SA, Esselman PC, Price LB, Cress ME, Conley KE. Large energetic adaptations of elderly muscle to resistance and endurance training. *J Appl Physiol.* 2001;90:1663–70.
117. Judge JO, Whipple RH, Wolfson LI. Effects of resistive and balance exercises on isokinetic strength in older persons. *J Am Geriatr Soc.* 1994;42(9):937–46.
118. Judge JO, Underwood M, Gennosa T. Exercise to improve gait velocity in older persons. *Arch Phys Med Rehabi.* 1993; 74(4):400–6.
119. Kallman DA, Plato CC, Tobin JD. The role of muscle loss in the age-related decline of grip strength: cross-sectional and longitudinal perspectives. *J Gerontol.* 1990;45:M82–8.
120. Kasch FW, Boyer JL, Schmidt PK, et al. Ageing of the cardiovascular system during 33 years of aerobic exercise. *Age Ageing.* 1999;28:531–6.
121. Katsanos C. Prescribing aerobic exercise for the regulation of postprandial lipid metabolism : current research and recommendations. *Sports Med.* 2006;36:547–60.
122. Katzmarzyk PT, Craig CL. Musculoskeletal fitness and risk of mortality. *Med Sci Sports Exerc.* 2002;34(5):740–4.
123. Kay SJ, Fiatarone Singh MA. The influence of physical activity on abdominal fat: a systematic review of the literature. *Obes Rev.* 2006;7:183–200.
124. Kelley GA. Exercise and regional bone mineral density in postmenopausal women: a meta-analytic review of randomized trials. *Am J Phys Med Rehabil.* 1998;77(1):76–87.
125. Kelley GA, Kelley KS, Tran ZV. Exercise and bone mineral density in men: a meta-analysis. *J Appl Physiol.* 2000;88:1730–6.
126. Kenney WL, Munce TA. Invited review: aging and human temperature regulation. *J Appl Physiol.* 2003;95:2598–603.
127. Keysor JJ. Does late-life physical activity or exercise prevent or minimize disablement? A critical review of the scientific evidence. *Am J Prev Med.* 2003;25(3 Suppl 2):129–36.
128. King AC, Taylor CB, Haskell WL. Effects of differing intensities and formats of 12 months of exercise training on psychological outcomes in older adults. *Health Psychol.* 1993; 12(4):292–300.
129. Kirwan JP, Kohrt WM, Wojta DM, Bourey RE, Holloszy JO. Endurance exercise training reduces glucose-stimulated insulin levels in 60- to 70-year-old men and women. *J Gerontol.* 1993;48:M84–90.
130. Klein CS, Marsh GD, Petrella RJ, Rice CL. Muscle fiber number in the biceps brachii muscle of young and old men. *Muscle Nerve.* 2003;28(1):62–8.
131. Klitgaard H, Mantoni M, Schiaffino S, et al. Function, morphology and protein expression of ageing skeletal muscle: a cross-sectional study of elderly men with different training backgrounds. *Acta Physiol Scand.* 1990;140:41–54.
132. Kohrt WM, Bloomfield SA, Little KD, Nelson ME, Yingling VR. American College of Sports Medicine. Position Stand. Physical activity and bone health. *Med Sci Sports Exerc.* 2004; 36(11):1985–96.
133. Kraemer WJ, Hakkinen K, Newton RU, et al. Effects of heavy- resistance training on hormonal response patterns in younger vs. older men. *J Appl Physiol.* 1999;87(3):982–92.
134. Kramer AF, Erickson KI, Colcombe SJ. Exercise, cognition, and the aging brain. *J Appl Physiol.* 2006;101(4):1237–42.
135. Kramer AF, Hahn S, Cohen NJ, et al. Ageing, fitness and neurocognitive function. *Nature.* 1999;400(6743):418–9.
136. Laidlaw DH, Kornatz KW, Keen DA, Suzuki S, Enoka RM. Strength training improves the steadiness of slow lengthening contractions performed by old adults. *J Appl Physiol.* 1999; 87(5):1786–95.
137. Lakatta EG, Levy D. Arterial and cardiac aging: major shareholders in cardiovascular disease enterprises: Part I: Aging arteries: a "setup" for vascular disease. *Circulation.* 2003;107:139–46.
138. Laurin D, Verreault R, Lindsay J, MacPherson K, Rockwood K. Physical activity and risk of cognitive impairment and dementia in elderly persons. *Arch Neurol.* 2001;58(3):498–504.
139. Lemmer JT, Hurlbut DE, Martel GF, et al. Age and gender responses to strength training and detraining. *Med Sci Sports Exerc.* 2000;32(8):1505–12.
140. Lexell J, Downham DY, Larsson Y, Bruhn E, Morsing B. Heavy-resistance training in older Scandinavian men and women: short- and long-term effects on arm and leg muscles. *Scand J Med Sci Sports.* 1995;5(6):329–41.
141. Li F, Harmer P, Fisher KJ, et al. Tai chi and fall reductions in older adults: a randomized controlled trial. *J Gerontol A Biol Sci Med Sci.* 2005;60(2):187–94.
142. Locke GR, Pemberton J, Phillips S. American Gastroenterological Association Medical Position Statement: guidelines on constipation. *Gastroenterology.* 2000;119(6):1761–6.
143. Lyons DM, Yang C, Eliez S, Reiss AL, Schatzberg AF. Cognitive correlates of white matter growth and stress hormones in female squirrel monkey adults. *J Neurosci.* 2004;24(14):3655–62.
144. Macaluso A, De Vito G, Felici F, Nimmo MA. Electromyogram changes during sustained contraction after resistance training in women in their 3rd and 8th decades. *Eur J Appl Physiol.* 2000; 82(5–6):418–24.
145. Makrides L, Heigenhauser GJ, Jones NL. High-intensity endurance training in 20- to 30- and 60- to 70-yr-old healthy men. *J Appl Physiol.* 1990;69:1792–8.
146. Malbut KE, Dinan S, Young A. Aerobic training in the 'oldest old': the effect of 24 weeks of training. *Age Ageing.* 2002; 31:255–60.
147. Marquis S, Moore MM, Howieson DB, et al. Independent predictors of cognitive decline in healthy elderly persons. *Arch Neurol.* 2002;59(4):601–6.

148. Martel GF, Roth SM, Ivey FM, et al. Age and sex affect human muscle fibre adaptations to heavy-resistance strength training. *Exp Physiol.* 2006;91(2):457–64.

149. Martin WH, Kohrt WM, Malley MT, Korte E, Stoltz S. Exercise training enhances leg vasodilatory capacity of 65-yr-old men and women. *J Appl Physiol.* 1990;69:1804–9.

150. Martinsen EW, Hoffart A, Solberg O. Comparing aerobic with nonaerobic forms of exercise in the treatment of clinical depression: a randomized trial. *Compr Psychiatry.* 1989;30(4):324–31.

151. Martinsen EW, Medhus A, Sandvik L. Effects of aerobic exercise on depression: a controlled study. *Br Med J (Clin Res Ed).* 1985;291(6488):109.

152. Masoro E. *Handbook of Physiology Section 11.* In: Masoro E, editor. New York (NY): Oxford University Press; 1995. p. 3–21.

153. Mather AS, Rodriguez C, Guthrie MF, McHarg AM, Reid IC, McMurdo ME. Effects of exercise on depressive symptoms in older adults with poorly responsive depressive disorder: randomised controlled trial. *Br J Psychiatry.* 2002;180:411–5.

154. McAuley E, Blissmer B, Marquez DX, Jerome GJ, Kramer AF, Katula J. Social relations, physical activity, and well-being in older adults. *Prev Med.* 2000;31(5):608–17.

155. McAuley E, Katula J. Physical activity interventions in the elderly: influence on physical health and psychological function. In: Schulz MPLR, Maddox G, editors. *Annual Review of Gerontology and Geriatrics.* New York (NY): Springer Publishing; 1998. p. 115–54.

156. McAuley E, Rudolph D. Physical activity, aging, and psychological well-being. *J Aging Phys Act.* 1995;3(1):67–98.

157. McDermott M, Liu K, Ferrucci L, et al. Physical performance in peripheral arterial disease: a slower rate of decline in patients who walk more. *Ann Intern Med.* 2006;144(1):10–20.

158. Meijer EP, Westerterp KR, Verstappen FT. Effect of exercise training on physical activity and substrate utilization in the elderly. *Int J Sports Med.* 2000;21(7):499–504.

159. Metter EJ, Conwit R, Tobin J, Fozard JL. Age-associated loss of power and strength in the upper extremities in women and men. *J Gerontol A Biol Sci Med Sci.* 1997;52A:B267–76.

160. Metter EJ, Talbot LA, Schrager M, Conwit RA. Arm-cranking muscle power and arm isometric muscle strength are independent predictors of all-cause mortality in men. *J Appl Physiol.* 2004; 96:814–21.

161. Michel BA, Lane NE, Bjorkengren A, Bloch DA, Fries JF. Impact of running on lumbar bone density: a 5-year longitudinal study. *J Rheumatol.* 1992;19:1759–63.

162. Miszko TA, Cress ME, Slade JM, Covey CJ, Agrawal SK, Doerr CE. Effect of strength and power training on physical function in community-dwelling older adults. *J Gerontol A Biol Sci Med Sci.* 2003;58(2):171–5.

163. Moritani T, deVries HA. Potential for gross muscle hypertrophy in older men. *J Gerontol.* 1980;35(5):672–82.

164. Mussolino ME, Looker AC, Orwoll ES. Jogging and bone mineral density in men: results from NHANES III. *Am J Public Health.* 2001;91:1056–9.

165. NCEP. Third Report of the National Cholesterol Education Program (NCEP) Expert Panel on Detection, Evaluation, and Treatment of High Blood Cholesterol in Adults (Adult Treatment Panel III): NIH Publication No. 01–3670. 2001.

166. NCHS. DATA 2010. *National Center for Health Statistics.* 2008.

167. Nelson ME, Rejeski WJ, Blair SN, et al. Physical activity and public health in older adults: recommendation from the American College of Sports Medicine and the American Heart Association. *Circulation.* 2007;116(9):1094–105.

168. Netz Y, Wu MJ, Becker BJ, Tenenbaum W. Physical activity and psychological well-being in advanced age: a meta-analysis of intervention studies. *Psychol Aging.* 2005;20(2):272–84.

169. Newton RU, Hakkinen K, Hakkinen A, McCormick M, Volek J, Kraemer WJ. Mixed-methods resistance training increases power and strength of young and older men. *Med Sci Sports Exerc.* 2002;34(8):1367–75.

170. NHLBI. *Global Initiative for Chronic Obstructive Lung Disease (GOLD). Global Strategy for the Diagnosis, Management, and Prevention of Chronic Obstructive Pulmonary Disease.* In: National Heart, and Blood Institute, editor. Bethesda (MD): NHBLI; 2001.

171. Norton R, Galgali G, Campbell AJ, et al. Is physical activity protective against hip fracture in frail older people? *Age Ageing.* 2001;30(3):262–4.

172. Ochala J, Lambertz D, Van Hoecke J, Pousson M. Effect of strength training on musculotendinous stiffness in elderly individuals. *Eur J Appl Physiol.* 2005;94(1–2):126–33.

173. Ogawa T, Spina RJ, Martin WH, et al. Effects of aging, sex, and physical training on cardiovascular responses to exercise. *Circulation.* 1992;86:494–503.

174. Okazaki K, Iwasaki K, Prasad A, et al. Dose-response relationship of endurance training for autonomic circulatory control in healthy seniors. *J Appl Physiol.* 2005;99:1041–9.

175. Olshansky SJ, Hayflick L, Carnes BA. Position statement on human aging. *J Gerontol A Biol Sci Med Sci.* 2002;57(8):B292–7.

176. Ostchega Y, Harris TB, Hirsch R, Parsons VL, Kington R. The prevalence of functional limitations and disability in older persons in the US: data from the National Health and Nutrition Examination Survey III. *J Am Geriatr Soc.* 2000;48:1132–5.

177. Oswald WD, Rupprecht R, Gunzelmann T, Tritt K. The SIMA- project: effects of 1 year cognitive and psychomotor training on cognitive abilities of the elderly. *Behav Brain Res.* 1996;78(1): 67–72.

178. Parkhouse WS, Coupland DC, Li C, Vanderhoek KJ. IGF-1 bioavailability is increased by resistance training in older women with low bone mineral density. *Mech Ageing Dev.* 2000;113(2): 75–83.

179. Paterson D. Physical activity, fitness, and gender in relation to morbidity, survival, quality of life, and independence in older age. In: Shephard R, editor. *Gender, Physical Activity, and Aging.* Boca Raton (FL): CRC Press; 2002. p. 99–120.

180. Paterson DH, Govindasamy D, Vidmar M, Cunningham DA, Koval JJ. Longitudinal study of determinants of dependence in an elderly population. *J Am Geriatr Soc.* 2004;52(10):1632–8.

181. Patla AE, Frank JS, Winter DA. Balance control in the elderly: implications for clinical assessment and rehabilitation. *Can J Public health.* 1992;83(Suppl 2):S29–33.

182. Pavot W, Diener E, Colvin CR, Sandvik E. Further validation of the Satisfaction with Life Scale: evidence for the cross-method convergence of well-being measures. *JPers Assess.* 1991;57(1): 149–61.

183. Pescatello L, Franklin B, Fagard R, Farquhar W, Kelley G, Ray C. American College of Sports Medicine. Position Stand. Exercise and hypertension. *Med Sci Sports Exerc.* 2004;36(3):533–53.

184. Petrella RJ, Cunningham DA, Paterson DH. Effects of 5-day exercise training in elderly subjects on resting left ventricular diastolic function and VO$_{2max}$. *Can J Appl Physiol.* 1997;22: 37–47.

185. Pollock M, Franklin B, Balady G, et al. American Heart Association Science Advisory. Resistance exercise in individuals with and without cardiovascular disease: benefits, rationale, safety, and prescription: an advisory from the Committee on Exercise, Rehabilitation, and Prevention, Council on Clinical Cardiology, American Heart Association; Position paper endorsed by the American College of Sports Medicine. *Circulation.* 2000;101(7):828–33.

186. Porter NM, Landfield PW. Stress hormones and brain aging: adding injury to insult? *Nat Neurosci.* 1998;1(1):3–4.

187. Proctor DN. Longitudinal changes in physical functional performance among the oldest-old: insight from a study of Swedish twins. *Aging Clin Exp Res.* 2006;18:517–30.

188. Proctor DN, Sinning WE, Walro JM, Sieck GC, Lemon PW. Oxidative capacity of human muscle fiber types: effects of age and training status. *J Appl Physiol.* 1995;78:2033–8.

189. Proctor DN, Dietz NM, Eickhoff TJ, et al. Reduced leg blood flow during dynamic exercise in older endurance-trained men. *J Appl Physiol.* 1998;85:68–75.

190. Racette SB, Evans EM, Weiss EP, Hagberg JM, Holloszy JO. Abdominal adiposity is a stronger predictor of insulin resistance than fitness among 50-95 year olds. *Diabetes Care.* 2006;29: 673–8.

191. Rafferty AP, Reeves MJ, McGee HB, Pivarnik JM. Physical activity patterns among walkers and compliance with public health recommendations. *Med Sci Sports Exerc.* 2002;34(8):1255–61.

192. Rantanen T, Guralnik JM, Foley D, et al. Midlife hand grip strength as a predictor of old age disability. *JAMA.* 1999;281: 558–60.

193. Reeves ND, Maganaris CN, Narici MV. Effect of strength training on human patella tendon mechanical properties of older individuals. *J Physiol.* 2003;548(Pt 3):971–81.

194. Reeves ND, Narici MV, Maganaris CN. Effect of resistance training on skeletal muscle-specific force in elderly humans. *J Appl Physiol.* 2004;96(3):885–92.

195. Reeves ND, Narici MV, Maganaris CN. In vivo human muscle structure and function: adaptations to resistance training in old age. *Exp Physiol.* 2004;89(6):675–89.

196. Rejeski WJ, Mihalko SL. Physical activity and quality of life in older adults. *J Gerontol A Biol Sci Med Sci.* 2001;56 Spec No 2:23–35.

197. Remme W, Swedberg K. Guidelines for the diagnosis and treatment of chronic heart failure. *Eur Heart J.* 2001;22(17): 1527–60.

198. Rhodes EC, Martin AD, Taunton JE, Donnelly M, Warren J, Elliot J. Effects of one year of resistance training on the relation between muscular strength and bone density in elderly women. *Br J Sports Med.* 2000;34(1):18–22.

199. Rico-Sanz J, Rankinen T, Joanisse DR, et al. Familial resemblance for muscle phenotypes in the HERITAGE Family Study. *Med Sci Sports Exerc.* 2003;35(8):1360–6.

200. Rider RA, Daly J. Effects of flexibility training on enhancing spinal mobility in older women. *J Sports Med Phys Fitness.* 1991;31:213–7.

201. Rogers MA, King DS, Hagberg JM, Ehsani AA, Holloszy JO. Effect of 10 days of physical inactivity on glucose tolerance in master athletes. *J Appl Physiol.* 1990;68:1833–7.

202. Rose DJ. Promoting functional independence in older adults at risk for falls. *J Aging Phys Act.* 2002;10:1–19.

203. Roth SM, Ivey FM, Martel GF, et al. Muscle size responses tostrength training in young and older men and women. *J Am Geriatr Soc.* 2001;49:1428–33.

204. Said CM, Goldie PA, Patla AE, Culham E, Sparrow WA, Morris ME. Balance during obstacle crossing following stroke. *Gait Posture.* 2008;27(1):23–30.

205. Salem GJ, Wang MY, Young JT, Marion M, Greendale GA. Knee strength and lower- and higher-intensity functional performance in older adults. *Med Sci Sports Exerc.* 2000;32(10):1679–84.

206. Saltin B. The aging endurance athlete. In: Sutton J, Brock RM, editors. *Sports Medicine for the Mature Athlete.* Indianapolis (IN): Benchmark; 1986. p. 59–80.

207. Samaras K, Kelly PJ, Chiano MN, Spector TD, Campbell LV. Genetic and environmental influences on total-body and central abdominal fat: the effect of physical activity in female twins. *Ann Intern Med.* 1999;130:873–82.

208. Schlicht J, Camaione DN, Owen SV. Effect of intense strength training on standing balance, walking speed, and sit-to-stand performance in older adults. *J Gerontol A Biol Sci Med Sci.* 2001;56(5):M281–6.

209. Schoenborn CA, Adams PF, Barnes PM, Vickerie JL, Schiller JS. Health behaviors of adults: United States, 1999-2001. *Vital Health Stat 10.* 2004;(219):1–79.

210. Schulman S, Fleg J, Goldberg A, et al. Continuum of cardiovascular performance across a broad range of fitness levels in healthy older men. *Circulation.* 1996;94(3):359–67.

211. Seals DR, Hurley BF, Schultz J, Hagberg JM. Endurance training in older men and women II. Blood lactate response to submaximal exercise. *J Appl Physiol.* 1984;57:1030–3.

212. Seals DR, Hagberg JM, Hurley BF, Ehsani AA, Holloszy JO. Endurance training in older men and women. I. Cardio-vascular responses to exercise. *J Appl Physiol.* 1984;57:1024–9.

213. Seals DR, Taylor JA, Ng AV, Esler MD. Exercise and aging: autonomic control of the circulation. *Med Sci Sports Exerc.* 1994;26(5):568–76.

214. Seeman TE, Berkman LF, Charpentier PA, Blazer DG, Albert MS, Tinetti ME. Behavioral and psychosocial predictors of physical performance: MacArthur studies of successful aging. *J Gerontol A Biol Sci Med Sci.* 1995;50:M177–83.

215. Sharman MJ, Newton RU, Triplett-McBride T, et al. Changes in myosin heavy chain composition with heavy resistance training in 60- to 75-year-old men and women. *Eur J Appl Physiol.* 2001;84(1-2):127–32.

216. Shchoenborn C, Adams PF, Barnes PM, Vickerie JL, Schiller JS. 1991-2001. In: VH Statistics, editor. *Health Behaviors of Adults: United States.* Washington (DC): National Center for Health Statistics; 2004. p. 39–54.

217. Shephard R. *Aging, Physical Activity, and Health.* Champaign (IL): Human Kinetics; 1997.

218. Short KR, Vittone JL, Bigelow ML, et al. Impact of aerobic exercise training on age-related changes in insulin sensitivity and muscle oxidative capacity. *Diabetes Care.* 2003;52:1888–96.

219. Sial S, Coggan AR, Hickner RC, Klein S. Training-induced alterations in fat and carbohydrate metabolism during exercise in elderly subjects. *Am J Physiol.* 1998;274:E785–90.

220. Sigal R, Kenny G, Wasserman D, Castaneda-Sceppa C. Physical activity/exercise and type 2 diabetes. *Diabetes Care.* 2004; 27(10):2518–39.

221. Simonsick EM, Lafferty ME, Phillips CL, et al. Risk due to inactivity in physically capable older adults. *Am J Public Health.* 1993;83(10):1443–50.

222. Singh M. Exercise and aging. *Clin Geriatr Med.* 2004;20:201–21.

223. Singh N, Clements KM, Fiatarone MA. A randomized controlled trial of the effect of exercise on sleep. *Sleep.* 1997;20(2):95–101.

224. Singh NA, Clements KM, Fiatarone MA. A randomized controlled trial of progressive resistance training in depressed elders. *J Gerontol A Biol Sci Med Sci.* 1997;52(1):M27–35.

225. Singh NA, Clements KM, Singh MA. The efficacy of exercise as a long-term antidepressant in elderly subjects: a randomized, controlled trial. *J Gerontol A Biol Sci Med Sci.* 2001;56(8): M497–504.

226. Sipila S, Multanen J, Kallinen M, Era P, Suominen H. Effects of strength and endurance training on isometric muscle strength and walking speed in elderly women. *Acta Physiol Scand.* 1996; 156(4):457–64.

227. Skelton DA, Young A, Greig CA, Malbut KE. Effects of resistance training on strength, power, and selected functional abilities of women aged 75 and older. *J Am Geriatr Soc.* 1995;43:1081–7.

228. Spina R. Cardiovascular adaptations to endurance exercise training in older men and women. *Exerc Sport Sci Rev.* 1999;27:317–32.

229. Spina RJ, Turner MJ, Ehsani AA. Exercise training enhances cardiac function in response to an afterload stress in older men. *Am J Physiol.* 1997;272:H995–1000.

230. Spirduso WW, Cronin DL. Exercise dose-response effects on quality of life and independent living in older adults. *Med Sci Sports Exerc.* 2001;33(6 suppl):S598-608; discussion S609–10.

231. Spirduso WW, Francis KL, MacRae PG. *Physical Dimensions of Aging.* Champaign (IL): Human Kinetics; 2005.

232. Stewart K, Hiatt W, Regensteiner J, Hirsch A. Exercise training for claudication. *N Engl J Med.* 2002;347(24):1941–51.

233. Stewart KJ, Bacher AC, Hees PS, Tayback M, Ouyang P, Jan de Beur S. Exercise effects on bone mineral density relationships to changes in fitness andfatness. *Am J Prev Med.* 2005;28(5):453–60.

234. Stratton J, Levy W, Cerqueira M, Schwartz R, Abrass I. Cardiovascular responses to exercise: effects of aging and exercise training in healthy men. *Circulation.* 1994;89:1648–55.

235. Sugawara J, Miyachi M, Moreau KL, Dinenno FA, DeSouza CA, Tanaka H. Age-related reductions in appendicular skeletal muscle mass: association with habitual aerobic exercise status. *Clin Physiol Funct Imaging.* 2002;22:169–72.

236. Suominen H. Muscle training for bone strength. *Aging Clin Exp Res.* 2006;18:85–93.

237. Taaffe DR, Pruitt L, Reim J, Butterfield G, Marcus R. Effect of sustained resistance training on basal metabolic rate in older women. *J Am Geriatr Soc.* 1995;43(5):465–71.

238. Tabbarah M, Crimmins EM, Seeman TE. The relationship between cognitive and physical performance: MacArthur Studies of Successful Aging. *J Gerontol A Biol Sci Med Sci.* 2002;57(4): M228–35.

239. Tanaka H, Dinenno FA, Monahan KD, Clevenger CM, DeSouza CA, Seals DR. Aging, habitual exercise, and dynamic arterial compliance. *Circulation.* 2000;102:1270–5.
240. Taylor AH, Cable NT, Faulkner G, Hillsdon M, Narici M, Van Der Bij AK. Physical activity and older adults: a review of health benefits and the effectiveness of interventions. *J Sports Sci.* 2004;22(8):703–25.
241. Thompson P, Buchner D, Pina I. Exercise and physical activity in the prevention and treatment of atherosclerotic cardiovascular disease: a statement from the Council on Clinical Cardiology (Subcommittee on Exercise, Rehabilitation, and Prevention) and the Council on Nutrition, Physical Activity, and Metabolism (Subcommittee on Physical Activity). *Circulation.* 2003;107(24): 3109–16.
242. Thompson PD, Crouse SF, Goodpaster B, Kelley D, Moyna N, Pescatello L. The acute versus the chronic response to exercise. *Med Sci Sports Exerc.* 2001;3(6 suppl):S438-45; discussion S452–3.
243. Tinetti ME, Baker DI, McAvay G, et al. A multifactorial intervention to reduce the risk of falling among elderly people living in the community. *N Engl J Med.* 1994;331(13):821–7.
244. Toth MJ, Beckett T, Poehlman ET. Physical activity and the progressive change in body composition with aging: current evidence and research issues. *Med Sci Sports Exerc.* 1999;31(11 suppl): S590–6.
245. Toth MJ, Gardner AW, Ades PA, Poehlman ET. Contribution of body composition and physical activity to age-related decline in peak VO$_2$ in men and women. *J Appl Physiol.* 1994;77:647–52.
246. Tracy BL, Ivey FM, Hurlbut D, et al. Muscle quality: II. Effects of strength training in 65- to 75-yr-old men and women. *J Appl Physiol.* 1999;86(1):195–201.
247. Trappe SW, Costill DL, Vukovich MD, Jones J, Melham T. Aging among elite distance runners: a 22-yr longitudinal study. *J Appl Physiol.* 1996;80:285–90.
248. Treuth MS, Hunter GR, Kekes-Szabo T, Weinsier RL, Goran MI, Berland L. Reduction in intra-abdominal adipose tissue after strength training in older women. *J Appl Physiol.* 1995;78(4): 1425–31.
249. Treuth MS, Hunter GR, Weinsier RL, Kell SH. Energy expenditure and substrate utilization in older women after strength training: 24-h calorimeter results. *J Appl Physiol.* 1995;78(6):2140–6.
250. Tsutsumi T, Don BM, Zaichkowsky LD, Takenaka K, Oka K, Ohno T. Comparison of high and moderate intensity of strength training on mood and anxiety in older adults. *Percept Mot Skills.* 1998;87(3 Pt 1):1003–11.
251. USDHHS. *Bone Health and Osteoporosis: A Report of the Surgeon General.* In: OotSG Department of Health and Human Services, editor. Rockville (MD): USDHHS; 2004.
252. USPSTF. Screening for obesity in adults: recommendations and rationale. *Ann Intern Med.* 2003;139(11):930–2.
253. Vandervoort A. Aging of the human neuromuscular system. *Muscle Nerve.* 2002;25:17–25.
254. Vincent KR, Braith RW. Resistance exercise and bone turnover in elderly men and women. *Med Sci Sports Exerc.* 2002; 34(1):17–23.
255. Vincent KR, Braith RW, Feldman FA, et al. Resistance exercise and physical performance in adults aged 60 to 83. *J Am Geriatr Soc.* 2002;50(6):1100–7.
256. Wallace RB. Bone health in nursing home residents. *JAMA.* 2000;284(8):1018–9.
257. Wang BW, Ramey DR, Schettler JD, Hubert HB, Fries JF. Postponed development of disability in elderly runners: a 13-year longitudinal study. *Arch Intern Med.* 2002;162:2285–94.
258. Weinert BT, Timiras PS. Invited review: theories of aging. *J Appl Physiol.* 2003;95:1706–16.
259. Welle S, Bhatt K, Shah B, Thornton C. Insulin-like growth factor-1 and myostatin mRNA expression in muscle: comparison between 62-77 and 21-31 yr old men. *Exp Gerontol.* 2002; 37(6):833–9.
260. West S, King V, Carey TS, et al. Systems to rate the strength of scientific evidence. *Evid Rep Technol Assess (Summ).* 2002; (47):1–11.
261. Westerterp K. Daily physical activity and ageing. *Curr Opin Clin Nutr Metab Care.* 2000;3:485–8.
262. Whitehurst MA, Johnson BL, Parker CM, Brown LE, Ford AM. The benefits of a functional exercise circuit for older adults. *J Strength Cond Res.* 2005;19:647–51.
263. Whitmer RA, Gunderson EP, Quesenberry CP Jr, Zhou J, Yaffe K. Body mass index in midlife and risk of Alzheimer disease and vascular dementia. *Curr Alzheimer Res.* 2007;4(2):103–9.
264. Williams P. Coronary heart disease risk factors of vigorously active sexagenarians and septuagenarians. *J Am Geriatr Soc.* 1998;46:134–42.
265. Wolf SL, Sattin RW, Kutner M, O'Grady M, Greenspan AI, Gregor RJ. Intense tai chi exercise training and fall occurrences in older, transitionally frail adults: a randomized, controlled trial. *JAm Geriatr Soc.* 2003;51(12):1693–701.
266. Wolff I, van Croonenborg JJ, Kemper HC, Kostense PJ, Twisk JW. The effect of exercise training programs on bone mass: a meta-analysis of published controlled trials in pre- and postmenopausal women. *Osteoporos Int.* 1999;9(1):1–12.
267. Wray DW, Uberoi A, Lawrenson L, Richardson RS. Evidence of preserved endothelial function and vascular plasticity with age. *Am J Physiol Heart Circ Physiol.* 2006;290:H1271–7.
268. Yaffe K, Barnes D, Nevitt M, Lui LY, Covinsky K. A prospective study of physical activity and cognitive decline in elderly women: women who walk. *Arch Intern Med.* 2001; 161(14):1703–8.
269. Yaffe K, Haan M, Blackwell T, Cherkasova E, Whitmer RA,West N. Metabolic syndrome and cognitive decline in elderly Latinos: findings from the Sacramento Area Latino Study of Aging study. *J Am Geriatr Soc.* 2007;55(5):758–62.

R

Randomized controlled trials (experimental studies), 24
Range-of-motion exercise, 16, 21
Rating of perceived exertion (RPE) values, 17
Reciprocal determinism, 53
Relevance, 125
Reliability, 125
Repetition maximum (RM) testing, 137
Resistance exercise training (RET), 19, 79–82, 211–214
  and endurance programs, BAM activities in, 90t
  program
    progression for, 84–85
    starting/resuming, 83–84
  on psychological health and well-being, 219
  types of, 82–83
Resistance training, 105
RET. *See* Resistance exercise training (RET)
Retention phase, 56, 57
Retinopathy, 108–109
Revised Physical Activity Readiness Questionnaire (rPAR-Q), 172, 173, 174
RM testing. *See* Repetition maximum (RM) testing

S

Safe and effective stretches, 92–93
Sarcopenia, 149
Sarcopenic obesity, 153
Self-concept, 59–60
Self-definition model, 60–63, 65
Self-efficacy, 64
  definition of, 54
  theory, 53–55

Self-reports, 128
Self-tracking
  and goal setting, 142
  with journaling, 143
  with new technologies, 143–144
  with pedometers, 142–143
  with social networking, 143
Senior fitness test, 132
  range of scores for men, 135t
  range of scores for women, 134t
  test items for, 133t
Senior Walking Environment Assessment Tool, 37
Seniors
  health for, 40–43
  physical activity for, 38–40
  walking program for, 44
Shuttle run tests, 140
Skeletal muscle mass, 153
Skinfold measurements, 139
Slow dance, 76–77
Smart phones and internet, 143–144
Social age, 5–6
Social and economic environmental factors, 42
Social desirability. *See* Self-reports
Social learning theory, 56
Social networking, self-tracking with, 143
Social persuasion, 54
SORT evidence strength taxonomy, 220–221t
Specificity of training principles, 216
Speed and agility testing, 140
Sprint tests, 140
Stair climb test, 138
Standard group exercise sessions, 95
Static balance activity, 177
Static postures, 89
Static stretches, types of, 92
Step counters, 79

Stepping exercises, session of, 89
Stiffer arteries, 103
Strength-related activity, 177
Stretching and flexibility training, 215–216
Stroke, 208t
Submaximal tests, 136
Successful aging, 8–9, 9–11t

T

Tai chi styles, 87
Test modification options, for older adults, 136
"Three-legged stool," concept, 156–157
Tran–Weltman equations, 140
Type 2 diabetes mellitus (T2DM), 107–109, 208t

V

Validity, 125
Valsalva maneuver, 138
Vandalism and graffiti, 40
Verbal persuasion, 54, 55
Vicarious experiences, 55
Vitamin D, 163
VO_{2max} (maximal oxygen uptake), 17

W

Walkability
  concept of, 36
  of neighborhood, 42
Weight-bearing exercises, 175
Weight loss
  in older adults, 164–166
  therapy, 165
Weight management, therapeutic options for, 165